Creative Nursing Leadership & Management

Carolyn Chambers Clark, EdD, ARNP, FAAN

Nursing and Health Services
Walden University
Minneapolis, Minnesota

D0073727

JONES AND BARTLETT PUBLISHERS

Sudbury, Massachusetts

BOSTON   TORONTO   LONDON   SINGAPORE

Welcome to *Creative Nursing Leadership & Management!*

Along with useful tables and figures, each chapter includes:

CHAPTER OBJECTIVES

These objectives provide instructors and students with a snapshot of the key information they will encounter in each chapter. They can serve as a checklist to help guide and focus study.

LEADERSHIP IN ACTION

These short vignettes help tie theory to practice, synthesize information, and enhance critical thinking abilities.

LEADERSHIP TIPS

These useful tips provide readers with specific ideas about how to implement theories and concepts.

LEADERSHIP CHALLENGE

These exercises test the readers' knowledge and ability to apply theory and information by answering leadership-related questions.

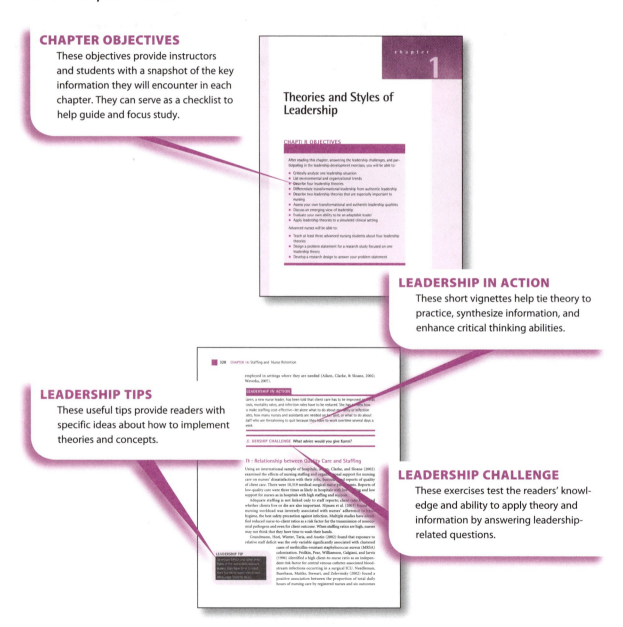

Visit **http://nursing.jbpub.com/leadership**

KEY TERMS

Found in the margins throughout each chapter, these terms will create an expanded vocabulary in nursing leadership and management. Visit **http://nursing.jbpub.com/leadership** to see these terms in an interactive glossary and use flashcards and word puzzles to nail the definitions!

RESEARCH BOXES

These boxes summarize current research studies and contain information focused on nursing leadership or management behaviors.

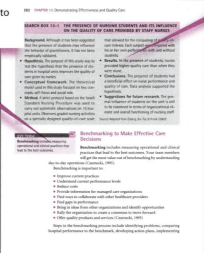

KEY TERM REVIEW

Key terms are listed and defined here for quick and easy reference.

LEADERSHIP DEVELOPMENT EXERCISES

Found at the end of each chapter, these exercises provide readers with active and interactive learning tasks that help to meet the behavioral objectives of nursing leadership.

Other key features include:

LEADERS SPEAK

Real-life nurses share their experiences, providing crucial information about what it takes to be a successful nursing leader.

GUIDED LEADERSHIP TIPS

Additional in-depth leadership tips guide the reader toward ideal leadership qualities.

for interactive exercises and additional review.

World Headquarters
Jones and Bartlett Publishers
40 Tall Pine Drive
Sudbury, MA 01776
978-443-5000
info@jbpub.com
www.jbpub.com

Jones and Bartlett Publishers Canada
6339 Ormindale Way
Mississauga, Ontario L5V 1J2
Canada

Jones and Bartlett Publishers International
Barb House, Barb Mews
London W6 7PA
United Kingdom

Jones and Bartlett's books and products are available through most bookstores and online booksellers. To contact Jones and Bartlett Publishers directly, call 800-832-0034, fax 978-443-8000, or visit our website www.jbpub.com.

Substantial discounts on bulk quantities of Jones and Bartlett's publications are available to corporations, professional associations, and other qualified organizations. For details and specific discount information, contact the special sales department at Jones and Bartlett via the above contact information or send an email to specialsales@jbpub.com.

The authors, editor, and publisher have made every effort to provide accurate information. However, they are not responsible for errors, omissions, or for any outcomes related to the use of the contents of this book and take no responsibility for the use of the products and procedures described. Treatments and side effects described in this book may not be applicable to all people; likewise, some people may require a dose or experience a side effect that is not described herein. Drugs and medical devices are discussed that may have limited availability controlled by the Food and Drug Administration (FDA) for use only in a research study or clinical trial. Research, clinical practice, and government regulations often change the accepted standard in this field. When consideration is being given to use of any drug in the clinical setting, the health care provider or reader is responsible for determining FDA status of the drug, reading the package insert, and reviewing prescribing information for the most up-to-date recommendations on dose, precautions, and contraindications, and determining the appropriate usage for the product. This is especially important in the case of drugs that are new or seldom used.

Production Credits
Executive Editor: Kevin Sullivan
Acquisitions Editor: Emily Ekle
Acquisitions Editor: Amy Sibley
Editorial Assistant: Patricia Donnelly
Production Director: Amy Rose
Associate Production Editor: Wendy Swanson
Associate Marketing Manager: Rebecca Wasley
Manufacturing and Inventory Control Supervisor: Amy Bacus
Composition: Shawn Girsberger
Cover Design: Anne Spencer
Cover and Interior Image: © Lee Torrens/ShutterStock, Inc.
Printing and Binding: Malloy, Inc.
Cover Printing: Malloy, Inc.

Library of Congress Cataloging-in-Publication Data
Clark, Carolyn Chambers.
   Creative nursing leadership and management / Carolyn Chambers Clark.
      p. ; cm.
   Includes bibliographical references and index.
   ISBN-13: 978-0-7637-4976-7 (pbk. : alk. paper)
   ISBN-10: 0-7637-4976-1 (pbk. : alk. paper) 1. Nursing services—Administration. 2. Leadership. I. Title.
   [DNLM: 1. Nursing, Supervisory. 2. Leadership. 3. Nursing Services—organization & administration. 4. Personnel Management—methods. WY 105 C592c 2008]
   RT89.C54 2008
   362.17'3068—dc22
                                    2007050707
6048

Printed in the United States of America
12 11 10 09   10 9 8 7 6 5 4 3

Dedication

For all the nursing leaders, past, current, and future

CCC

Contents

Contributors to Part V: Nurse Leaders Speak

Marion Anema, PhD, RN
Associate Director, Nursing Programs
Western Governors University
Wimberley, TX

Robin Arnicar, RN
Past Director of Nursing
Maryland Long-Term Care Facility

Ellen Cram, PhD, RN
Associate Professor
University of Iowa College of Nursing
Iowa City, IA

M. Louise Fitzpatrick, EdD, RN, FAAN
Connelly Endowed Dean and Professor
College of Nursing
Villanova University
Villanova, PA

Jane E. Hirsch, RN, MS, CNAA-BC
School of Nursing
University of California, San Francisco
San Francisco, CA

Jeanne Jacobson, RN, MA
Educator
Metro State University and St. Catherine's College
St. Paul, MN

Bonnie T. Mackey, PhD, AHN-BC
Director
Mackey Health Institute
West Palm Beach, FL

Shirley A. Smoyak, RN, PhD, FAAN
Editor
Journal of Psychosocial Nursing and Mental Health
    Services
Professor II
Division of Continuous Education and Outreach
Rutgers, The State University of New Jersey
New Brunswick, NJ

Sandra Swearingen, PhD, RN
Nursing Leadership Development
Florida Hospital
Orlando, FL

Ann Marriner Tomey, PhD, RN, FAAN
Professor Emerita
Indiana State University College of Nursing
Terre Haute, IN

Sharon M. Weinstein, MS, RN, CRNI, FAAN
President
Global Education Development Institute
Hawthorn Woods, IL

Gracie S. Wishnia, PhD, RN C
Associate Professor, Gerontology
Spalding University
Louisville, KY

Acknowledgments

I want to thank all my teachers and mentors, both formal and informal, past and present, whose wisdom has helped me shape this book.

Thanks go out to learners who asked the right questions and prompted me to use my critical thinking skills to provide the answers—or direct them to find their own solutions. This process has helped me consider unique and creative aspects of nursing leadership.

At Jones and Bartlett, thanks to Emily Ekle and Wendy Swanson who have been especially helpful, providing just the right amount of structure and support to help this book blossom.

Thanks to my husband, Tony, who has always supported my creative projects and given me the time and space to bring them to fruition.

Introduction

Health care changes daily, challenging current models of nursing leadership and moving organizations and institutions to more fluid and mobile models of work. Technology is moving us at such a pace that what was completed only last year in a hospital or medical center is now a walk-in procedure in a healthcare practitioner's office or clinic.

Nursing used to be about caring for sick patients, fixing what was wrong so that they could return to their lives. The challenge of nursing now relates more to a wellness approach—accessing, informing, guiding, teaching, counseling, linking, and collaborating with clients to change their lifestyles. If nurses fail in this process, clients will look up their diagnosis and medications on the Internet, demand prescriptions from their healthcare workers based on advertisements they see on television, and expect to participate, if not control, their own care.

Nurse leaders must be in the forefront, collaborating with staff and helping them move forward. Highly decentralized, Internet-moderated distance learning for clients is becoming more common. Nursing service delivery is moving toward community-driven, clinic-based ambulatory settings. Greater integration and cooperation with other disciplines is necessary for cost-efficient and effective treatment.

Health services are becoming more population centered, not disease-related diagnostic categories of care. Nurse leaders must find creative ways to serve populations and become more community based to form integrated clinical-economic systems.

Alternative and complementary approaches must be seamlessly integrated into existing clinical options for clients. Nurses cannot be poised to help clients if they are stressed from work conditions or if they do not care for themselves. Nursing leaders must help staff nurses use these alternative and complementary approaches to reduce stress and conflict so they have energy and clear minds to help clients, and such leaders must devise ways to integrate these approaches into client care.

Nursing leaders must also be able to understand employee values, beliefs, and motivations and how current nursing leadership roles can be creatively redesigned to engage those staff members.

This text reflects many of these changes, adopting the term *client* throughout. All theories, procedures, and critical-thinking situations apply to hospital and nonhospital settings. Alternative and complementary approaches that work for staff as clients appear in the chapters on managing stress, time, conflict, and violence.

Purpose and Audience

This text intends to introduce basic theories and practices that affect leadership and show you how to apply them creatively in today's ever-changing healthcare environment. It breaks new ground by providing application exercises, Leadership in Action situations, Leadership Tips, and Leadership Challenge questions in each chapter to help you integrate the material into your clinical and leader persona, building your critical-thinking abilities with each topic.

Although this book is designed to present a foundation of leadership and management principles, more advanced leadership exercises related to teaching and research appear at the end of each chapter, and the Nurse Leaders Speak section, written by nurse leaders, provides information from which both basic and more advanced learners can benefit.

The impetus for writing this book comes from teaching both graduate and undergraduate learners and recognizing the need for a text that demystifies the leadership process by showing learners how to apply concepts and theory.

Organization and Coverage

The organizational framework for this book groups the 23 chapters and Nurse Leaders Speak section into the following parts:

- Part I, "Theories of Leadership and Management," provides basic leadership and management theories.
- Part II, "Basic Skills to Creatively Lead and Manage," addresses role transitioning, managing stress and time, critical thinking, decision making, problem solving, communicating effectively, managing conflict, delegating, and acting legally, ethically, and politically.
- Part III, "Advanced Skills to Creatively Lead and Manage," focuses on motivating and team building, budgeting, demonstrating effectiveness, changing and innovating, and using information technology.
- Part IV, "Creatively Managing Human Resources," reviews the essence of staffing and retaining staff, recruiting and interviewing, establishing a healthy environment, developing staff, evaluating staff performance, coaching and mentoring, reducing workplace violence, and planning for succession.

■ Part V, "Nurse Leaders Speak," provides examples of how real-life nurse leaders solved leadership challenges and offers copious data for discussion, research, and evaluation.

Unique Text Features

In addition to traditional text features (chapter objectives, chapter summaries, and references), this book contains other important features that aid comprehension and integration of information.

Leadership in Action vignettes help tie theory to practice. Short vignettes appear near the beginning of each chapter and sometimes throughout chapters. They are the basis of leadership challenges that will help you synthesize information and enhance your critical-thinking abilities. Contributed leadership vignettes appear in Part V of the text, where seasoned nurse leaders reveal the secrets of how they handled leadership situations and how their decisions affected outcomes.

Leadership Challenges help you test your knowledge and your ability to apply theory and information. As previously mentioned, each chapter begins with a vignette presenting a nurse leader in a situation related to the chapter's focus. You are then asked to answer challenging questions throughout the chapter about what the leader did or should do and to provide a rationale for your answer.

Leadership Tips provide you with specific ideas about how to use theory and concepts with staff.

Leadership Development Exercises appear at the end of every chapter. These exercises provide you with active and interactive learning tasks that help you meet the behavioral objectives and include such activities as interviewing a nurse leader, role-playing leadership situations, working with a small group of colleagues on a critical-thinking activity, consulting with a more skilled researcher, teaching a group of less skilled nurse leaders, and even developing a research statement and design. This kind of interactive learning will help you integrate theory and concepts in a way that stays with you and becomes part of your leadership repertoire.

Boxes contain summaries of relevant research studies, or provide other types of information that you can directly apply to leadership situations

Key Terms are defined throughout each chapter and placed in boxes near the point in the text that further describes them. In addition, all key terms appear at the end of every chapter to reinforce learning.

Both students and instructors will find **online resources** at http://nursing.jbpub.com/leadership. Features include an instructor's manual, PowerPoint slides, and a TestBank to faciliate and ease the work of instructors. Students can enhance their learning with interactivities such as flash cards, crossword puzzles, a dynamic glossary, Web links, and all of the exercises from the text for easy downloading and printing.

A Note to Nursing Faculty

This book was written from the viewpoint of interactive learning. Leadership Challenges, Leadership in Action, Boxes (research and otherwise that appear as figures) found throughout the text, and Nurse Leaders Speak (the final section of the book) can form the basis of much of classroom activities. Learners can be prompted to answer the challenges, discuss a specific Leadership in Action situation, or Nurse Leaders Speak topic individually or in small groups. In the latter case, each small group can present their findings to the larger group in the second half of the class period.

Leadership Development Exercises found at the end of each chapter provide both beginning and advanced situations. Again, these situations can form the basis of individual, dyadic, or small group activity in or out of class. These exercises can also be used as test questions for essay-related formats or assigned as papers or projects for portions of a total grade and/or as extra credit activities.

All best wishes in your leadership activities,

Carolyn Chambers Clark, EdD, ARNP, FAAN

Part I

Theories of Leadership and Management

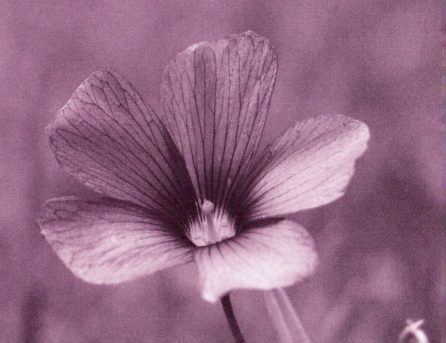

Theories and Styles of Leadership

CHAPTER OBJECTIVES

After reading this chapter, answering the leadership challenges, and participating in the leadership development exercises, you will be able to:

- Critically analyze one leadership situation
- List environmental and organizational trends
- Describe four leadership theories
- Differentiate transformational leadership from authentic leadership
- Describe two leadership theories that are especially important to nursing
- Assess your own transformational and authentic leadership qualities
- Discuss an emerging view of leadership
- Evaluate your own ability to be an adaptable leader
- Apply leadership theories to a simulated clinical setting

Advanced nurses will be able to:

- Teach at least three advanced nursing students about four leadership theories
- Design a problem statement for a research study focused on one leadership theory
- Develop a research design to answer your problem statement

Introduction

Nurse leaders empower themselves and others to help achieve organizational goals. Nurse leaders at all levels, from students to the chief executive officer, are in key positions to participate in decision making that affects client care. This means you have the opportunity to exhibit nursing leadership qualities in your clinical work. This book will help you begin to broaden your outlook from a single client to a nursing unit and beyond.

Effective nurse leaders use leadership theory and principles to guide their actions. This chapter introduces such theories and suggests ways to use them in nursing situations to empower staff.

This chapter, and all others, begins with a short "Leadership in Action" vignette of a real-life nursing situation and contains a series of leadership challenges, tips, and development exercises to help you understand theories and apply them in clinical settings. When you come to a challenge question, take a moment to think about what you just read, and answer it. This will help you anchor leadership information in your mind, making it accessible for use later on.

LEADERSHIP IN ACTION

Mrs. Moore, an LPN, has been working in an outpatient clinic for 15 years. Head nurses, physicians, and administrators have come and gone, but Mrs. Moore has stayed. She is a verbal, well-organized, and defiant member of the nursing team. Mrs. Moore does things her way and rarely follows policy. She has helped many staff members and has friends throughout the city who keep her apprised of upcoming changes. As an informal leader with a great deal of influence, she typifies the reality that exists in many nursing arenas. Although she has little formal power or influence, she can be thought of as a nurse leader and part of a sphere of healthcare influence.

LEADERSHIP CHALLENGE What kind of leadership challenges might Mrs. Moore present for a new nurse leader?

What Is Creative Nursing Leadership?

Leadership is one of the major factors, sometimes the only factor, that determines whether an organization succeeds or fails (Simkins, 2005). As a nurse leader, you will be called on to use all your knowledge and problem-solving skills to find creative solutions to healthcare situations, such as the one presented by Mrs. Moore.

Creative leadership involves not just imitating what is already in effect; it includes producing or inventing new solutions to challenging situations and using imagination and skill to apply relevant theory and concepts.

Environmental trends make creative nursing leadership a necessity. As nursing situations and the world itself become more complex, so does being a leader. To function as a creative nurse leader, you must familiarize yourself with the many theories and forms of leadership.

> **KEY TERM**
>
> **Creative leaders** produce or invent new solutions by using imagination, skill, and relevant theory and concepts.

As you've probably noticed, leaders don't necessarily have to be formally appointed. Mrs. Moore, the LPN at the beginning of this chapter, is a good example. You can be an informal and creative leader in whatever position you are in—even if you are a student. You can demonstrate creative leadership when you use your knowledge, personal power, and individual traits to teach a client a skill, to show a family how to do aftercare, to help a client communicate effectively with a physician, or to petition politicians to promote health and wellness.

To be a creative nurse leader, you need to be aware of healthcare trends that can affect your practice. What are some of these trends? Consider the following:

- Advances in information technology
- A focus on quality
- Globalization
- Growth in service-based organizations

Organizational changes also demand creative nursing leadership. Some of the changes that can challenge you are the increased diversity of staff and clients, the movement from formal leadership to self-managed teams, and nurse leaders who also serve as sponsors, team leaders, and internal consultants.

What kind of creative nursing leadership do these trends and organizational changes require? Nurse leaders who hope to succeed may need to be especially creative when they assume roles that demonstrate the following competencies:

- Technology master
- Problem solver
- Ambassador
- Change maker
- Great communicator
- Team player

LEADERSHIP CHALLENGE Which of these roles, if any, does Mrs. Moore, the LPN, exemplify?

As you witness these changes, rather than mourning what has been lost, seize the moment to facilitate staff and consumers into the 21st-century healthcare climate. A knowledge of leadership theories can help you understand what you observe and prepare you to become a creative nursing leader.

Leadership Theories

Although in the real-world leadership and management skills may intertwine, this chapter focuses on nursing leadership. Take a look at the various theories of leadership that have been put forth over the years, and see what ideas they provide for nursing leadership in this century. The most well-known leadership theories are:

- The great man theory
- Trait theory
- Behavioral theory
- Role theory
- The leadership grid
- Lewin's leadership styles
- Likert's leadership styles
- Hersey and Blanchard's situational leadership theory
- Vroom and Yetton's normative leadership
- Path-goal theory of leadership
- Leader-member exchange theory
- Transformational leadership
- Authentic leadership
- Collective leadership (Syque, 2006)

The Great Man Theory

> **KEY TERM**
>
> The **great man theory** states that leaders are born, not made.

Theories of leadership began with the **great man theory.** This theory was formulated after studying men who were already leaders. Most of them were rich and born into leadership. The main tenet of this theory is that leaders are born, not made (Syque, 2006).

Trait Theory

> **KEY TERM**
>
> **Trait theory** assumes that leaders are born with traits particularly suited to leadership.

The next leadership theory to find followers was **trait theory**. Tenets of this theory are:

- People are born with inherited traits.
- Some traits are particularly suited to leadership.

- People who make good leaders have the right (or sufficient) combination of traits.

Stogdill (1974) reviewed 163 studies conducted between 1949 and 1970. The negative trait findings he unearthed caused leadership researchers to reject the relevance of traits and turn to other theories. In 1983, McCall and Lombardo returned to trait theory and found four primary traits by which leaders could succeed or "derail," including:

1. Staying calm under pressure
2. Admitting errors and owning up to mistakes rather than covering them up
3. Persuading others without resorting to negative or coercive tactics
4. Being an expert in a broad range of areas rather than having a narrow-minded approach

LEADERSHIP CHALLENGE **What can you take from contemporary trait theory to help you with Mrs. Moore?**

Behavioral Theory

Behavioral theory proponents assume that leaders are made, not born. These theorists believed anyone can learn to be a leader. Rather than study capabilities or inborn traits, behavioral theorists study what leaders do. This approach opened the floodgates to leadership development once these researchers showed that simple assessment procedures weren't the only way to examine leadership ability (Syque, 2006).

> **KEY TERM**
> **Behavioral theory** proponents assume leaders are made, not born.

Role Theory

Role theory (Merton, 1957; Pfeffer & Salancik, 1975) was based on the assumptions that individuals:

> **KEY TERM**
> **Role theory** describes how expectations frame behavior.

- Define roles for themselves and others based on social learning and reading
- Form expectations about the roles that they and others will play
- Subtly encourage others to act within role expectations
- Will act within the role they adopt

Within organizations, formal and informal information about leadership values, culture, training, and modeling shapes expectations and behavior. When expectations do not match behavior, **role conflict** can occur. For example, when a nursing student steps out of the student role to become a staff nurse or when a nurse struggles to take over the head nurse role, conflict can result until these people learn new behavior patterns.

> **KEY TERM**
> **Role conflict** occurs when expectations don't match behavior.

The Leadership Grid

Back in 1961, Blake and Mouton developed a grid to chart leaders' concern about the work to be done compared to their concern for their people. The task-versus-person preference grid appeared in many other studies, including the Michigan and Ohio State leadership studies. Although these are important dimensions, they have one shortcoming: they don't address all aspects of leadership. The next theory that was developed, participative leadership, focused on more aspects of the leadership role.

Lewin's Leadership Styles

A group of psychologists led by Lewin (1939) focused their theory on leadership styles. They identified three leadership styles: autocratic, democratic, and laissez-faire.

KEY TERM

Autocratic leaders cause the worst level of discontent because they make decisions without consulting anyone.

Autocratic leaders make decisions without consulting anyone. In Lewin's experiments, this approach caused the worst level of discontent and can lead to revolution.

Autocratic leadership sometimes happens in healthcare situations when the administration decides on a change without consulting nursing. Revolution may not result, but low morale, bad feelings, and undercover retaliation can occur.

KEY TERM

Democratic leaders involve others in their decisions.

Democratic leaders involve people in their decisions, although they may make the final decision. Participants in settings that have a democratic leader may appreciate being consulted, but they may be confused when confronted by a wide range of opinions with no clear way to reach a decision.

LEADERSHIP TIP

When using the democratic style of leadership, provide staff with examples of specific ways to reach a decision.

LEADERSHIP IN ACTION

Roberta M., a nurse leader, decided to implement democratic leadership because she believed it would help her staff grow more independent and would help them stop complaining about staffing assignments. When she announced that the staff would now fill out the staffing assignments, some of the staff members cheered while others looked shocked and unsure. At the end of the week, when Roberta asked for the staffing assignments, she was surprised to find the sheet had not been filled out.

LEADERSHIP CHALLENGE How do you think Roberta could have averted problems in implementing a democratic leadership style?

Laissez-faire leaders are minimally involved in decision making. This style of leadership works best when people are capable and motivated to decide and are not hindered by a central coordinator. When laissez-faire leadership is used, people may not work in a coherent manner or put in the energy they would if they were actively led.

KEY TERM

Laissez-faire leaders are minimally involved in decision making.

LEADERSHIP CHALLENGE Which one of Lewin's leadership styles may help you with Mrs. Moore, the LPN in the Leadership in Action vignette at the beginning of this chapter?

Likert's Leadership Styles

In 1967, Likert published his leadership findings. He identified four main styles of leadership for decision making. In the **exploitative authoritative style,** the leader uses threats and other fear-based methods to achieve conformance. People's concerns are ignored, and communication comes from the top down. Adam is an example.

KEY TERM

In the **exploitative authoritative style**, the leader uses threats and fear to achieve conformance.

LEADERSHIP IN ACTION

Adam, a new nurse leader, was worried that his staff might not provide enough education for clients. As a result, he tightened up their job descriptions and told them that they'd have to keep detailed records of their performance or they would not progress to the next level of achievement. His staff didn't think that Adam supported them, and some even thought of his words as a threat. When they asked for more information, they were ignored.

LEADERSHIP CHALLENGE What could Adam do to begin to reverse the pattern that he has established? Give a theoretical rationale for your answer.

In the **benevolent authoritative style,** the leader is concerned for people and forms a benevolent dictatorship. Rewards are dispensed, and appropriate performance is praised. The leader listens to people's concerns, although what others hear is often rose colored. Some decisions may be delegated, but most are still made by the leader. Martha T. exemplifies the benevolent authoritative style.

KEY TERM

In the **benevolent authoritative style**, the leader shows concern but sugarcoats information and maintains control of decisions.

LEADERSHIP IN ACTION

Martha T., a nurse leader, showed a high degree of concern for her staff and gave them verbal and nonverbal rewards for their progress. When administration decided to change the performance appraisal method, Martha sugarcoated the decision and told staff that it would be a small change that would work to their benefit. When the staff tried out the new system and found that it required much more time and effort without additional compensation, they were angry at Martha, and several of them quit.

KEY TERM

A **consultative leader** listens to everyone but still makes the major decisions.

Another type of leadership is exemplified by the consultative style. A **consultative leader** makes the major decisions and offers somewhat rose-colored information, but information flows upward from the staff and the leader listens to people. Lucy C.'s leadership style provides an example.

LEADERSHIP IN ACTION

Lucy C., a seasoned nurse leader, believed in being a consultant to her staff. She listened to them and let the administration know where her staff stood on various issues. She prided herself on telling staff members that what they said counted. When a new administrator took over, he no longer listened to Lucy C.'s reports of staff wishes. She decided not to mention that fact to staff members because she believed they had enough to worry about with client care.

Staff members were shocked when they found out that they no longer had the hospital administrator's ear. More than that, they felt that their nurse leader had made a decision not to tell them about the change in administration. They complained that what Lucy did affected them and that she should have told them about the change.

Although Lucy tried to smooth over the bad feelings, several staff members harbored resentment toward her, and the new administrator countered with increasing noncooperative behaviors.

LEADERSHIP CHALLENGE   **What suggestions would you have for Lucy to help restore staff trust in her?**

KEY TERM

A **participative leader** increases collaboration, and seeks to involve other workers in the process of decision making.

Another kind of leadership style focuses on staff participation. A **participative leader** makes maximum use of participative methods, engages people in making decisions, and helps make sure everyone works well together at all levels (Likert, 1967; Syque, 2006).

LEADERSHIP IN ACTION

Kimberly T., a nurse leader, believed in the participative leader model and put it into action with her staff. She encouraged everyone to be involved in decisions that affected them and regularly asked how people were getting along, what obstacles they faced, and how she could involve staff even more in decision making.

LEADERSHIP CHALLENGE **Explain how participative leadership may help you with Mrs. Moore.**

The level of participation may vary depending on the type of decision being made. For example, deciding how to reach goals may be highly participative; decisions about performance evaluations may not. The downside of participative leadership is that it can lead to feelings of betrayal and cynicism when managers ask for input and then ignore it (Coch & French, 1948; Syque, 2006; Tannenbaum & Schmidt, 1958).

LEADERSHIP CHALLENGE **Which one of Likert's leadership styles may help you with Mrs. Moore, the LPN in the Leadership in Action vignette at the beginning of this chapter? Give a theoretical rationale for your answer.**

Hersey and Blanchard's Situational Leadership Theory

Hersey and Blanchard (1999) realized that encouraging staff to participate in leadership may not solve all problems. In some cases, a situational leadership approach may work best. Before choosing a response, a **situational leader** takes into account:

> **KEY TERM**
>
> A **situational leader** takes into account followers' motivation and capability and other factors within a particular situation.

- The motivation and capability of followers
- The situation in which decisions take place
- The fact that followers may affect leaders and vice versa
- Stress and mood
- Available resources and support
- Distant events, such as a family argument (Maier, 1963; Tannenbaum & Schmidt, 1958)

According to Hersey, Blanchard, and Johnson (2008) leaders should adapt their style to their followers' development levels or maturity, based on those followers' competence and motivation. Hersey and Blanchard described four leadership styles that matched followers' development levels. They believed leaders should put greater or less focus on the task or the relationship between the leader and follower depending on the follower's development level. The developmental levels they focused on were:

- *High-task, low-relationship focus.* When the follower cannot do the job and is unwilling or afraid to try, the leader steps in and tells the person what to do, providing a working structure for the follower, and determines the source of the lack of motivation.

LEADERSHIP IN ACTION

Linda K., a nurse leader, noticed that one of her staff members was having difficulty finishing the assigned tasks and diagnosed the problem as high task, low relationship. Linda stepped in and asked the nurse what was preventing her from completing her assignments. It became clear that the nurse was new to the unit and needed more structure and direction. Linda paired the new nurse with a more seasoned nurse who gave the newcomer specific directions. Within a day, the new nurse had learned the procedures and was able to complete her assignments.

- *High-task, high-relationship focus.* When the follower can do the job to some extent but is overconfident, the leader listens, advises, and coaches.

LEADERSHIP IN ACTION

Laura F., a nurse leader, noticed that one of the staff members took on a task for which he was not prepared. She diagnosed the problem as a high-task, high-relationship focus. Laura spoke with the staff member and reported her observations. She suggested that the staff member attend a continuing education class that afternoon to prepare him to take on the task in a more prepared fashion. The staff member thanked the nurse leader the next day and told her that he hadn't realized all that was involved with the procedure.

- *Low-task, high-relationship focus.* When the follower can do the job but refuses to do it, the leader listens, praises, and makes the follower feel good when he or she shows the necessary commitment.

LEADERSHIP IN ACTION

Leslie O., a nurse leader, noticed that a staff member who had been working on the unit for a long time was a very skilled nurse but that he refused to complete certain tasks. Leslie diagnosed the problem as a low-task, high-relationship focus. The nurse leader spoke with the staff member and asked him what prevented him from doing the tasks. The staff member told her that the previous nurse leader had yelled at him for the way he'd done the tasks even though he'd followed accepted procedures. Leslie told him that she was confident he could do the procedures and encouraged him to try a dry run. She praised him when he completed the tasks efficiently and safely. After that, the staff member stopped refusing to complete the tasks. The nurse leader continued to praise the staff member monthly just to ensure that he didn't revert to his earlier pattern.

- *Low-task, low-relationship focus.* When the follower can do the job and is motivated, the leader gets out of the way and doesn't interfere except to provide occasional recognition and praise.

LEADERSHIP IN ACTION

Gloria U., a nurse leader, was pleased with the nursing staff. One nurse was especially excellent. She worked well and appeared to be highly motivated. Gloria didn't interfere with the staff nurse's tasks except to compliment her work at least once a week.

LEADERSHIP CHALLENGE Which of Blanchard and Hersey's leadership styles may help you with Mrs. Moore, the LPN in the Leadership in Action vignette at the beginning of this chapter? Give a theoretical rationale for your answer.

Normative Leadership

Normative leadership is a variant of situational leadership. Vroom and Yetton (1973) noted that situational factors could yield unpredictable leader behavior, so they defined the norms, or rules, of leader behavior using rational logic and didn't spend long hours observing leader behavior.

> **KEY TERM**
>
> A **normative leader** chooses a decision procedure, ranging from autocratic to group-based, depending on decision acceptance and follower knowledge.

They defined different decision procedures based on the theory that participation increases acceptance of a decision and that, when there are many alternatives, the selection procedure—including autocratic, consultative, and group-based methods—is important. This model is most apt when opinions about the decision are clear and accessible.

- *Autocratic decision procedures.* In this format, the leader decides alone and does not share the problem with followers. There are two cases for autocratic decision procedures: one is when followers do not have useful information and the leader does; the other is when followers possess useful information and the leader asks for it but still decides alone. Neither of these are good choices when followers are unlikely to accept an autocratic decision, when the leader sees decision quality as important but the followers don't, or when followers aren't given an opportunity to resolve their differences.

LEADERSHIP IN ACTION

Kim G., a new nurse leader, learned that the hospital administrator planned to institute a new procedure. She called a staff meeting and asked for staff feedback on the procedure but then decided how to institute the procedure on her own. When the staff found out that Kim had made an autocratic decision, they were upset because they didn't get a chance to resolve their differences. Later, Kim found the previous nurse leader had never made an autocratic decision with this group and that the staff were unlikely to accept one.

LEADERSHIP CHALLENGE **Why do you think Kim's action backfired? Give a theoretical rationale for your answer.**

- *Consultative decision procedures.* In this category, the leader shares the problem either with people individually or with the group, listens to ideas, and then decides alone. Individual sharing is not appropriate when staff members are apt to disagree with one another because it doesn't offer people a chance to resolve differences.

LEADERSHIP IN ACTION

Kelly A., a seasoned nurse leader, usually allowed her group to come to consensus on decisions, but when the administration decided on a new procedure and there was no hope of changing it, she shared the problem with staff members individually and then made a consultative decision.

LEADERSHIP CHALLENGE **Did Kelly make the right decision? Give a theoretical rationale for your answer.**

- *Group-based decision procedures.* In this category, the leader either shares problems with followers as a group and then decides alone or seeks and accepts a consensus. Group-based decisions work especially well when decision acceptance and/or decision quality are important or when the leader lacks the information or skills to make the decision alone.

LEADERSHIP IN ACTION

Denise F., a novice nurse leader, was just learning about making leadership decisions. When the hospital administrator sent her a memo about implementing a new electronic charting system, she called the whole staff together to help decide the best way to implement this system.

LEADERSHIP CHALLENGE **Did Denise make a good decision? Give a theoretical rationale for your answer.**

Path-Goal Theory of Leadership

Path-goal theory helps leaders:

- Clarify the path toward the goal
- Remove roadblocks
- Increase rewards along the way (House & Mitchell, 1974)

KEY TERM

Path-goal theory helps clarify the path to a goal, removes roadblocks, and increases rewards along the way.

This theory offers three leadership styles depending on follower needs:

1. *Supportive leadership is the best choice when work is stressful, boring, and/or hazardous.* Making the environment more friendly is the goal. The leader strives to increase followers' self-esteem and make the job more interesting.

2. *Directive leadership is the best choice when the task is unstructured and/or complex and followers are inexperienced.* Telling followers what needs to be done and giving appropriate guidance along the way are the goals. Rewards are increased as needed, and role ambiguity is decreased by providing clear instructions, which strengthens followers' sense of security and control of the situation.

LEADERSHIP CHALLENGE Which of the path–goal leadership styles may help you with Mrs. Moore, the LPN in the Leadership in Action vignette at the beginning of this chapter?

---

3. *Achievement-oriented leadership is the best choice when the task is complex.* With this style, the leader knows the right and best way of achieving a goal; the follower is dependent but is believed to be able to succeed. This style also assumes the leader and follower are completely rational, which may be a big assumption.

KEY TERM

Leader-member exchange theory explains how group leaders maintain their position by exchanging informal agreements with their members.

Leader-Member Exchange Theory

Leader-member exchange theory, also called LMX or vertical dyad linkage theory, explains how group leaders maintain their position by exchanging informal agreements with their members. In this approach:

- Leaders have an inner circle of trusted assistants and advisers whom they give responsibility, decision influence, and access to resources, but leaders ensure that those consulted do not strike out on their own.
- The in-group works harder, is more committed to task objectives, and shares more administrative duties.
- The out-group is given low levels of influence or choice.

Successful in-group members are similar to the leader, and they are good at seeing situations from the leader's viewpoint. The out-group may react aggressively to the leader's treatment of the in-group but limit complaining to conversations in the restroom and at the water cooler.

The theory is useful when trying to understand the inner workings of a team. To be successful as a team member:

- Work hard to join the inner circle by seeking to understand and support the leader's viewpoint. Be loyal.
- Take on more than your share of administrative and other tasks.
- Pick your arguments carefully. (Graen & Uhl-Bien, 1995)

If you are the leader, pick your inner circle with care, and reward members' loyalty (Graen & Uhl-Bien, 1995).

LEADERSHIP CHALLENGE Which portions of leader–member exchange theory may help you with Mrs. Moore, the LPN in the Leadership in Action vignette at the beginning of this chapter?

Leadership in the Nursing Context

It is clear so far that the definition of leadership depends on whom you ask. Attempts to define leadership in a nursing context first focused on the traits of the nurses involved (McBride, Fagin, Franklin, Huba, & Quach, 2006). Two executive nurse fellows in the Robert Wood Johnson Foundation's Executive Nurse Fellows Program interviewed a dozen nurse leaders and concluded that the nurse leaders did share common characteristics (Houser & Player, 2004). Those characteristics were as follows:

- Thoughtful
- Responsive
- Committed
- Creative
- Resilient
- Visionary
- Scholarly
- Courageous
- Innovative

Positive traits may not be enough. The idea that leadership means influencing followers to do what is necessary to achieve organizational and societal goals may even be archaic (Tan, 2006). Two types of leadership are particularly relevant for nurse leaders: transformational leadership and authentic leadership.

The Importance of Transformational Leadership

Fagin (2000) applauded nurse leaders' ability to respond capably to managerial challenges but bemoaned their lack of vision and ability to shape a changing environment through a transformational process.

Transformational Leadership Defined

Transformational leadership follows three assumptions:

1. People will follow a leader who inspires them.

KEY TERM

Transformational leaders use vision, passion, personal integrity, ceremonies, rituals, and enthusiasm to shape a changing social architecture by being proactive, serving as a catalyst for innovation, functioning as a team member, and encouraging organizational learning.

2. A leader with vision and passion can achieve great things but must maintain personal integrity, be willing to stand up and be counted, and use ceremonies, rituals, and other types of cultural symbolism to maintain motivation.

3. The best way to get things done is to inject enthusiasm and energy into the effort.

Some of the negatives of transformation leaders are:

- They may believe that passion and enthusiasm are more important than truth and reality.
- Their energy can wear out their followers.
- They may see only the big picture, not the details.
- They may become frustrated when an organization doesn't want to be transformed. (Syque, 2006)

Burns's (1978) view of transformational leadership is that it appeals to social values and encourages people to collaborate, rather than work as individuals who compete with one another. Transformational leaders give people an uplifting sense of being connected to a higher purpose, enhancing their sense of meaning and identity.

How Transformation Happens

According to the Institute of Medicine (2004), nurse leaders transform the work environment for nurses by:

- Balancing the tension between production and efficiency
- Creating and sustaining trust through the organization
- Managing the process of change
- Involving workers in decision making
- Establishing the organization as a learning organization

Research backs up this model. Findings from focus groups and a review of literature on healthy work environments indicated that nursing leaders must prioritize efforts to improve the culture in the work environment. Three elements emerged to help nursing leaders set the tone and standard of practice for healthy work environments:

1. Effective communication
2. Collaborative relationships
3. Shared decision making among nurses (Heath, Johanson, & Blake, 2004)

LEADERSHIP CHALLENGE Which portions of transformational theory may help you with Mrs. Moore, the LPN in the Leadership in Action vignette at the beginning of this chapter?

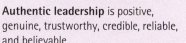

The Emergence of Authentic Leadership

Authentic leadership is another kind of positive leadership that is genuine, trustworthy, credible, reliable, and believable (George, 2003; Kouzes & Posner, 1991, 2003; Luthans & Avolio, 2003; Shirey, 2006). Authentic leaders have:

- Purpose
- Values
- Heart
- Positive relationships
- Self-discipline (George, 2003; Shirey, 2006)
- Credibility (Kouzes & Posner, 1991, 2003)
- Ability to encourage others

Purpose for an authentic leader includes developing a better understanding of one's personal passion and finding a way to express it in the work setting (Covey, 2004). Values are exemplified through an authentic leader's actions, including speaking the truth. Actions are based on doing right despite the challenges that result (Shirey, 2006).

Heart is exemplified by authentic leaders who show they care for themselves and for others. Authentic leaders know that workers flourish when they are encouraged again and again. Heart is about encouraging others so that they will actually achieve higher levels of performance, not just dream about doing so. Authentic leaders recognize and reward the good in people because it keeps hope alive. Such leaders have courage and impart it to others, train and coach people to exceed their current capacities, give specific feedback, and publicly recognize a job well done, always pointing out that people's work is important and has meaning (Kouzes & Posner, 1991).

Relationships are close between authentic leaders and those followers who believe in them. This psychological engagement is key to a healthy work environment (Shirey, 2006) and can reduce chronic stress and burnout in the workplace (Maslach, Schaufeli, & Leiter, 2001).

Self-discipline means authentic leaders find a balance between their personal and professional lives. They engage in personal renewal and reflective practices (meditation, prayer, personal hobbies, etc.) that make them a better person first and a better leader second (Shirey, 2006).

Credibility means authentic leaders do what they expect others to do. They model the way, inspire a shared vision through their own action, and enable others to act (Kouzes & Posner, 2003).

The heart of leadership is encouragement. Authentic leaders encourage people to perform at their best. Authentic leaders realize that people are starving for recognition, and they hone their encouraging skills by:

- *Setting clear standards.* An authentic leader knows that commitment flows from personal values in action. Goals become concentrated in our minds and shape who we are and what we do. Feedback about our goals and how we attain them keeps us engaged.
- *Expecting the best.* An authentic leader holds high expectations of each and every person. An authentic leader talks about and provides positive images that create positive possibilities.
- *Paying attention.* An authentic leader pays attention to others and puts them first, spending time with them by being physically present. An authentic leader looks for the good in others, not for problems.
- *Personalizing recognition.* An authentic leader realizes recognition can hurt when it is not personalized. An authentic leader is thoughtful, knows what achievers like, and provides a personalized sign of recognition.
- *Telling the story.* An authentic leader knows the story of the work is the reality that teaches, mobilizes, and motivates. An authentic leader is a great storyteller.
- *Celebrating together.* An authentic leader celebrates when goals are achieved. An authentic leader knows that celebrations build community and reinforce values.
- *Setting the example.* An authentic leader goes first and shows the way. An authentic leader lives out the motto "Do what you say you will do" and finds a caring voice. (Kouzes & Posner, 2003)

LEADERSHIP CHALLENGE Which traits of authentic leadership, if any, does Mrs. Moore, the LPN in the Leadership in Action vignette at the beginning of this chapter, demonstrate?

Authentic Leadership and Healthy Work Environments

In 2005, the American Association of Critical-Care Nurses (AACN) made a commitment to promote healthy work environments that are:

- Safe
- Healing
- Humane
- Respectful for patients, their families, and nurses

Becoming an authentic leader is not an easy task. It requires positive organizational supports that encourage this kind of leadership. To that end, a 2005 AACN document identified authentic leadership as one of the six standards that are crucial to creating and sustaining healthy work environments in nursing. (The other standards were skilled communication, true collaboration, effective decision making, appropriate staffing, and meaningful recognition.)

So important is authentic leadership that the president of AACN called it the "glue" that holds together a healthy work environment (McCauley, 2005). The

American Organization of Nurse Executives (2002) also supports healthy work environments and produced a two-volume series of exemplars. A total of 21 hospitals and 61 individuals participated in the organization's survey, contributing experiences, best practices, and lessons for strengthening the nursing work environment. The resulting report focuses on six key organizational success factors: leadership development and effectiveness, empowered collaborative decision making, work design and service delivery innovation, values-driven organizational culture, recognition and reward systems, and professional growth and accountability.

Alternative Leadership Models

The **traditional model of leadership** holds that:

- Leadership resides in individuals.
- Leadership is hierarchically based and linked to office.
- Leadership means doing things to followers.
- Leadership is different from and more important than management.
- Leaders are different from followers.
- Leaders make a crucial difference to organizational performance.
- Effective leadership is generalizable to other situations.

An emerging view of **collective leadership** provides new thinking about what leadership is. In this view:

- Leadership is a property of social systems, which means it influences and is influenced by other properties (e.g., resources, healthcare workers and their relationships, clients, cultural values, organizational purposes and objectives, and information and knowledge).
- Leadership is a process of creating something significant, like a vision or common understanding.
- Leadership is a complex process of mutual influence.
- Leadership is within everyone's grasp; the designated leader is a participant in the process of leadership.
- Leadership is only one of many factors that can influence organizational performance.
- Context emerges as crucial; it's important to know the setting in which leadership occurs.
- Leadership development involves the whole community, and everybody takes responsibility. (Simkins, 2005)

> **KEY TERM**
>
> The **traditional model of leadership** holds that leadership resides in individuals, is linked to office, involves doing things to followers, is different from management, and changes organizational performance.

> **KEY TERM**
>
> In the **collective** view, **leadership** is a property of a social system, can occur anywhere, is a complex process of mutual influence, is within everyone's grasp, is only one factor influencing organizational performance, and is viewed in context.

Context includes such things as autonomy, professional control, and accountability. Leadership helps nurses become more autonomous, in control, and accountable. But leadership is not a linear, easily understood process. It is complex and ever changing, and it interacts with other parts of the healthcare system.

To make sense of leadership in nursing:

- Make sense of the role and purposes of the healthcare organization within a dynamic and conflicting policy environment
- Make sense of the ways leadership roles are changing and should change
- Make sense of the ways power and authority are and should be constituted and distributed across the organization
- Make sense of other worlds, those that lie outside of our interprofessional and organizational boundaries
- Use leadership development to understand the process of sense-making itself (Simkins, 2005)

LEADERSHIP CHALLENGE Does Mrs. Moore, the LPN in the Leadership in Action vignette at the beginning of this chapter, demonstrate any of the qualities of alternative leadership models?

None of these processes can be easily resolved. Each needs to be addressed through a complex view of what works, of what is practical and ethical, which always depends on the values of and wisdom of the group involved.

Summary

This chapter explored leadership theories and suggested ways you can use this information as a nurse leader. Once you finish the leadership development exercises that follow, you will have critically analyzed one leadership situation, identified environmental and organizational trends, differentiated between transformational and authentic leadership, chosen several leadership theories that are especially important to you, assessed your own transformational and authentic leadership qualities, discussed an emerging view of leadership, evaluated your ability to be an adaptable leader, and applied leadership theories to a simulated clinical setting.

Looking Ahead

The rest of this book helps you explore some of these leadership issues. Part 2 delves into basic skills to creative leadership and management, and Part 3 explores advanced leadership and management skills. Part 4 focuses on creatively managing human resources. Key terms and leadership development exercises are listed here and in the other chapters of this book to help you integrate knowledge.

Key Term Review

- **Authentic leadership** is leadership that is positive, genuine, trustworthy, credible, reliable, and believable.
- **Behavioral theory** proponents assume that leaders are made, not born, and that anyone can learn to be a leader.
- In the **collective view of leadership,** leadership is a property of a social system, can occur anywhere, is a complex process of mutual influence, is within everyone's grasp, is only one factor influencing organizational performance, and is viewed in context.
- **Creative leaders** produce or invent new solutions by using imagination, skill, and relevant theory and concepts.
- Theories of leadership began with the **great man theory** that leaders are born, not made.
- **Leader-member exchange theory,** also called LMX or vertical dyad linkage theory, explains how group leaders maintain their position by exchanging informal agreements with their members.
- The **leadership grid** charts leaders' concern for the work to be done compared to their concern for their people.
- Lewin, Lippit, and White identified three leadership styles: **autocratic, democratic,** and **laissez-faire.**
- Likert identified four main styles of leadership for decision making: **exploitative authoritative**, **benevolent authoritative**, **consultative leader,** and **participative leader.**
- A **normative leader** chooses a decision procedure, ranging from autocratic to group-based, depending on decision acceptance and follower knowledge.
- The theory of **participative leadership** holds that involvement in decision making improves team members' understanding and commitment to action.
- **Path-goal theory** helps clarify the path to a goal, removes roadblocks, and increases rewards along the way.
- **Role conflict** occurs when expectations don't match behavior.
- **Role theory** describes how expectations frame behavior.
- A **situational leader** takes into account followers' motivation and capability and other factors within a particular situation.
- The **traditional model of leadership** holds that leadership resides in individuals, is linked to office, involves doing things to followers, is different from management, and changes organizational performance.
- **Trait theory** holds that people are born with traits particularly suited for leadership.
- **Transformational leaders** use vision, passion, personal integrity, ceremonies, rituals, and enthusiasm to maintain motivation.

Leadership Development Exercises

■ **Leadership Development Exercise 1-1**

Write down your vision of the future of nursing. Explain how you can influence the future by pursuing a specific desired end. Chart the exact steps toward attaining your vision.

■ **Leadership Development Exercise 1-2**

Discuss your vision of the future of nursing with at least three other nursing colleagues. Listen to their visions. Did your vision change as a result of listening to their visions? Write down how it changed and what new things and ways of visioning you learned about.

■ **Leadership Development Exercise 1-3**

Write down three ways you maintain a belief in your capabilities and the essential goodness of things. Write about three ways you've learned to view challenges as opportunities.

■ **Leadership Development Exercise 1-4**

Discuss your ways of maintaining optimism with at least three other nursing colleagues. Write down what you learned from listening to their ideas, and chart a plan for implementing at least two of their ideas in the next month. Monitor your success, and write about it.

■ **Leadership Development Exercise 1-5**

Write about three times in the past when you were able to adapt to different people, situations, and approaches and how you revised your plan to suit changed circumstances.

■ **Leadership Development Exercise 1-6**

Discuss with at least three other nursing colleagues the way you adapted to changed circumstances, identifying the tactics you used. Listen to their three adaptations, and write down what you learned from the discussion that you might be able to use in future situations.

■ **Leadership Development Exercise 1-7**

Pretend you're the nursing director of a medical center or the head nurse of a unit. Answer the following questions based on one or more theories you read about in this chapter (identifying each theory with each answer):

a. What specific actions would you take to challenge the status quo when it reduces client and/or nurse wellness?
b. What specific actions would you take to encourage others to do the same?
c. What specific actions would you take to champion new initiatives that enhance nursing care?
d. What specific actions would you take to champion new initiatives that enhance the work environment for nurses?

■ Leadership Development Exercise 1-8

Share your ideas for championing new initiatives (and the theory behind them) with at least three other nursing colleagues, and listen to their ideas. Write down what you learned from listening to your colleagues that adds new dimensions or new ideas to yours.

Advanced Leadership Development Exercises

■ Leadership Development Exercise 1-9

Follow these steps to organize an in-class simulation for extra credit:

a. Fourteen students volunteer to lead a 5-minute group session with 8–12 other students, who simulate the behavior of staff members. Each leader chooses a leadership theory and a discussion point from the following lists to use with their group.

Theories:

- The great man theory
- Trait theory
- Behavioral theory
- Role theory
- The leadership grid
- Lewin's leadership styles
- Likert's leadership styles
- Hersey and Blanchard's situational leadership theory
- Vroom and Yetton's normative leadership
- Path-goal theory of leadership
- Leader-member exchange theory
- Transformational leadership
- Authentic leadership
- Collective leadership

Discussion Points:

- Who is going to represent the unit on a centerwide safety committee?

- What should the policy for unit violence be?
- What should the unit's uniform policy be?
- Should seniority or documented behavior factor more in promotions?

b. The nurse educator writes the numbers from 1 to 14 on slips of paper and puts them in a hat. The volunteer leaders each draw a slip of paper to decide who'll go first.

c. Enough chairs to seat the first group are pulled into the center of the room to form a circle.

d. A timekeeper is chosen to make sure that the group is warned when 4 minutes are up and when 5 minutes are up.

e. The group leader raises the discussion question and then acts according to the chosen leadership theory.

f. When time is called, the nurse educator asks the students in the group to identify which leadership theory was being demonstrated and to give examples of how the leader modeled that theory.

g. The rest of the class is asked to join in the discussion and give any examples that were missed by the group.

h. The nurse educator leads a discussion about the pros and cons of the chosen leadership style.

■ **Leadership Development Exercise 1-10**

Assess your leadership qualities by answering the items and scoring your responses on pages 27 and 28.

Assessing My Transformation and Authentic Self

Directions: *For each item, check whether you* never, sometimes, *or* always *practice or believe in the approach.*

		Never	Sometimes	Always
1.	I demonstrate care for others through sincere, practical deeds.	___	___	___
2.	I maintain consistency between words and actions.	___	___	___
3.	I'm willing to admit when I'm wrong and move past it.	___	___	___
4.	I treat other people as equal partners.	___	___	___
5.	I'm willing to spend time building professional relationships with others.	___	___	___
6.	I focus on doing what is right, not what other people tell me to do.	___	___	___
7.	I'm driven by a sense of a higher calling.	___	___	___
8.	I find a sense of meaning in my everyday work.	___	___	___
9.	I promote values that transcend self-interest and profit.	___	___	___
10.	I focus on finding a sense of purpose and direction.	___	___	___
11.	I make sure everyone has a clear understanding of our shared vision.	___	___	___
12.	I lead by positive personal example.	___	___	___
13.	I allow myself to experiment and be creative.	___	___	___
14.	I am trustworthy and trust others.	___	___	___
15.	I am reliable; when I say I'll do something, I do it.	___	___	___
16.	I work to empower others.	___	___	___
17.	I support clear communication and collaboration.	___	___	___
18.	I make sure everyone who's involved gets a say in decisions affecting them.	___	___	___
19.	I act to encourage a feeling of physical and emotional safety wherever I am.	___	___	___
20.	I provide others with meaningful recognition for their achievements.	___	___	___
21.	I try to bring a sense of family and cheer to fellow students and workers.	___	___	___
22.	I allow others to be true to their core values, preferences, and emotions.	___	___	___
23.	I share my life stories with colleagues so we understand each others' perspectives.	___	___	___
24.	I reduce my stress by engaging in meditation, prayer, hobbies, and other stress-reducing activities.	___	___	___
25.	I show others my principles, values, and ethics through my actions.	___	___	___

Assessing My Transformation and Authentic Self *(continued)*

Scoring: *The more instances of* always *you checked, the more you are in tune with transformational and authentic leadership values. For each* sometimes *or* never, *make a plan to participate in new activities to learn the skills or attitude change you need to become a transformational and authentic leader.*

Write your plan here:

Item #:___ Plan:

Item #:___ Plan:

Item #:___ Plan:

Item #:___ Plan:

Item #:___ Plan:

Item #:___ Plan:

Item #:___ Plan:

Item #:___ Plan:

Item #:___ Plan:

Item #:___ Plan:

Item #:___ Plan:

Item #:___ Plan:

Item #:___ Plan:

Item #:___ Plan:

Item #:___ Plan:

Item #:___ Plan:

Item #:___ Plan:

Item #:___ Plan:

References

American Association of Critical-Care Nurses. (2005). *AACN standards for establishing and sustaining healthy work environments.* Retrieved September 20, 2007, from www.aacn.org/AACN/pubpolcy.nsf/vwdoc/workenv

American Organization of Nurse Executives. (2002). *Healthy work environments. Volume 1. Striving for excellence.* www.aone.org/aone/keyissues/jhwe_excellence.html

Blake, R. R., & Mouton, J. S. (1961). *Group dynamics: Key to decision making.* Houston, TX: Gulf.

Burns, J. M. (1978). *Leadership.* New York: Harper & Row.

Coch, L., & French, J. R. P. (1948). Overcoming resistance to change. *Human Relations, 1,* 512–533.

Covey, S. R. (2004). *The 8th habit: From effectiveness to greatness.* New York: Free Press.

Fagin, C. M. (2000). *Essays on nursing leadership.* New York: Springer.

George, B. (2003). *Authentic leadership: Rediscovering the secrets to creating lasting value.* San Francisco: Jossey-Bass.

Graen, G. B., & Uhl-Bien, M. (1995). Relationship-based approach to leadership: Development of leader-member exchange (LMX) theory of leadership over 25 years: Applying a multilevel multi-domain perspective. *Leadership Quarterly, 6,* 219–247.

Heath, J., Johanson, W., & Blake, N. (2004). Healthy work environments: A validation of the literature. *Journal of Nursing Administration, 34,* 524–530.

Hersey, P., & Blanchard, K. H. (1999). *Leadership and the one minute manager.* New York: William Morrow.

Hersey, P., Blanchard, K. H., & Johnson, D. E. (2008). *Management of organizational behavior: Leading human resources* (9th ed.). Upper Saddle River, NJ: Prentice Hall.

House, R. J., & Mitchell, T. R. (1974, Fall). Path-goal theory of leadership. *Contemporary Business, 3,* 81–98.

Houser, B. P., & Player, K. N. (2004). *Pivotal moments in nursing: Leaders who changed the path of a profession.* Indianapolis, IN: Sigma Theta Tau International.

Institute of Medicine. (2004). *Keeping patients safe: Transforming the work environment of nurses.* Washington, DC: National Academies Press.

Kouzes, J. M., & Posner, B. Z. (1991). *The leadership challenge: How to get extraordinary things done in organizations.* San Francisco: Jossey-Bass.

Kouzes, J. M., & Posner, B. Z. (2003). *Encouraging the heart: A leader's guide to rewarding and recognizing others.* San Francisco: Jossey-Bass.

Lewin, K., Lippit, R., & White, R. K. (1939). Patterns of aggressive behavior in experimentally created social climates. *Journal of Social Psychology, 10,* 271–301.

Likert, R. (1967). *The human organization: Its management and value.* New York: McGraw-Hill.

Luthans, F., & Avolio, B. (2003). Authentic leadership development. In K. S. Cameron, J. E. Dutton, & R. E. Quinn (Eds.), *Positive organizational scholarship.* San Francisco: Berrett-Koehler.

Maier, N. R. F. (1963). *Problem-solving discussions and conferences: Leadership methods and skills.* New York: McGraw-Hill.

Maslach, C., Schaufeli, W. B., & Leiter, M. P. (2001). Job burnout. *Annual Reviews in Psychology, 52,* 397–422.

McBride, A. B., Fagin, C. M., Franklin, P. D., Huba, G. J., & Quach, L. (2006). Developing geriatric nursing leaders via an annual leadership conference. *Nursing Outlook, 54*(4), 226–229.

McCall, M. W., Jr., & Lombardo, M. M. (1983). *Off the track: Why and how successful executives get derailed.* Greensboro, NC: Center for Creative Leadership.

McCauley, K. (2005). President's note: All we needed was the glue. *AACN News, 22,* 2.

Merton, R. K. (1957). *Social theory and social structure.* New York: Free Press.

Pfeffer, J., & Salancik, G. R. (1975). Determinants of supervisory behavior: A role set analysis. *Human Relations, 28,* 139–153.

Shirey, M. R. (2006). Authentic leaders creating healthy work environments for nursing practice. *American Journal of Critical Care, 15*(3), 256–267.

Simkins, T. (2005). Leadership in education. *Educational Management Administration & Leadership, 33*(1), 9–26.

Stogdill, R. (1974). *Handbook of leadership.* New York: Free Press.

Syque. (2006). *Leadership theories.* Retrieved December 1, 2006, from http://changing minds.org/disciplines/leadership/theories/leadership_theories.htm

Tan, P. (2006). Nurturing nursing leadership: Beyond the horizon. *Singapore Nursing Journal, 33*(1), 33–38.

Tannenbaum, A. S., & Schmidt, W. H. (1958, March/April). How to choose a leadership pattern. *Harvard Business Review, 36,* 95–101.

Vroom, V. H., & Yetton, P. W. (1973). *Leadership and decision-making.* Pittsburgh, PA: University of Pittsburgh Press.

Theories and Styles of Management

CHAPTER OBJECTIVES

After reading this chapter, answering the leadership challenges, and participating in the leadership development exercises, you will be able to:

- Critically analyze one management situation
- Describe the relationship between leadership and management
- Describe four management theories that can be applied to nursing
- Assess your own management qualities
- Identify management values and beliefs
- Simulate conveying an unpopular decision to staff
- Develop a personal philosophy of management
- Join an online nursing support group
- Interview two staff members about how their organization could be improved
- Participate in an in-class simulation to help employees achieve a balance between work and family life

Advanced nurses will be able to:

- Teach at least three advanced nursing students about four management theories
- Design a problem statement for a research study focused on one management theory
- Develop a research design to answer your problem statement

Introduction

Although management and leadership can overlap and you must have both sets of skills to be effective, management is more concerned with accomplishing specific tasks; leadership is a broader concept (Hersey, Blanchard, & Johnson, 2008). This chapter focuses on how you can apply management theories, which are often developed in business contexts, to nursing situations.

First, read how a new nursing manager became involved in nurse management issues.

LEADERSHIP IN ACTION

Jenny Overbrook, a new nurse manager, is unsure of how to relate to her staff and encourage them to accomplish their tasks. She's heard a lot of stories about the staff on her unit and isn't sure whether she should trust them. Some of the nurses have been on the unit for years. When she talks to them about accomplishing their work, they tell her that they have tried everything and that nothing is going to change, no matter what she does. There are also some new nurses who are not confident of their clinical skills; others have a lot of good ideas, but Jenny is not sure what to do with their comments.

Taking a position as a nurse manager is challenging. You will use Jenny's situation to examine some of the many management theories that can guide you in this role.

LEADERSHIP CHALLENGE   Should Jenny, the head nurse, first concentrate on leadership or on management theory and skills? Give a rationale for your answer.

The Management Process

In 1925, Henri Fayol, an engineer, first identified management functions. As an administrative theorist, he looked at productivity improvements from the top down and focused on the job, not on the worker. Fayol believed that management was an acquired skill, something that could be learned, and included a body of principles that could be administered in a rational way. These principles included:

- *Division of work.* Output increases when workers specialize. In a nursing context, this translates into a medication nurse, a head nurse, technicians, physicians, and other roles. Each person has a job to do. If everyone tried to do everything, less work would get done.

- *Authority and responsibility.* Managers and leaders delegate power to others so an organization can balance authority and responsibility for tasks.
- *Unity of command.* Each person in an organization reports to only one supervisor.
- *Unity of direction.* A group's objectives are directed by one manager implementing one plan.
- *Discipline.* Each organization has rules and regulations for employees to follow. Discipline is used to improve effectiveness in the organization.
- *Subordination of individual interests to the general interest.* The interests of the organization as a whole are more important than the interests of one employee or group of employees.
- *Centralization.* The authority for making decisions is centralized to management or decentralized to subordinates. The degree of centralization varies depending on the type of situation.
- *Scalar chain.* The span of control indicates the number of subordinates that an immediate supervisor manages and shows communication channels.
- *Remuneration.* Workers are paid fairly for their services. If they're not, they may leave work early or arrive late, exhibiting their grievance.
- *Order.* To run an organization efficiently, staff and resources must be at the right place at the right time.
- *Equity.* Workers are treated in a fair and equitable manner.
- *Stability of personnel.* High staff turnover is inefficient. Planning and policies can reduce staff turnover.
- *Initiative.* Staff develop and carry out positive organizational plans.
- *Esprit de corps.* Leaders promote team spirit to ensure that the organization works in harmony. (Kannan, 2004a)

Although some of these ideas are quite old, many are still in use today.

LEADERSHIP CHALLENGE   Which of Fayol's ideas have you observed in clinical units? Provide specific examples.

Fayol's five functions of managers are planning, organizing, commanding, coordinating, and controlling. These were revised somewhat and are now taught as planning, organizing, staffing, directing, and controlling (Kannan, 2004b).

Although these functions appear to be independent, they are really interactive and make up the **management process.**

KEY TERM

The **management process** includes planning, organizing, staffing, directing, and controlling functions.

For example, if planning is awry, that will affect all other management functions. If a unit is understaffed, that will affect the nurse leader's ability to plan, organize, direct, and control. The interactive nature of management functions explains why a nurse leader must provide all five functions in a way that not only betters the organization but also motivates employees.

Planning includes everything that has to do with determining:

- Mission/philosophy
- Goals/objectives
- Policies/rules
- Procedures
- Scheduled changes
- Fiscal/budget actions

To plan effectively, a nurse manager must study the organization's resources, strengths, and weaknesses and access the opportunities and challenges it faces (Kannan, 2004b).

Organizing provides the structure required to execute the plan. Organizing includes everything needed to:

- Carry out plans
- Assign the duties and activities to specific positions and people to provide client care

LEADERSHIP CHALLENGE Based on what Jenny knows now, which of the organizing subfunctions should she focus on at this time? Give a rationale for your answer.

- Group activities to meet goals
- Delegate authority
- Establish horizontal and vertical authority-responsibility relationships
- Work within the system (Kannan, 2004b)

Staffing involves selecting the right person to execute each planned task. Staffing transforms a plan into action. It includes everything that has to do with:

- Recruiting
- Interviewing
- Hiring
- Orientation
- Staff development

Directing includes everything needed to:

- Motivate
- Manage conflict
- Delegate
- Communicate
- Collaborate

KEY TERM

Directing staff includes motivating, managing conflict, delegating tasks, communicating, monitoring/overseeing, and collaborating.

The nurse manager guides the team by training, coaching, instructing, and indicating what to do, when to do it, and how to do it. Directing also includes monitoring team members to ensure high standards of practice and efficiency. The function of directing includes giving orders and instructions; supervising or overseeing people at work; enhancing motivation by creating a willingness in others to work toward specific objectives; communicating or establishing an understanding with employees about what the plans are and how they ought to be implemented; and influencing others.

LEADERSHIP CHALLENGE Based on what Jenny knows now, which of the directing subfunctions should she focus on at this time? Give a rationale for your answer.

Controlling includes everything related to:

- Performance appraisals
- Fiscal accountability
- Quality control
- Legal and ethical issues
- Professional and collegial control

KEY TERM

Controlling helps keep the team on course by using performance appraisals, fiscal accountability, quality control, legal and ethical approaches, and professional and collegial control.

Control mechanisms help keep the team on course by removing obstacles whenever possible or by finding a new course if the present one is not working. Control systems help identify who isn't performing or who is functioning at a very low level of performance.

The process of controlling involves:

- Establishing standards for measuring work performance
- Measuring performance and comparing it with standards
- Identifying the reasons for the discrepancy between standards and performance
- Taking corrective action to ensure that goals are attained (Kannan, 2004b)

LEADERSHIP CHALLENGE Based on what Jenny knows now, which of the controlling subfunctions should she focus on at this time? Give a rationale for your answer.

Although not everyone's list of essential management functions includes innovation as an important quality of management, Kannan (2004b) insists that a conventional approach leads to routine results. Innovative approaches lead to more successes. The innovative organization endures and the process of **innovating** encourages the flow of innovative proposals and suggestions.

Historical Development of Management Theories

It has been claimed that management began evolving at the turn of the 19th century, but surely the Egyptians, Asians, Mayans, Romans, Greeks, and other empire builders could not have constructed roads, palaces, and magnificent buildings without management skills.

Weber's Theory of Bureaucracy and Authority

Max Weber, a German sociologist and philosopher, lived from 1864 to 1920. He studied social change and the effect of rationality on capitalism and religious thought. He defined three types of authority:

1. Traditional authority, which is invested in a hereditary line or determined by a higher power
2. Rational-legal authority or bureaucracy, which is enforced by regulations
3. Charismatic authority, which rests on the appeal of leaders (Kannan, 2004d)

According to Kannan (2004c), an **ideal bureaucracy** has a hierarchy of authority and written rules of conduct, provides for promotion based on achievement, has a specialized division of labor, and is efficient.

Bureaucracies that go awry do so because they do not respond to their customers' needs, are corrupted by power-wielding officials, fall prey to manipulative specialists, or experience a shift in power from leaders to bureaucrats (Kannan, 2004c).

Scientific Management Theory

Frederick Taylor developed his **scientific management theory** in the late 1800s. A product of his environment—which included large industrialized organizations, with ongoing routine tasks that produced a variety of products—Taylor analyzed and timed movements with a stopwatch to increase production. He coined the term *time study*. Workers were rewarded and punished, and Taylor refused to compromise in his approach. He believed his theory could be applied to all problems, whether they were related to managers or workers. He justified his approach with hundreds of experiments to demonstrate the rules and laws that govern scientific management (Kannan, 2004a).

> **KEY TERM**
>
> **Scientific management theory** heralded the analysis and timing of routine movements to increase production.

This approach worked for organizations with assembly lines and other mechanistic, routinized activities. Taylor studied things such as the optimum shovel size for coal, the best surface for digging coal, and the ideal size and type of coal. Ford Motor Company embraced Taylor's work and adopted the production line as the way to produce its vehicles (McNamara, 2006; Taylor, 1911).

The four objectives of scientific management were to:

1. Develop a science for each element of work
2. Scientifically select, train, and develop workers instead of letting them choose their own work and train themselves
3. Encourage cooperation between workers and management so work was carried out according to scientifically developed procedures
4. Create a division of labor in equal shares between workers and management, which led to a hierarchy, abstract rules, and impersonal relationships between staff (Kannan, 2004d)

Scientific management focused on job productivity and was widely criticized because it ignored the human side of the organization, treated workers like machines, exploited employees, was narrow in scope, and led to monotonous jobs and worker discontent (Kannan, 2004a).

LEADERSHIP CHALLENGE   How can Jenny, the new nurse manager, use Taylor's organizational framework with her staff? Give a rationale for your answer.

Taylor also contributed to organizational theory. The framework he used included:

- Clearly defined authority
- Delineated responsibility
- Separating planning from operations
- Incentives for workers
- Task specialization
- Intervening only when employees fail to perform (Kannan, 2004a)

> **LEADERSHIP TIP**
>
> If you focus only on getting the job done efficiently and effectively, you may foment employee discontent.

Motion Study/Efficiency Theory

Frank and Lillian Gilbreth, a husband-and-wife team of psychologists, developed **efficiency theory.** They studied faster and more efficient ways to do jobs, prepare employees for the next level, and train successors.

LEADERSHIP CHALLENGE Which of the Gilbreths' goals could Jenny use with her staff? Choose one and give a rationale for your choice.

They were more sophisticated in their approach to workers than Taylor and examined more incentive payments. The Gilbreths also studied physicians and the way in which operations and operating room procedures were organized. Although ignored by the medical hierarchy when presented to the AMA in 1915, by the 1930s, the Gilbreths' recommendations about laying out surgical instruments and standardizing surgical techniques were accepted practice (The Science Museum, 2004).

After Frank died, Lillian, who had by then become an industrial psychologist, was known as "the mother of modern management." She established domestic economy and home economics as scientifically taught subjects in colleges across the United States and Europe (The Science Museum, 2004).

Mayo's Hawthorne Experiments

Elton Mayo's work contradicted the prevailing theory of Frederick Taylor that the worker was motivated solely by self-interest.

Even when Mayo cut rest breaks and returned female employees to longer working hours, productivity rose. When he checked into the process, he found that women, exercising freedom that they didn't have on the factory floor, formed a social group and included the observer who tracked their productivity as a group. The women joked, talked, and met after work (Accel-Team, 2003b).

Mayo discovered what seems obvious now. Workplaces are social environments, and employees are motivated by doing things of social value. The women felt better about themselves when their boss singled them out to have a friendly relationship with their supervisor. When that supervisor discussed changes in advance with the women, they felt like part of the team. This enhanced their cooperation and loyalty, even when their rest breaks were taken away. The fact that they were singled out to be special participants in the study reinforced these feelings. This led to greater productivity and an effort to continue the behavior they believed would help them gain more attention. This phenomenon was called the **Hawthorne effect,** after the workplace, the Hawthorne Works, which was owned by Western Electric. The findings of the Hawthorne studies took their place in the human relations school of management and have been recycled as quality circles, participatory management, and team building.

KEY TERM

The **Hawthorne effect** refers to feeling part of a special team that is under study.

Mayo's findings included:

- Work is a group activity, not an individual one.
- The social world of adults is patterned around work.
- The physical conditions of work aren't as important to employees as the need for recognition, security, and a sense of belonging.
- An employee complaint is often a symptom of the worker's low or unrecognized status in the organization.
- Employee attitudes and effectiveness are affected by social demands.
- Informal groups in the workplace control individual employees' work habits and attitudes.
- Group collaboration must be planned and developed. (Accel-Team, 2003b)

LEADERSHIP CHALLENGE How can Jenny use the Hawthorne effect with her staff? Why should she or shouldn't she use it? Give a rationale for your answer.

This was the first in a series of theories called the **human relations approach to management,** which included six propositions:

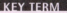

KEY TERM

The **human relations approach to management** focuses on motivating staff through teamwork to fulfill individual and organizational goals and encourages the staff's coordination and cooperation.

1. People, not machines or economics, are the focus.
2. People exist in an organizational environment rather than an organized social context.
3. Motivating staff is important.
4. Such motivation should be directed toward teamwork and requires the staff's coordination and cooperation.
5. Teamwork can fulfill individual and organizational goals.
6. Individuals and organizations strive for efficiency by achieving maximum results with minimum inputs. (Kannan, 2004e)

McGregor's Theory X and Theory Y

Douglas McGregor formulated two models of individuals at work based on social science research findings.

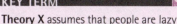

KEY TERM

Theory X assumes that people are lazy and must be controlled and threatened.

In McGregor's **Theory X:**

- The average human being tries to avoid work.
- Because of humans' dislike for work, they must be controlled and threatened to get them to work hard.
- Humans desire security and direction and hate responsibility.

In McGregor's **Theory Y**:

- Work is as natural as play or rest.
- People will work hard if they are committed to their organization's aims.
- If a job is satisfying, employees will be committed to their organization.
- People can learn to accept responsibility.
- Employees can use imagination, creativity, and ingenuity to solve work problems.
- The intellectual potential of the average worker is only partially utilized.

The way nurse managers use Theory Y in their interactions with employees is by finding ways to:

- Help employees commit to their organization's aims
- Make jobs satisfying so employees will be committed to the organization
- Teach employees how to accept responsibility
- Help employees use their imagination, creativity, and ingenuity to solve work problems
- Teach employees how to use more of their potential (Accel-Team, 2003a)

LEADERSHIP CHALLENGE Should Jenny, the new manager, use Theory X or Theory Y with her staff? Give a rationale for your choice.

McClelland's Achievement Motivation Theory

David McClelland studied people with a high need for achievement and a high need for affiliation. He learned that it is possible to learn to be achievement oriented. People with a high need for achievement:

- Prefer a moderate degree of risk because they believe their efforts and abilities can influence the outcome; this **aggressive realism** is the mark of a successful entrepreneur
- Get a bigger kick out of winning or solving a problem than they get from money or praise
- View money as a way of assessing their progress and comparing themselves with others
- Desire concrete feedback on how well they're doing

- Are not interested in comments about how cooperative or helpful they are
- Always try to think of better ways of doing things
- Help organizations grow faster and be more profitable

Employees with high-affiliation needs:

- Are more concerned about the environment
- Want to know how people feel about them, not how well they're doing (Accel-Team, 2006b)

> **LEADERSHIP TIP**
>
> To motivate achievement-oriented employees, give concrete feedback about how well they're doing, give them problems to solve, and reward them for finding better ways of doing things.

LEADERSHIP CHALLENGE Jenny learns that two staff members are more concerned with affiliation than with achievement. What should she do to motivate those two staff members? Give a rationale for your answer.

Argyris's Theory of Humanistic and Democratic Values

Chris Argyris, through his **theory of humanistic and democratic values,** postulated that bureaucratic values lead to poor, shallow, and mistrustful relationships. Without interpersonal competence or a psychologically safe environment, the organization breeds mistrust, intergroup conflict, rigidity, disgruntled and discouraged employees, and poor problem solving. To increase interpersonal competence, intergroup cooperation, and flexibility to get the job done:

> **KEY TERM**
>
> The **theory of humanistic and democratic values** holds that interpersonal competence must be encouraged in work systems to increase organizational success in problem solving.

- Promote humanistic and democratic values
- Treat people as human beings and give them an opportunity to develop to the fullest potential
- Make work exciting and challenging
- Use clear, rational, and logical communication; effectiveness decreases as behavior becomes more emotional and increases when relevant behavior becomes conscious, discussible, and controllable and when rewards and penalties emphasize rational behavior and achieving objectives (Accel-Team, 2006)

> **LEADERSHIP TIP**
>
> To increase organizational success in problem solving, make work exciting and challenging, give employees an opportunity to develop to their fullest potential, use clear and logical communication, discuss issues and problems in a clear and open manner, and emphasize rational behavior and achieving objectives when providing rewards or penalties.

The Behavioral Science Approach to Management

A group of psychologists and sociologists improved on the human relations approach by hoping not just to study employees but to predict behavior. This approach is called the **behavioral science approach to management.** Motivation, leadership, communication, group dynamics, and participative management are important to the approach. This approach helps secure better employee performance and the willing pursuit of organizational goals. Proponents of this approach include Abraham Maslow and Chris Argyris, whose theories were discussed earlier, as well as Douglas McGregor and Frederick Herzberg, whose theories are discussed here.

Maslow's Hierarchy of Needs

Maslow reinforced the idea that human beings are motivated by complex needs. He constructed a **hierarchy of basic needs,** including:

- Physiological needs (hunger, thirst, sleep)
- Safety
- Love and belonging (associating happily with people, belonging to one or more groups, and having friends)
- Esteem (self-respect, reputation, recognition, and appreciation)
- Self-actualization (drive for self-development, creativity, fulfillment, and job satisfaction)

LEADERSHIP CHALLENGE How can Jenny use Maslow's hierarchy of needs with her staff? Give a rationale for your answer.

Maslow arranged basic needs in order of importance, ranging from physiological needs to self-actualization. He believed that people had to fulfill basic needs before they could move to higher needs, such as self-actualization. Maslow's theory helps explain the Hawthorne experiment findings (Accel-Team, 2002).

Herzberg's Motivational Theory

Frederick Herzberg (1923–2000), clinical psychologist and pioneer of "job enrichment," is regarded as one of the most original thinkers in **motivational theory** and management. He established the Department of Industrial Mental Health at Case Western Reserve University when he served as professor of management there. The absence of any serious challenge to his work validates its importance (Chapman, 2006).

Herzberg (1971) found that job satisfaction and job dissatisfaction are not opposites; they are on completely different continua, are produced by different

factors, and have their own dynamics. He also found that certain factors called "motivators" truly motivate but that other
factors tend to lead to dissatisfaction. Motivators include:

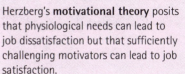

KEY TERM

Herzberg's **motivational theory** posits
that physiological needs can lead to
job dissatisfaction but that sufficiently
challenging motivators can lead to job
satisfaction.

- Achievement
- Recognition
- The work itself
- Responsibility
- Advancement
- Personal growth

He called certain factors in the environment "hygiene factors." Hygiene factors include basic needs for food, warmth, shelter, and safety.

Herzberg found that money wasn't a motivator, and other surveys and research
studies have backed that up by showing that many other factors are more important motivators than money (e.g., Chapman, 2006). Doing something meaningful or worthwhile outranks pay as the reason to stay in a job (Internet Center
for Management and Business Administration, 2006). Real motivators are more
concerned with the actual job and include:

- How interesting the job is
- How much opportunity the job provides for earning extra responsibilities,
  gaining recognition, and being promoted (tutor2u, 2006)

Herzberg believed that jobs should be sufficiently challenging and that
employees need to be challenged. If a job doesn't use an employee's full ability,
Herzberg thought the task should be automated or given to someone who has a
lower level of skill (Internet Center for Management and Business Administration, 2006).

Hertzberg believed that managers should adopt a democratic approach to
management and improve the content and nature of tasks by:

- Giving workers a greater variety of tasks to perform,
  thereby making the job more interesting
- Fostering a great sense of achievement in workers by
  giving them a wider range of more complex, interesting,
  and challenging tasks
- Delegating more power to employees so they can make
  their own decisions about their work

LEADERSHIP TIP

A good leader provides interesting and challenging tasks and
delegates power to employees.

LEADERSHIP CHALLENGE How can Jenny, the new nurse manager, use
Herzberg's theory to help build a viable work team? Give a rationale for your
answer, and list the steps you would use to implement the theory.

The Systems Theory Approach to Management

KEY TERM

Systems theory provides a way to examine the interdependent and interrelated parts (boundaries, outputs, feedback, equifinality) of an organization and to deal with change by establishing system objectives called "performance criteria," by identifying wider systems in the environment, by creating formal subsystems, and by integrating the subsystems within the system.

The **systems theory** approach to management, developed in the early 1950s, examined management as a set of distinguishable but interdependent and interrelated parts known to operate in a logical manner to achieve goals. Open systems have flexible boundaries allowing for dynamic interchanges (e.g., nurse-doctor relationships, healthcare planning activities). Closed systems have rigid boundaries that permit minimal or no exchange (e.g., wheelchairs, unit-dose medications). Conflict is viewed as an opportunity, with openness on one side of the boundary and closedness on the other. The transfer of energy, people, information, or materials occurs at the interface between one system and another. Massive environmental changes could produce a crisis, disrupting the dynamic equilibrium.

A steady state is regained when the structure or processes of subsystems are reorganized to a higher level of functioning. According to Watzlawick, Beavin, and Jackson (1967), feedback can lead to change and adaptation (positive) or maintain a steady state (negative).

All systems have a hierarchy of components (Bertalanffy, 1976). Socially, people are organized into groups, groups are organized into departments, and so on. The hierarchical structure of a healthcare system, for example, has the shape of a pyramid, with an administrator at the top, a few managers or supervisors at the middle levels, and many healthcare providers and consumers at the bottom. As the hierarchy's complexity increases, order is needed to coordinate activities and processes.

System outputs include such things as enhanced quality of life or productivity. In a systems frame of reference, there is no direct cause-and-effect relationship. Final states can be reached from different starting points along various pathways; this is called "equifinality."

Systems theory concepts provide a view of management that considers the interaction between people and the organization in the context of the larger society. Management in this context is the process of linking together individuals or work groups around specific problems or issues of the work environment (Bennis, 1966).

Systems theory resembles the scientific method: it includes developing hypotheses, designing a controlled experiment, and collecting and analyzing data. Systems theory uses science to obtain results that can be used to affect the control of an organization. For managers, this means:

- Defining the organization as a system
- Establishing system objectives called "performance criteria"

- Identifying wider systems in the environment
- Creating formal subsystems
- Integrating the subsystems within the system

Decades of management theory and practice in the workplace focused on only one aspect of management. Systems theory helps managers examine the effects of the tremendous change facing organizations and how they operate, recognize the various parts of the organization and the interrelations of its parts, and coordinate central administration with programs.

LEADERSHIP CHALLENGE How can Jenny use systems theory with her staff? Give a rationale for your answer.

This constituted a major advancement. In the past, managers focused on only one part of an organization at a time, which could lead to an organization with a wonderful central administration and terrific staff but departments that couldn't relate to each other or synchronize (McNamara, 2006).

Summary

This chapter focused on major theories and styles of management and described the relationship between leadership and management. Once you finish the leadership development exercises that follow, you will have critically analyzed one management situation, assessed your management qualities, simulated conveying an unpopular decision to staff, developed a personal philosophy of management, joined an online nursing support group, interviewed two staff members about how their organization could be improved, and participated in an in-class simulation to help employees achieve a balance between work and family life. All these learning experiences will help you apply management theory to nursing leadership situations.

Key Term Review

- McClelland's **achievement motivation theory** suggests that to motivate achievement-oriented employees, managers should provide concrete feedback about how well they're doing, should give them problems to solve, and should reward them for finding better ways of doing things.
- **Aggressive realism** means that successful entrepreneurs prefer a moderate degree of risk because they believe their efforts and abilities can influence the outcome.
- The **behavioral science approach to management** used motivation, leadership, communication, group dynamics, and participative management to achieve organizational goals.
- **Controlling** helps keep the team on course by using performance appraisals, fiscal accountability, quality control, legal and ethical approaches, and professional and collegial control.
- **Directing** staff includes motivating, managing conflict, delegating tasks, communicating, monitoring/overseeing, and collaborating.
- The **Hawthorne effect** refers to feeling part of a special team that is under study.
- Maslow's **hierarchy of basic needs** implies that lower level needs (i.e., physiological needs and safety) must be satisfied before higher level needs (i.e., belonging, esteem, and self-actualization) can be met.
- The **human relations approach to management** focuses on motivating staff through teamwork to fulfill individual and organizational goals and encourages the staff's coordination and cooperation.
- Weber believed that an **ideal bureaucracy** has a hierarchy of authority and written rules of conduct, provides for promotion based on achievement, has a specialized division of labor, and is efficient.
- **Innovating** means the nurse leader encourages the flow of innovative proposals and suggestions.
- The **management process** includes the interacting functions of planning, organizing, staffing, directing, and controlling.
- **Motion study/efficiency theory** provided a framework for studying faster and more efficient ways to do jobs, including surgery.
- Herzberg's **motivational theory** posits that managers should give workers a greater variety of tasks to make the job more interesting; should foster a sense of achievement by giving workers a wider range of more complex, interesting, and challenging tasks; and should delegate more power to employees so they can make their own decisions about their work.

- **Organizing** provides the structure needed to carry out plans and assign the duties.
- **Planning** includes determining mission, philosophy, goals, objectives, policies, rules, procedures, scheduled changes and fiscal/budget actions.
- Taylor's **scientific management theory** heralded the analysis and timing of routine movements to increase production.
- **Staffing** uses recruiting, interviewing, hiring, orientation and staff development to select the right person to execute each planned task
- **Systems theory** provides a way to examine the interdependent and interrelated parts (boundaries, outputs, feedback, equifinality) of an organization and to deal with change by establishing system objectives called "performance criteria," by identifying wider systems in the environment, by creating formal subsystems, and by integrating the subsystems
- Argyris's **theory of humanistic and democratic values** holds that interpersonal competence must be encouraged in work systems to increase organizational success in problem solving.
- McGregor's **Theory X** says that people are inherently lazy; his **Theory Y** assumes that people want to work and can learn to meet organizational goals.

Leadership Development Exercises

■ Leadership Development Exercise 2-1

Being a nurse manager means you will sometimes have to choose to adhere to certain of your values and beliefs and compromise on others. To prepare for this eventuality, answer the following questions:

a. What values and beliefs are most important to me?
b. On which of these will I never compromise?
c. For which am I willing to fight? How will I do that?

■ Leadership Development Exercise 2-2

Being a nurse manager is not a cut-and-dry affair. You can always learn from others by talking about how they handled difficult work situations and deciding whether what they learned may be helpful to you. Talk with at least three other nurses or nursing students, and ask them:

a. How they make difficult decisions and what goes into their decision
b. How they handle the aftereffects of a decision
c. What about their decision-making method works for them
d. What doesn't work for them

Write about which of these ideas you plan to incorporate into your approach to nursing management and how you will implement them.

Make a specific plan: By next week, I will implement _____.

By the end of the month, I will implement _____.

■ **Leadership Development Exercise 2-3**

The situation: You are a nurse manager who has to communicate an unpopular decision to your staff.

  a. What management theories might help you do that?
  b. How will you allow enough time for people to process the message and express their feelings?
  c. How will you take ownership of the decision without becoming defensive or angry? (Be sure to write down specific steps.)
  d. How will you show that you are listening and understanding? (Write down specific things that you will say and do.)
  e. What is the worse-case scenario, and what will you do if that happens?
  f. What else can you do to influence a positive outcome?
  g. Devise a simulation to play out this situation so that you demonstrate a–f.

Simulation directions:

  a. Gather together 4–10 learners.
  b. Give each person a role to play throughout the simulation. Suggested roles include a complaining RN, a "nothing's ever going to change around here" staff member, a teased or teasing LPN, an aggressive RN, a joking LPN, and so forth. Make one person the timekeeper to watch the clock, make sure the simulation moves along, and give everyone a 2-minute and a 1-minute warning: "You have 2 more minutes (or 1 more minute) to finish this step."
  c. Consult with your group for 5 minutes about possible unpopular decisions. During that time, choose one unpopular decision that you will tell group members about in the simulation.
     Alternative step: Choose the unpopular decision in advance, based on consultation with one or more nursing leaders you know or have observed.
  d. To begin the simulation, tell the group the unpopular decision using the suggestions implied or stated in the management theory (or theories) you have chosen. Group members should act out their role; and should act according to the chosen theory (or theories).
  e. At the end of 15 minutes, the timekeeper will call time, and you should ask the group to tell you:

     • Which management theory (or theories) you portrayed

- Which of your comments worked the best
- Which of your comments or behaviors weren't effective
- Anything else they wish to share about the simulation

■ Leadership Development Exercise 2-4

Being an advocate for your staff is part of your job as a nurse manager. Explain—and be very specific—about what you'd say and do to:

a. Decide how and when to support your staff's decisions despite opposition
b. Teach staff how to take risks and learn new skills
c. Protect staff from fear of failure
d. Avoid getting drawn into personal agendas

■ Leadership Development Exercise 2-5

a. Develop a personal philosophy of management, and write it down.
b. Communicate your philosophy to three other nurses or nursing students.
c. Ask them to tell you their philosophies.
d. Revise your philosophy as needed once you've completed a–c.
e. Set up a feedback schedule so you can obtain evaluations from those three people to make sure you live out your philosophy.

■ Leadership Development Exercise 2-6

Discuss with at least three other nursing colleagues the way you managed a situation, and ask them to tell you:

a. Which management theory you used
b. What might have been a more effective theory to use

■ Leadership Development Exercise 2-7

Go to Google and search for "nursing support groups" and related phrases.

a. Visit at least two groups and participate.
b. Pose a leadership/management question that you're burning to ask.
c. Read what others write or say.
d. Come up with at least one concrete management tip to share with the class.

Advanced Leadership Development Exercises

■ Leadership Development Exercise 2-8

Interview two staff members at your school or at a clinical site. Ask questions about how the organization could be improved, including:

a. What are your high-priority work needs?

b. Is the organization meeting your work needs?

c. What family concerns do you need help with from the organization?

d. What exactly do you wish the organization would do to meet your needs?

e. How do you suggest administrators do that?

Once you have this information, share it with your classmates, and ask for suggestions on what to do with the information and how to use it.

■ **Leadership Development Exercise 2-9**

Develop an in-class simulation to hold a university or hospital contest to generate ideas for how employees can achieve a better balance between work life and family life while maintaining a high rate of client satisfaction and worker productivity.

a. Form a group of employees and managers to build a work and family life plan based on the best suggestions.

b. Simulate a meeting to launch the plan and publicly recognize the employees who made major contributions by sharing their ideas for building balance.

c. Have the role-playing group draw roles out of a hat.

d. Be sure to include basic roles, such as a nurse manager (who chooses one of the management theories and portrays it throughout), a hospital administrator (who pooh-poohs all new ideas), a student nurse, staff participants, and a client ombudsperson (who supports the nurse manager).

e. Play out the recognition meeting (consider giving prizes or awarding play money to participants).

f. Be sure to discuss various ways to measure the meeting's effectiveness and how to make necessary improvements in the manager's behavior.

References

Accel-Team. (2002). *Abraham Maslow's hierarchy of needs.* Retrieved December 7, 2006, from http://www.accel-team.com/human_relations/hrels_02_maslow.html

Accel-Team. (2003a). *Douglas McGregor: Theory X and Theory Y.* Retrieved December 7, 2006, from http://www.accel-team.com/human_relations/hrels_03_mcgregor.html

Accel-Team. (2003b). *Elton Mayo's Hawthorne experiments.* Retrieved December 7, 2006, from http://www.accel-team.com/motivation/hawthorne_03.html

Accel-Team. (2006a). *Chris Argyris.* Retrieved December 7, 2006, from http://www.accel-team.com/human_relations/hrels_061_argyris.html

Accel-Team. (2006b). *David McClelland: Achievement motivation.* Retrieved December 7, 2006, from http://www.accel-team.com/human_relations/hrels_06_mcclelland.html

Bennis, W. (1966). *Beyond bureaucracy: Essays on the development and evolution of human organizations.* New York: McGraw-Hill.

Bertalanffy, L. V. (1976). Introduction. In H. H. Werley, A. Zuzich, M. Zajkowski, & A. D. Zagornik (Eds.), *Health research: The systems approach.* New York: Springer.

Chapman, A. (2006). *Frederick Herzberg motivational theory*. Retrieved December 21, 2006, from http://www.businessballs.com/herzberg.htm

Fayol, H. (1925). *General and industrial management*. London: Pittman.

Hersey, P., Blanchard, K. H., & Johnson, D. E. (2008). *Management of organizational behavior: Leading human resources* (9th ed.). Upper Saddle River, NJ: Prentice-Hall.

Herzberg, F. (1971). Managers or animal trainers? *Management Review, 60,* 2–5.

Internet Center for Management and Business Administration. (2006). *Herzberg's motivation theory*. Retrieved December 22, 2006, from http://www.netmba.com/mgmt/0b/motivation/herzberg

Kannan, R. (2004a). *Evolution of management thought: Henri Fayol: Administrative theory of management*. Retrieved December 7, 2006, from http://www.geocities.com/kstability/learning/management/administrative-management.html

Kannan, R. (2004b). *The functions of management*. Retrieved December 22, 2006, from http://www.geocities.com/kstability/learning/management/function.html

Kannan, R. (2004c). *Evolution of management thought: Weber's theory of bureaucracy & authority*. Retrieved December 7, 2006, from http://www.geocities.com/kstability/learning/management/bureaucracy.html

Kannan, R. (2004d). *Evolution of management thought: Frederick Winslow Taylor: Theory of scientific management*. Retrieved December 7, 2006, from http://www.geocities.com/kstability/learning/management/evolution2.html

Kannan, R. (2004e). *Human relations management & behavioural approach to management*. Retrieved December 7, 2006, from http://www.geocities.com/kstability/learning/management/behavioural.html

McNamara, C. (2006). *Brief overview of contemporary theories in management*. Retrieved December 8, 2006, from http://www.managementhelp.org/mgmnt/cntmpory.htm

The Science Museum. (2004). *Lillian Gilbreth*. Retrieved December 8, 2006, from http://www.makingthemodernworld.org.uk/people/BG.0129/

Taylor, F. W. (1911). *The principles of scientific management*. New York: Harper & Row.

tutor2u. (2006). *Theories of motivation: Herzberg*. Retrieved December 22, 2006, from http://www.tutor2u.net/business/gcse/people_motivation_theories.htm

Watzlawick, P., Beavin, J. H., & Jackson, D. D. (1967). *Pragmatics of human communication*. New York: Norton.

Part II

Basic Skills to Creatively Lead and Manage

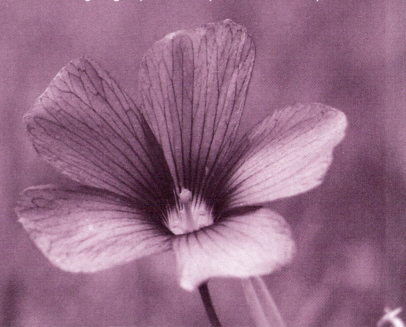

Role Transitioning

CHAPTER OBJECTIVES

After reading this chapter, answering the leadership challenges, and participating in the leadership development exercises, you will be able to:

- Critically analyze one role transitioning situation
- List the assumptions of role theory
- Describe four paths to nursing leadership/management
- Identify ways a nurse can transition to a leadership role

Advanced nurses will be able to:

- Teach at least three nursing students about role transition
- Design a problem statement for a research study focused on role transition
- Develop a research design to answer your problem statement

Introduction

Transitioning to new roles is a frequent occurrence for nurses. This chapter focuses on role theory, paths to nursing leadership, and transitioning to a leadership role.

Sarah, a new nurse manager, was promoted because of her clinical skills, but she's not sure she wants the job. She has butterflies in the pit of her stomach and a stack of notes that she's written to herself about her priorities, her goals, her vision for the unit, and more. Keeping her staff happy is at the top of her to-do list, but so far, they don't want to listen to her. Why? They used to be her colleagues and would catch a cup of coffee together on break, share pictures of their kids, and complain about the head nurse. Now Sarah's the head nurse, and she has to give them orders.

LEADERSHIP CHALLENGE What advice do you have for Sarah?

Role Theory

Role theory may help explain what's happening to Sarah. Some of the assumptions of role theory are that people (Role theory, 2006):

- Define roles for themselves and others based on social learning and reading
- Form expectations about the roles they and others will play
- Subtly encourage others to meet those role expectations
- Act within the roles they adopt

LEADERSHIP TIP

Formal and informal information about what the leader's role should be appears in memos and reports, during training sessions and rounds, in modeling by upper-level nurse leaders, and more.

LEADERSHIP CHALLENGE Which role theory assumptions apply to Sarah?

Transitioning to a new role means acquiring knowledge, skills, and abilities that may differ from the ones you used in a clinical role (Nugent and colleagues, 2004; Vriesendorp & Buxbaum, 2006). This transition can be challenging.

KEY TERM

Role conflict can occur when the leader's expectations differ from the group's expectations.

Role conflict can occur when group members have different expectations of their leaders. Role conflict can also occur when the nurse leader has an idea about what to do that differs from rest of the group's expectations.

KEY TERM

Role transition is the process of moving from one role to another.

Role transition is the process of moving from one role to another. In the Leadership in Action vignette at the beginning of this chapter, is Sarah in role transition or role conflict?

Paths to Nursing Leadership

Why do nurses enter leadership and management positions? See **Box 3-1** for some ideas.

Because nursing care environments have become more technological and more complex, client care has become more complicated. Assuming a management role can affect your family life, relationships with employees, and self-image.

Barriers and Enablers of a Successful Transition to Nurse Manager

Nurse leaders are a vital link in stemming nursing shortages. Moving to a management position can elicit feelings of stress, confusion, and being unprepared for the job (Heller et al., 2004).

Hudson (2005) interviewed 13 nurse leaders and found they often "did" management but continued to "be" nurses. They flourished as clinical nurses but floundered as nurse managers. According to the interviewees, this schism affected attitude, job satisfaction, and performance. See **Box 3-2** for a summary of the themes Hudson found for nurse managers.

Hudson found that while the nurse managers she interviewed changed jobs, they didn't acquire a new set of attitudes and beliefs and they reported suffering high levels of stress and tension in both their personal and professional lives. Hudson attributed such feelings to the nature of the nurses' work, which includes tedious, nonemotional activities, such as doing payroll, making a budget, dealing with human resource issues, and going to meetings.

BOX 3-1   PATHS TO LEADERSHIP

Bondas (2006) explored why nurses want to take nursing leadership and management positions. She used a semistructured questionnaire with a strategic sample of 68 Finnish nurses who were all active in leadership positions. She applied analytic induction to generate a theory and found that the nurses took four different paths that varied according to their education, primary commitment, and situational factors: the Path of Ideals (in which the nurse leader created a caring culture and an ideal unit); the Path of Chance (chance factors lead to a leadership position); the Career Path (which provided the nurse leader with more power); and the Temporary Path (in which the nurse accepted the position but had the option to withdraw). Bondas found that current nursing education does not equip future nurse leaders to use evidence-based practices or leadership, organizational, or economic skills. She counseled that healthcare organizations need nurse leaders who enter with a combination of the Path of Ideals and the Career Path.

BOX 3-2   THEMES IN HUDSON'S RESEARCH

Hudson (2005) found that nurse managers have or experience:
- A passion for nursing
- Beliefs about management
- Expectations of others
- Identity conflict/role ambiguity
- Self-confidence/self-efficacy
- Fulfillment

All 13 of Hudson's nurse leaders reported a lack of autonomy and power and thought they were highly "directed" and supervised in their roles—that is, they were told what to do and when and how to do it. These nurses appeared to transfer their care-taking orientation from clients to staff and reported over-whelming responsibilities in keeping the staff happy, fighting for the staff, and protecting the staff. Some participants carried a beeper 24/7 so the staff could reach them and even missed family events to help the staff.

Participants in Hudson's study also reported a sense of isolation; they felt lost without a clear reference group with which to identify. Many talked about returning to the bedside if the management position didn't work out. Several spoke of going through "clinical withdrawal" because they missed client contact and saving lives.

Miller and Rahn (2002) found that identity commitment was strongest when "being" and "doing" corresponded to attitude and action. Hudson's findings suggest that staff nurses who aren't willing to make a change in identity and let go of attitudes about working directly with clients may have difficulty ceasing to be clinical nurses and transitioning to being a manager.

Another important finding of Hudson's study was that *none* of the participants in the study received formal management training or apprenticeships in advance or during their transition.

LEADERSHIP CHALLENGE Based on Hudson's study, what kind of training would you offer Sarah, the nurse in the Leadership in Action vignette at the beginning of this chapter?

Hudson pointed out the need for two specific levels of training for transitioning nurse managers: one focused on managerial skills and competencies (the "doing" of management), and the other focused on the nature of feeling (the "being" of management). Nurses who are transitioning to managerial positions must change their thoughts *and* feelings because both influence attitudes and behaviors (Bandura, 1997).

Outstanding clinicians do not necessarily make good nurse managers. Hudson's study showed that the selection and training of nurse managers might heighten commitment to the role. She pointed out that in other work contexts

> ### GUIDED LEADERSHIP TIP
> ## USING BANDURA'S SOCIAL COGNITIVE THEORY
>
> Social cognitive theory posits that factors such as economic conditions, socioeconomic status, and educational and familial structures do not affect human behavior directly. Instead, they affect it to the degree that they influence people's aspirations, self-efficacy beliefs, personal standards, emotional states, and other self-regulatory influences. The implications of Bandura's social cognitive theory are that, as a nurse leader, you:
>
> - Take care to model positive behaviors, attitudes, and emotional reactions when teaching supervisees
>
> - Provide a learning environment that allows supervisees to extract meaning from it
> - Use social persuasion based on attainable success to help supervisees create and develop high self-efficacy beliefs
> - Remove real or imagined social or resource constraints to encourage supervisees to perform well
> - Help supervisees use self-reflection and self-evaluation to alter their thinking and behavior toward high self-efficacy
> - Provide learning incentives

management is considered a discipline requiring formal preparation and ongoing training, not learned "on the job" as nurse managers may be expected to do.

The passionate nature of nursing may make the transition to the less emotional, more cognitive realm of management difficult. The profession needs to rethink how nurses are managed—and who is chosen to transition to the management role. Nurse managers and leaders must be strongly committed to the job if the nursing profession, now facing an escalating decline in numbers, can rebound to meet healthcare demands.

> **LEADERSHIP TIP**
>
> It's critical to receive formal management training as a way to move from being a nurse to being a manager or leader.

LEADERSHIP CHALLENGE Based on what you just read, if you could ask Sarah, the new nurse manager in the Leadership in Action vignette at the beginning of this chapter, one question, what would it be?

The Need for Formal Training and Mentorship During Transitions

Members of the Nursing Leadership Institute at Florida Atlantic University (2002) echoed Hudson's comments. They identified critical leadership competencies for nursing managers as part of their research and stated that the nurse manager role has no defined career path and is rarely a career choice for nurses.

They concluded that there is a critical need to provide new nurse managers with formal orientation and mentoring early in their career transition. They also stated that the nurse manager role must receive the same attention from academic institutions that advanced practice roles receive.

Certain variables have been associated with a positive transition to nursing leadership, including:

- Letting go of deeply held attitudes and habits and altering identity (e.g., changing daily routines, habits, and self-image) and style of interaction (Hill, 2003)
- Tuning into opinions and expectations of others (Beyer & Hannah, 2002)
- Mastering task environments and innovating with roles (Ashforth & Saks, 2000)
- Using prior knowledge and skills in the new role (Ashforth & Saks, 1995)

Butler and Hardin-Pierce (2005) presented factors that may assist with a positive transition to a nurse manager or nurse leader role, including:

- Timely provision of constructive feedback on performance (Buckenham, 1997)
- Appropriate advice and guidance (Coeling, 1995; Vance, 1992)
- Continuing staff development opportunities (Kiat, 1996)

LEADERSHIP CHALLENGE How could Sarah use these suggestions to help with her transition to becoming a leader? Give a rationale for your answer.

Box 3-3 shows a leadership model that can help emerging nurse leaders.

BOX 3-3   STAFF NURSE PERCEPTION OF NURSE LEADERS

Problem focus: Krugman and Smith (2003) developed a leadership model over 4 years to help emerging nurse leaders.

Method: Survey instruments included Kouzes and Posner's Leadership Practice Inventory, which was used to measure nurse leaders' and other staff members' perceptions of nurse leadership, and the McClosky Mueller Satisfaction Scale, which was used to measure the job satisfaction of nurse leaders and staff. Krugman and Smith collected data pre-implementation, postimplementation, and at other points over the 4 years.

Results: Leader RNs reported significantly more favorable perceptions of the leadership's abilities than the staff did. Job satisfaction data showed nurse leaders reported higher satisfaction with scheduling, praise and recognition, control, and responsibility than staff nurses.

Nurse manager goals may also hold the key to understanding success when transitioning to a new role. Johansson, Porn, Theorell, and Gustafsson (2007) studied first-line nurse managers' goal profiles—that is, those managers' prioritization of goals. Action theory and confirmatory theory guided the study.

In a case study format, the researchers used interviews, observations, a job description, and policy documents to carry out a hermeneutic interpretation data analysis.

They found that each nurse manager had three goals. In order of priority, those goals were:

1. An accepted and well-controlled nurse goal
2. An accepted and well-controlled administrator goal
3. A leadership goal that the nurse had not accepted nor maintained control over

Both leadership and administrative goals were based on a job description, but the nurse goal was personally chosen and based on self-identity and goal fulfillment. This study contributed to a new understanding of the first-line nurse manager's identity based on goal acceptance and goal control. The researchers stated that this action-theoretic approach could be a valuable key for understanding leadership, or its lack, in clinical practice.

How Action Learning May Help with Transitions

One method that may be helpful in transitioning to a nurse manager role is **action learning.** Action learning is a method usually used to work on complex organizational problems in teams of 6–10 people, but the method can also be used with dyadic (two-person) groups. Kalliath and Kalliath (2006)

> **KEY TERM**
>
> **Action learning** is both a process and a powerful program for helping with nurses' transitions to a manager status.

reported what happened when two colleagues used the process. Taking on a new role can cause feelings of being overwhelmed and even a fear of failure. Sources of support for the transition can be a peer, colleague, mentor, or supervisor, as long as both individuals make a serious commitment to help each other in learning and retooling for the new role. Both partners learn as the process stimulates fresh ideas and deepens insights (Kalliath & Kalliath, 2006).

Action learning is both a process and a powerful program for solving real problems; participants focus on what and how they are learning, which can benefit them and the organization as a whole (Marquardt, 1999).

If you are transitioning to a managerial role, you can implement action learning by using the other person as a:

- Sounding board
- Support to generate possible solutions

- Helper to plan implementation steps
- Person to provide feedback about the results of actions taken

Proponents of action learning state that the process is enriched when participants engage in questioning and reflecting (Marquardt, 1999). Some questions to raise during the transition phase include:

- Am I getting what I want from this role?
- Where am I now compared to where I want to be?
- How can I get to where I want to be and achieve?

LEADERSHIP CHALLENGE Explain in what ways Sarah could use action learning to more smoothly transition to being a leader.

Survey on Nurse Manager Preparation

The results of a survey of nurse executives and nurse managers (Denning & Associates, 2004) provides hope that nurse managers may soon be better prepared for their role. Almost all nurse executives in the study reported preparing new nurse managers with on-the-job training. More than four-fifths reported using workshops, and almost two-thirds used continuing education classes. Others used personal mentoring, but more than 6 executives in 10 reported not having enough resources. At the top of their wish list was more emphasis on leadership development and transitioning from a clinical to a supervisory role, including:

- Curriculum-based study
- In-class speakers
- Study guides
- Web-based programs

LEADERSHIP CHALLENGE How could Sarah use these survey findings to smooth out her transition?

Leadership Transition Checklist

When planning to take a leadership position, gather the following helpful items; it may ensure a smoother transition:

- Information about the organization's history, hierarchy, flowcharts, mission, policies, and procedures

- Current leader's goals and objectives for the present year
- Job descriptions for all staff, including the leader
- Status reports for current projects
- Contacts, addresses, phone numbers, and e-mail addresses
- Financial information and records, including copies of completed requisitions
- Review of failures and lessons learned
- Master calendar of meetings, programs, and events
- Organization's Web address
- Leadership development resources
- Information about mentoring opportunities or other programs to help staff and leaders develop their leadership skills
- List of delegated tasks and who is responsible for them
- List of things the current leader wished someone would have told him or her a year ago
- List of important people in the organization whom you should meet
- Tips on how to run meetings, keep records, complete budgets
- Information on where to find needed forms and files
- Minutes of meetings
- List of the unique qualities of staff members and their evaluations

Summary

This chapter provided information about role theory and paths to nursing leadership. You've explored the need for formal training and mentorship during a transition and read about how action learning may help, how nurse managers prepare, and how gathering the items in a leadership transition checklist may make things easier. Read over the key terms and complete the leadership development exercises to gain a complete understanding of role transitioning.

Key Term Review

- **Action learning** is one process to help nurses transition to a manager role.
- **Role conflict** can occur when a leader's expectations differ from the group's expectations.
- **Role transition** is the process of moving from one role to another.

Leadership Development Exercises

- **Leadership Development Exercise 3-1**

List four assumptions of role theory.

- **Leadership Development Exercise 3-2**

Discuss the four paths to nursing leadership/management with at least two other nursing colleagues. Come to a consensus on which path would be the best to pursue. Give a rationale for your answer.

- **Leadership Development Exercise 3-3**

Discuss with at least two other colleagues ways to embrace those attitudes and beliefs that are necessary to become a nurse leader. Using Hudson's and Johansson's findings, come up with a specific plan for helping nurses transition to nurse leader roles.

- **Leadership Development Exercise 3-4**

Using the action learning information in this chapter, devise a specific action learning program to help a nurse transition to a leadership role. Give a rationale for your answer.

- **Leadership Development Exercise 3-5**

Search the Web, and find at least one curriculum-based study, study guide, or Web-based program to help nurses transition from a clinical to a supervisory role. Share your findings with the class.

- **Leadership Development Exercise 3-6**

Using the leadership transition checklist, see how much of the information you can gather for a unit on which you practice or have practiced. Tell the class what you learned from conducting this search.

- **Leadership Development Exercise 3-7**

Pretend you're a staff nurse preparing to take a leadership role.

   a. What are your concerns, and what information do you need?
   b. Search the Web for that information.
   c. Report your findings to the class.

■ **Leadership Development Exercise 3-8**

Organize an in-class simulation in which four to six students volunteer to simulate the situation presented in the opening Leadership in Action vignette.

a. Bring your chairs to the center or front of the room, and form a circle.

b. Use the leadership transition checklist if a nursing supervisor will be a part of the simulation. (In this case, the nurse leader can ask the staff to leave and discuss some of the items on the leadership transition checklist with the supervisor.)

c. *Optional:* Add a student to play the outgoing nurse leader who comes in after the nurse leader has presented her ideas to the staff and is either supportive or competitive (the simulation group decides which).

d. Choose a timekeeper to warn the simulation group when 5, 10, and 15 minutes are up. (A 15-minute simulation is suggested.)

e. The student playing the new nurse leader should present his or her ideas.

f. The students playing staff members should pay little attention to the new nurse leader until they are asked for their ideas about halfway into the simulation.

g. The nurse in transition should raise some of the issues in the Leadership Transition Checklist with the supervisor.

h. When time is called, the simulation players should describe their feelings and reactions and what they learned from the simulation with the class.

i. The class members then ask questions and identify any leadership concepts they observed. They give suggestions for adding additional elements that could be played out in future simulations.

Advanced Leadership Development Exercises

■ **Leadership Development Exercise 3-9**

Teach at least three advanced nursing students about role transition.

■ **Leadership Development Exercise 3-10**

Design a problem statement for a research study focused on role transition. Make sure it is specific, focused, and doable. Obtain feedback from at least three classmates or nurse leaders skilled in research methods.

■ **Leadership Development Exercise 3-11**

Develop a research design to answer your problem statement. Consult with at least three classmates or nurse leaders skilled in research methods. Revise your design, if necessary.

References

Ashforth, B. E., & Saks, A. M. (1995). Work-role transitions: A longitudinal examination of the Nicholson model. *Journal of Occupational & Organizational Psychology, 68*, 157–165.

Ashforth, B. E., & Saks, A. M. (2000). Personal control in organizations: A longitudinal investigation with newcomers. *Human Relations, 53*, 311–325.

Bandura, A. (1997). *Self-efficacy: The exercise of control.* New York: Freeman.

Beyer, J. M., & Hannah, D. R. (2002). Building on the past: Enacting established personal identities in a new work setting. *Organization Science: A Journal of the Institute of Management Sciences, 13*, 636.

Bondas, T. (2006). Paths to nursing leadership. *Journal of Nursing Management, 14*, 332–339.

Buckenham, J. (1997, June). The socialization of the graduate nurse. Paper presented at the "Hit the Ground" conference, Melbourne, Australia.

Butler, K. M., & Hardin-Pierce, M. (2005). Leadership strategies to enhance the transition from nursing student role to professional nurse. *Nursing Leadership Forum, 9*, 110–117.

Coeling, H. (1995). Commentary on supportive communication among nurses: Effects on commitment, burnout and retention. *AONE's Leadership Prospectives, 3*(1), 33.

Denning, D. R., & Associates. (2004). *Nurse executive/nurse manager survey, evaluation results.* Retrieved January 9, 2007, from http://www.moln.org/files/NurseSurveyRevised4-29-2004.ppt

Heller, B. R., Drenkard, K., Esposito-Herr, M. B., Romano, C., Tom, S., & Valentine, N. (2004). Educating nurses for leadership roles. *Journal of Continuing Education in Nursing, 35*, 203–213.

Hill, L. (2003). *Becoming a manager.* Boston: Harvard Business School Press.

Hudson, P. C. (2005). *Barriers and enablers of a successful transition to nurse manager.* Unpublished manuscript, Case Western Reserve University.

Johansson, G., Porn, I., Theorell, T., & Gustafsson, B. (2007). A first-line nurse manager's goal-profile. *Journal of Clinical Nursing, 16*(1), 149–159.

Kalliath, P., & Kalliath, T. (2006). *Applying action learning concepts to role transition in a dyadic group setting.* Retrieved January 12, 2007, from http://www.education.up.ac.za/alarpm/PRP_pdf/Kalliath&Kallaith.pdf

Kiat, K. (1996). NYP nursing graduates in the first year. *Professional Nurse* (Singapore), *23*(3), 22.

Krugman, M., & Smith, V. (2003). Charge nurse leadership development and evaluation. *Journal of Nursing Administration, 33*(5), 284–292.

Marquardt, M. (1999). Six essential elements of effective action learning. In M. Marquardt, *Action learning.* Palo Alto, CA: Davies-Black.

Miller, J., & Rahn, W. (2002). Identity based feelings, beliefs and actions how being influences doing. Paper presented at the annual scientific meeting of the International Society of Political Psychology, Berlin, Germany.

Nugent, K. E., Childs, G., Jones, R., & Cook, P. (2004). A mentorship model for the retention of minority students. *Nursing Outlook, 52*, 89–94.

Nursing Leadership Institute. (2002). *Identification of critical leadership competencies for nursing managers: Research project update.* Boca Raton, FL: Florida Atlantic University. Retrieved January 9, 2007, from http://www.fau.edu/nli/identification.pdf

Role theory. (2006). Retrieved January 8, 2007, from http://changingminds.org/disciplines/leadership/theories/role_theory.htm

Vance, C. (1992). Managing the politics of the workplace. *Imprint, 39*(1), 18.

Vriesendorp, A., & Buxbaum, A. (2006). Planning for leadership transition. *The Manager, 15*(1), 1–31.

Managing Stress

CHAPTER OBJECTIVES

After reading this chapter, answering the leadership challenges, and participating in the leadership development exercises, you will be able to:

- Explain the nature of stress at work
- Describe the health consequences of stressful work
- Explain how to use hardiness theory to reduce stress
- List three ways to use Bandura's self-efficacy theory to reduce stress
- Try out different stress reduction measures

Advanced nurses will be able to:

- Teach peers stress reduction measures
- Develop a problem statement for a research study related to stress
- Develop a research design to answer your problem statement

Introduction

This chapter explores stress, the source of job stress, the effect of stress on nurses and nurse leaders, two theories that may be helpful, and methods for reducing stress.

The Leadership in Action vignette that follows will be used in this chapter to explore aspects of stress.

LEADERSHIP IN ACTION

Roberta, an RN working in a medical center, had been plagued by a loss of appetite, frequent colds, restless sleep, aching muscles, lower back pain, hypertension, and exhaustion since her brother was diagnosed with multiple sclerosis. About that time, she was asked to work extra shifts. She tried to ignore her symptoms, but when she snapped at a client and her supervisor overheard it, Roberta was counseled to get help from a mental health clinical nurse specialist who consulted on her unit. Roberta didn't want to meet with this clinical specialist, but she felt the pressure from her supervisor. Roberta finally made an appointment and talked with the clinical specialist about her stress.

"Since the reorganization, it just doesn't feel safe around here," Roberta told her nurse colleague. "They're firing people and expecting the rest of us to take up the slack. I don't know how long I can keep up these 12-hour shifts. I swear, I wake up in a cold sweat, remembering someone who died on my shift or how I had to rush through pouring meds and may have made a mistake. People are calling in sick just to get a break from the pressure. They don't care that that leaves us alone to deal with everything. I'd complain to my supervisor, but then I'm caught between families, who think we're not giving their loved ones good care, and my supervisor, who tells me that my stress is all my fault. Sooner or later, someone is going to have to make changes in the way the place is run. It's just too stressful."

LEADERSHIP CHALLENGE Is Roberta's stress personal or organizational? Give a rationale for your answer.

Stress Defined

When the term *stress* was coined by Hans Selye, he used it to describe a series of responses in animals that were subjected to severe physical and emotional threats that resulted in stomach ulcers, hypertension, heart attacks, arthritis, kidney damage, and other disorders. Selye (1978) defined stress as the "non-specific response of the body to any demand for change."

Stress quickly became a popular buzzword. It is estimated that 75% to 90% of all visits to primary care physicians are for stress-related complaints. It is difficult to name an illness in which stress does not play a contributing role (Rosch, 1998b).

Rosch (1998b), Selye's protégé, who based his conclusions on some of his mentor's writings, said, "Stress, in addition to being itself, was also the cause of itself, and the result of itself." To clarify stress's relationship to itself, Selye coined the word **stressor** to refer to the cause of stress (Rosch, 1998b).

KEY TERM
A **stressor** is a cause of stress.

Selye later defined stress as "the rate of wear and tear on the body," which Rosch (1993) pointed out is also the definition of aging. As a result of these different meanings, it is difficult for scientists to define, let alone measure, stress (Rosch, 1998a).

Some experts use the term *stress* to refer to the disorder that results from repeated insults and disruption of homeostasis, such as a heart condition (Rosch, 1998a). Other authors use the term to refer to the feeling of pressure they feel; they may say, "I'm stressed out," for example, when what they may mean is "I feel pressured."

To add to the confusion, stress can also be mental stress. Free radicals can create stress, especially if a person has low levels of antioxidant vitamins and high levels of free radicals. Not only dietary factors but also emotional stress can affect the tenuous balance of pro-oxidative and antioxidative influences (Biesalski, Jentzsch, & Kirschbaum, 1994).

Stress has also been used to describe a wide range of distressful emotions (anxiety, panic, depression) and disturbing external events or stressors (observing people die, trying to keep clients alive, working too many hours, violence in the workplace, and being responsible for life-and-death decisions, to name a few).

LEADERSHIP CHALLENGE **Which of the many definitions of stress most closely describes Roberta's situation? Give a rationale for your answer.**

One thing that all animal and clinical research confirms is that the feeling or perception of having little control is always distressful, and that is what is perceived as **stress** (Rosch, 1998c). Whether the perception of having little control is internally or externally produced may not matter.

KEY TERM
Stress is the feeling or perception of having little control.

Can Stress Be Quantified?

KEY TERM
The **social readjustment rating scale** ranks and rates 43 stressful life-change events.

Holmes and Rahe (1967) developed a **social readjustment rating scale**, popularly known as the "Holmes-Rahe scale." It ranks and rates 43 stressful life-change events. Death of a spouse takes the top of the list at 100 points. The first work-related incident—"fired at work"—appears at 47. Other work-related stressors include a change in responsibility (29), an outstanding personal achievement (25), trouble with a boss (23), and a change in working conditions (20).

LEADERSHIP CHALLENGE Why might work-related stress rank so far down the list of stressful life-change events? Give a rationale for your answer.

The problem with the Holmes-Rahe scale is that an outstanding personal achievement, change in responsibility, or even a change in working conditions could be a positive experience, not a stressful one.

The Nature of Stress

Because of the difficulty of defining *stress*, the term has come to mean a subjective phenomenon that differs for each person. What is distressing for one person can be pleasurable to others. For example, some nurses may perceive a code as an exhilarating challenge, and others may find it highly stressful. The code itself is not inherently stressful. It depends on how each individual perceives the event.

An unpleasant event or threat—such as having to constantly deal with an intimidating boss, coworker, or client—may be identified as stressful by some people. Others may only be aware of how they react to such situations, and this can range from anxiety and depression to palpitations, agita and stomach upset, diarrhea, sweaty palms, and dozens of other emotional and physical responses (Rosch, 1998b). No matter how stress is identified, it is clear that job stress is on the upswing (Sauter et al., 1999).

Stress and Health

Stress sets off an alarm system. The brain responds by preparing the body for action. The nervous system is aroused, and hormones are released that quicken the pulse, deepen respiration, sharpen the senses, and tense the muscles—all of which characterize a fight-or-flight response.

This response is helpful when people need to run from physical danger. And short-lived or infrequent episodes of stress pose little risk. When stress becomes long term, however, danger awaits. The body is kept in a constant state of activation, increasing the wear and tear to biological systems. Fatigue and damage are the ultimate result, and the body's ability to repair and defend itself is seriously compromised. **Box 4-1** provides information about chronic conditions and job stress.

Because it has such wide-ranging effects, job stress is of utmost importance to nurse leaders and managers.

Job Stress

Job stress can be defined as the harmful physical and emotional responses that occur when a job's requirements do

KEY TERM

Job stress results from a mismatch between a worker's capabilities, resources, or needs and the job's requirements.

BOX 4-1   WHAT THE RESEARCH SHOWS ABOUT STRESS AND HEALTH

The National Institute for Occupational Safety and Health (NIOSH) examined the effects of stress on health:

Cardiovascular disease. Numerous studies suggest that psychologically demanding jobs that provide employees with little control over the work process increase the risk of cardiovascular disease.

Musculoskeletal disorders. Research conducted by NIOSH and other organizations has shown that job stress increases the risk of back and upper-extremity musculoskeletal disorders.

Psychological disorders. Several studies suggest that depression and burnout are due in part to high job stress, although economic and lifestyle differences may also contribute.

(Sauter et al., 1999)

not match the worker's capabilities, resources, or needs. Job stress can lead to poor health and injury. Job stress is the opposite of challenge, which energizes the worker psychologically and physically and motivates learning and job mastery (Sauter et al., 1999).

There are two schools of thought about job stress. Views differ on the importance of worker characteristics versus working conditions as the primary cause of job stress (Cox & Griffiths, 1996; Sauter et al., 1999). Focusing on worker stress leads to prevention strategies based on the individual (Rosch, 1993).

According to the National Institute for Occupational Safety and Health, excessive workload demands and conflicting expectations argue for identifying working conditions as the key source of job stress and for championing job redesign as a primary prevention strategy (Sauter et al., 1999). But often a mix of individual and organizational factors combine to create job stress.

Some job conditions that can lead to stress appear in **Box 4-2**.

LEADERSHIP CHALLENGE Using Box 4-2, suggest at least four changes you would make if you were the nurse leader on Roberta's unit.

Stress and Nurses

Nurses work in high stress and even dangerous environments. In an online health and safety survey of 4,826 nurses (from every age group, experience level, and type of care facilities) conducted by the American Nurses Association (ANA), over 70% of respondents cited the acute and chronic effects of stress and overwork as one of their top three health and safety concerns. Yet nurses continue to

BOX 4-2   STRESSFUL JOB CONDITIONS

The design of tasks. Heavy workload, infrequent rest breaks, long work hours, and hectic and routine tasks that have little inherent meaning, do not use worker skills, and provide little sense of control can increase stress.

Example: Roberta works to the point of exhaustion, and her work allows little chance for creativity, self-initiative, or rest.

Management style. Lack of worker participation in decision making and poor communication in the organization can add to stress.

Example: Roberta cannot make a decision without consulting her supervisor, and her boss is insensitive to her need to visit her brother.

Interpersonal relationships. The social environment is nonsupportive, and coworkers and supervisors seem unconcerned with helping.

Example: Roberta's physical isolation reduces opportunities to interact with coworkers and receive help from them.

Work roles. Job expectations are conflicting and changeable. There is too much responsibility, and staff must wear too many hats.

Example: Roberta is often caught in impossible situations trying to satisfy both client family members and her supervisor.

Career concerns. Opportunities for growth, advancement, or promotion are few. Job insecurity is in the air. Change is rapid, and workers cannot prepare for what's next.

Example: Since the reorganization of the hospital, Roberta is worried about her future and what will happen next; a neighboring hospital was closed down after profits fell, and the staff was split up and sent to various hospitals throughout the city.

Environmental conditions. Some of the dangerous work conditions nurses may be exposed to include noise, air pollution, ergonomic problems, infections, and radiation.

Example: Roberta is exposed to infections, air pollution, and radiation at work.

(Sauter et al., 1999)

be pressed harder, with more than two-thirds working some type of mandatory or unplanned overtime every month. Ten percent reported working overtime eight times a month (ANA, 2001).

But stress not only affects nurses. Seventy-five percent of nurse respondents reported the quality of nursing care at their facility had declined over the past 2 years, and 56% thought that the time they had available for client care had decreased (ANA, 2001).

Four years later, a survey of 76,000 nurses conducted through ANA's National Database of Nursing Quality Indicators, found that 82% of RNs reported working overtime, with most respondents reporting that overtime had increased on their unit during the past year and 26% reporting being floated to hospital units within the past 2 weeks (ANA, 2005).

American nurses are not the only ones to suffer from job stress. The National Survey of the Work and Health of Nurses, conducted by the Canadian Institute for Health Information and Health Canada (2005) with 19,000 Canadian respondents, found that many nurses regularly worked overtime and that many had more than one job. This groundbreaking study indicated that psychosocial and interpersonal factors (including work stress, low autonomy, and lack of respect) are strongly associated with health problems among Canada's 314,900 nurses. The Canadian study found the proportion of nurses who reported a high level of work stress (as determined by the level of job strain, physical demands, and support from coworkers and supervisors) was greater than that for employed people overall.

Job strain results when the psychological demands of a job exceed the worker's discretion in deciding how to do the job. Nearly one-third (31%) of nurses in Canada were classified as having high job strain. Job strain was strongly related to fair or poor physical and mental health and to lengthy or frequent absences from work for health-related reasons. Seventeen percent of nurses who perceived high job strain reported taking 20 or more sick days in the past year, compared with 12% of nurses who reported less job strain. Nearly half (46%) of the Canadian nurses reported that their employer expected them to work overtime, and 3 in 10 did work paid overtime. Half of them regularly worked unpaid overtime, averaging 4 hours per week.

> **KEY TERM**
>
> **Job strain** results when the psychological demands of a job exceed the worker's discretion in deciding how to do the job.

LEADERSHIP CHALLENGE What is the relationship between job strain and taking sick days? Give a rationale for your answer.

A groundbreaking study of 10,000 nurses and 230,000 patients from 168 hospitals in Pennsylvania from 1998 to 1999 verified the dangerous and unhealthy results of nurse short-staffing and how it increases client mortality, nursing dissatisfaction, and nursing burnout (Aiken, Clarke, Sloane, Sochalski, & Silber, 2002). See **Box 4-3** for more information.

LEADERSHIP CHALLENGE What is the relationship between staffing, patient death, and burnout? Give a rationale for your answer.

Stress and the Work Environment

While employers may believe that stressful working conditions are a necessary evil and that workers must be pressured to set aside health concerns for health

BOX 4-3   STAFFING, CLIENT MORTALITY, NURSE BURNOUT, AND JOB DISSATISFACTION

Aiken, Clarke, Sloane, Sochalski, and Silber (2002) found that each additional client assigned to a nurse resulted in:

- A 30-day mortality increase of 7%
- A failure-to-rescue rate increase of 7%
- A nursing job dissatisfaction increase of 15%
- A burnout rate increase of 23%

In fact, when nurses had eight clients instead of four, their caseload had a 31% higher chance of dying within 30 days of admission.

Other findings of the Aiken study included:

- Forty-three percent of the nurses surveyed were burned out and emotionally exhausted.
- Nurses who reported being burned out were four times as likely to report that they were leaving their jobs in the next year.

corporations to remain profitable, research findings challenge those assumptions. Studies like the ones just described show that stressful working conditions are actually associated with increased absenteeism, tardiness, and workers' intentions to quit their jobs. All these factors have a negative effect on the bottom line (Sauter et al., 1999).

LEADERSHIP CHALLENGE What motivates hospital owners or boards to continue these kinds of behaviors given the studies that are emerging? Provide a rationale for your answer. (Hint: Don't overlook the connection between the bottom line and job stress effects.)

Creating a healthy work environment for nursing practice is crucial to maintaining an adequate nursing workforce (American Association of Critical-Care Nurses, 2005). Being a nurse is associated with multiple and conflicting demands imposed by leaders, managers, and medical and administrative staff. The stressful nature of the profession often leads to burnout, disability, and high absenteeism.

The stress of healthcare environments has been linked to a shortage of registered nurses, projected to number just 400,000 by 2020 (Shirey, 2006a). In addition to the stresses of being a nurse that have already been discussed, there are other societal stresses that create even more job stress. New sources of stress are developing at what seems like supersonic speeds along with changes in society. These new sources include technostress, restructuring, and disconnectedness.

Technostress

KEY TERM

Technostress results from difficulties in dealing with computer technologies or from an unusual attraction to them.

In 1984, Craig Brod, a Silicon Valley psychiatrist, impressed with the steady increase in stress-related disorders resulting from the activities in this fast-paced and hectic community, coined the term *technostress*. He even wrote a book: *Technostress: The Human Cost of the Computer Revolution*. Technostress resulted from difficulties in dealing with computer technologies or from an unusual attraction to them.

According to Brod, technostress is related to technophobia, or a fear of new and constantly upgraded computer software and hardware devices as well as the computers themselves. Technostress can also stem from a preoccupation with computer-related activities and information overload.

Technology is all around—from computers to cell phones, pagers, iPods, BlackBerrys, electronic monitoring devices, video terminals, and more—and was supposed to make life less difficult (Leggiere, 2002). Rather than reduce the work-week, technology has increased it. Nurses are now tied to the workplace 24/7, on weekends, on holidays, and even on vacations (D'Anna, 2006). There is no rest period allowed anymore. The requirement to be constantly alert can only result in increased stress.

A part of technology enhancement in health care is the movement toward placing individual client records online (Detmer, Steen, & Dick, 1997). This can lead to additional mental stress for nurses who may be asked to add another task to their already-full day and may be especially stressful for those who are not computer savvy.

Working with computers can also lead to physical stress. Repetitive stress injuries, such as carpal tunnel syndrome, are now the most costly workplace injury. They account for one-third of the more than $60 billion in workers' compensation payments annually (Rosch, 2000).

Restructuring

Companies, including healthcare corporations, that have eliminated jobs are more likely to see increases in disability claims ranging from back pain to gastrointestinal disorders than firms that haven't cut jobs. What is being saved in payroll costs through downsizing may be eaten up in stress-related disability costs. Simply removing people without eliminating the work they did could cost *more* in the long run.

Today's organizations test the theory that employees can work forever with no time to recover. Administrators try to convince employees that they can work and work without letting up for a second. This false urgency can result in numerous errors and in activity without purpose or awareness (Robinson, 2003).

Overworked and overstressed healthcare professionals make mistakes that can be fatal. A report from the Institute of Medicine (Kohn, Corrigan, & Donaldson, 1999) revealed that errors in hospitals cause up to 100,000 deaths a year. Nurses throughout the country report fears that they may have made mistakes because of the fast pace at which they must work (Robinson, 2003).

For nurse leaders, the dilemma is doubly challenging. On one hand, employees are experiencing greater stress (Shirey, 2006b); on the other, they have less time to attend stress management training (Shimko, Meli, Restrypo, & Oehlers, 2000).

Disconnectedness

As nurses become too busy or too tired for healthy relationships, stress increases. Nurses are working more now and enjoying it less. They may be so overloaded that they cannot maintain those close family and friend relationships that are so crucial to reducing stress. In many households, family members have their own television sets and cell phones, which cuts down on those social support opportunities that are so important to stress reduction (Charles, 2001).

Satisfaction in life comes from close relationships, a sense of belonging, positive attitudes, managing expectations, high self-esteem, work goals that are congruent with personal values, and an active leisure lifestyle (Charles, 2003). When these elements are not available because of job requirements, stress overload and burnout can occur.

Burnout

KEY TERM

Burnout is a stage of exhaustion that can result from unrelieved work stress or from an erosion of the soul.

Burnout, a term coined by Freudenberger and Richelson (1980), is a debilitating psychological condition brought about by unrelieved work stress. Signs of burnout include:

- Depleted energy and emotional exhaustion
- Lowered resistance to illness
- Increased depersonalization in interpersonal relationships
- Increased dissatisfaction and pessimism
- Increased absenteeism and work inefficiency

Burnout was further described by Maslach and Leiter (1997). They defined burnout as a disconnect between expectations about work versus the realities of what is actually experienced. Burnout is a disconnect between what nurses are and what they have to do. Burned out people can be too depleted to give of themselves in a creative and cooperative fashion (Montague, 1994). This can be a real problem for nurses whose role is to provide care.

Burnout represents an erosion in values, dignity, spirit, and will—an erosion of the human soul. Maslach and Leiter do not fault the worker, but rather the work environment.

In a presentation at the New York Academy of Medicine in November 2006, Mason and Smith reported that, 41% of US nurses are dissatisfied with their jobs, 30% to 40% have experienced burnout, and 17% aren't even working in nursing anymore. Many of these nurses have a remote, indifferent, or impersonal relationship with their clients rather than a caring one.

Burnout can be considered a crisis of caring. Nurses are caring individuals and tend to work harder at caring than some other professionals. As they become more successful at caring, they are apt to be noticed and asked to do even more for the cause.

This can put additional demands on their time and energy.

Burnout is both a physical and an emotional exhaustion during which the professional no longer has any positive feelings, sympathy, or respect for clients. Over time, unless nurses take care of themselves, they may experience burnout. Nurses are at a greater risk for burnout than people in other professions. The very fact that nurses care about other people puts them at a greater risk than if they did not care because strong emotion takes more energy and can be depleting.

LEADERSHIP TIP

To reduce stress, make sure the workload is evenly distributed.

According to Maslach and Leiter (1997), the six systemic sources of burnout are:

1. Work overload
2. Lack of control
3. Insufficient reward
4. Unfairness
5. Breakdown of a sense of community
6. Value conflict

Some of the negative behavioral effects of burnout include:

- Rudeness
- Sarcasm
- Criticism and insults
- Irrational anger or isolation and introversion
- Eating too much or too little
- Abusing alcohol and drugs
- Suffering physical symptoms, such as hypertension and frequent headaches
- Downhill spiral of relationships with family, friends, and colleagues
- Fading dedication and commitment to the organization

Working to exhaustion and not stopping to engage in restorative activities can lead to burnout and force the body to take its own break (D'Anna, 2006). Pain, chronic illness, and other conditions can be messages from the body to pay attention, stop, and restore.

Rest and sleep are two ways the body takes a restorative break. Sixty-three percent of American adults don't get the recommended 8.5 hours of sleep, and that includes nurses. Researchers at the National Sleep Foundation found a direct relationship between the amount of hours worked and a corresponding loss of sleep (Robinson, 2003).

Nurses who stop to rest or sleep can combat stress and burnout. Many nurses don't even stop for lunch, let alone for a break. Yet it has been known since the early 1900s that even a 5-minute rest or break increases worker output and that a 10-minute break increases it even more (D'Anna, 2006).

LEADERSHIP TIP

To reduce burnout, make sure you and your staff take allotted breaks.

Box 4-4 provides an assessment tool for you to evaluate your level of burnout. Although the progression Box 4-4 presents is sobering, the model provides hope that taking action can break the cycle. It is always possible to strengthen your coping skills and return to an earlier stage. The wise course of action is to involve yourself in positive self-care to prevent anything after stage 1 from developing. Hardiness can assist with that effort.

Hardiness: A Personal Theory of Stress Protection

Dr. Suzanne Ouellette Kobasa (1984) researched the ability of humans to survive stress. She found that **psychological hardiness,** or the ability to survive stress, is composed of three ingredients:

1. A commitment to self, work, family, and other important values
2. A sense of personal control over one's life
3. The ability to see change in one's life as a challenge to master

Kobasa tested executives, lawyers, women in gynecologist offices, supervisors, US Army officers, and college students. Her results were the same for each population: biology is not destiny.

BOX 4-4   STAGES OF BURNOUT

Stage 1: Honeymoon. This stage is marked by high job satisfaction, commitment, energy, and creativity. If positive and adaptive patterns of coping are developed, it's possible to remain in the honeymoon stage indefinitely.

Stage 2: Balancing act. A noticeable increase in job dissatisfaction, work inefficiency, avoiding making necessary decisions, losing stuff at work, general and deep muscle fatigue, sleep disturbances (because of thoughts about work), and escapist activities (eating, drinking, smoking, zoning out) is experienced.

Stage 3: Chronic symptoms. The stage 2 symptoms intensify and include chronic exhaustion, physical illness, anger, and depression.

Stage 4: Crisis. The symptoms become more critical, and the physical symptoms intensify and/or increase in number; this may include obsessing about work frustrations, allowing pessimism and self-doubt to dominate thinking, and developing an escapist mentality.

Stage 5: Enmeshment. The symptoms of burnout are so embedded in a person's life that he or she is more likely to be labeled as having a significant mental or physical illness than burnout.

(Based on Veninga & Spradley, 1981)

A hardy personality is more important than a strong constitution. It is possible to come from a family with chronic illness and do better under stress if you are hardy than if you had come from a healthy family and have fewer inner resources (Kobasa, 1984).

Exercise is a good antidote to stress but may be short term. Jogging after an argument can help you that evening, but the next morning, your stress levels may rise if you reencounter the stress-provoking situation. Hardiness skills may be long-term inoculations against stressors. Two studies even found that hardiness is more powerful than optimism and religiousness in coping with stress (Maddi, 2006).

Judkins, Massey, and Huff (2006) provided evidence for the importance of hardiness. They discovered that intense job-related demands affected job performance and increased the use of sick time. They found that managers with high hardiness skills and low stress used less sick time than managers with low hardiness skills and high stress.

In another study of hardiness, Judkins, Reid, and Furlow (2006) investigated the development of a model hardiness training program to reduce stress and increase hardiness among nurse managers. Thirteen nurse managers at an urban hospital completed pretests for hardiness levels before undergoing a 2.5-day hardiness training program. Posttests were completed after the initial training, after each of 6 weekly sessions, and after 6 and 12 months. Findings suggested that the hardiness program and intermittent follow-up increased and sustained hardiness levels in nurse managers and may have had a positive effect on staff turnover rates (Judkins, Reid, & Furlow, 2006).

Three helpful techniques for increasing hardiness are:

1. Focusing on body signals that something is wrong
2. Restructuring stressful situations
3. Compensating through self-improvement (Kobasa, 1984)

Focusing

KEY TERM

Focusing helps individuals recognize signals from their body that stress is interfering with comfort.

Focusing is a technique developed by Eugene Gendlin (1978) that can help you recognize signals from your body that stress is interfering with comfort. Gendlin found that executives are so used to pressure in their temples, tightened necks, or stomach knots that they have stopped noticing these signals that something is wrong.

A beginning focusing question might be "Where is tension located in my body?" Those who have learned to tune out body signals can begin with a progressive relaxation tape to help them identify the location of stress and tension.

Reconstructing Stressful Situations

The second technique for enhancing hardiness is reconstructing stressful situations. This is accomplished by thinking about a recent episode of distress and writing about:

- Three ways it could have gone better
- Three ways it could have gone worse

This exercise will increase your ability to put the situation in perspective, which is useful for reducing stress.

Compensating through Self-Improvement

The third technique Kobasa found useful for enhancing hardiness was compensating through self-improvement. This approach works most effectively for stressors that cannot be avoided, such as an illness, an intimidating or unfair boss, or an unexpected change or loss. You can balance the feeling of lost control that results from such unexpected events by taking on a new challenge. Learning a new skill or teaching someone else can reassure you that you can still cope with life adequately.

LEADERSHIP CHALLENGE Which signs of burnout have you observed in healthcare situations? If you were the leader of that unit, what would you do to help the burned-out nurses? (Hint: How could you use hardiness theory?) Give a rationale for your answer.

In addition to hardiness theory, nurse leaders can also benefit from the use of Bandura's theory of self-efficacy.

Bandura's Theory of Self-Efficacy

KEY TERM

Bandura's **theory of self-efficacy** focuses on the belief in one's ability to perform adequately.

Bandura (1977, 1986, 1997, 2001, 2004) developed a social cognitive theory that has been widely used and accepted. Bandura (1986) wrote that individuals possess self-beliefs that can enable them to exercise control over their thoughts, feelings, and actions.

Self-efficacy, or the belief in one's ability to perform adequately, has proved to be a more consistent predictor of behavioral outcomes than others (Bandura, 2004). Learners with high self-efficacy expect more of themselves and put forth the effort to get it. They approach difficult tasks as challenges rather than as situations to avoid.

Certain environmental characteristics can cause even highly self-efficacious and well-skilled learners not to behave in concert with their beliefs and abilities if they:

- Lack the incentive
- Lack the necessary resources
- Perceive social constraints

Bandura (1977) believed that learning would be laborious and hazardous if people had to rely only on themselves. Luckily, employees have nurse managers to model appropriate behavior for them. This vicarious learning permits individuals to learn novel behaviors without going through the arduous task of trial-and-error learning.

Bandura (1977) emphasized the importance of modeling behaviors, attitudes, and emotional reactions. He believed that it was the human ability to symbolize that allowed learners to:

- Extract meaning from the environment
- Construct guides for action
- Solve problems cognitively
- Support well-thought-out courses of action
- Gain new knowledge by reflective thought
- Communicate with others at any distance in time and space
- Use self-reflection to make sense of their experiences
- Engage in self-evaluation and alter their thinking and behavior accordingly (Bandura, 1986)

LEADERSHIP CHALLENGE Based on what you know about Bandura's work, how could you, as a nurse leader, use this theory? Give a rationale for your answer.

A series of principles underlie Bandura's social cognitive theory:

- The highest level of observational learning is achieved by first organizing and rehearsing the modeled behavior symbolically and then enacting it overtly.
- Coding modeled behavior into words, labels, or images results in better retention of information than does simply observing.
- Individuals are more likely to adopt a modeled behavior if it results in outcomes they value, if others admire the role model, and if the behavior has functional value.
- Self-efficacy beliefs are paramount; motivation levels, affective states, and actions are based more on what people believe than on what is objectively true (1997).

Jason, a seasoned nurse leader, had been using Bandura's social learning theory for many years. Just recently, he'd been promoted to a new nursing leadership position. He'd observed that several of the staff exhibited signs of high stress and possibly even burnout. He spent some time planning what to do and decided to call a staff meeting to discuss Bandura's theory and explain how journal writing has reduced his own job stress. Once the meeting began, he asked employees to think about their job and to write about any unsafe or unpleasant aspects of their job, whether they had too much work to do, whether they had adequate control over their duties, and whether they were able to use all their skills and talents to the fullest in their work.

LEADERSHIP CHALLENGE If you were Jason, what would you do with the information about workplace stress that he had asked employees to write about? Give a rationale for your answer.

Devon, a seasoned nurse manager, planned to model the most effective way to obtain an intake interview, allow employees to practice small segments of the interview process, and provide each with a certificate of achievement once they did a full interview.

LEADERSHIP CHALLENGE Think of at least two other ways you could use self-efficacy theory to reduce job stress with employees. Give a rationale for your answer.

Individual Approaches to Job Stress

Hardiness and Bandura's theory of self-efficacy can certainly help nurses combat job-related stress. Other individual approaches to job stress include employee assistance programs and nutrition.

Employee Assistance Programs

After Roberta, the RN in this chapter's opening Leadership in Action vignette, shared her job stress concerns with the mental health clinical nurse specialist, she was directed to an employee assistance program (EAP) that provided stress management. Stress management programs teach workers about the nature and sources of stress, the effects of stress on health, and personal skills to reduce stress, such as relaxation exercises.

EAPs also counsel employees on their work and personal problems. Stress management training can rapidly reduce stress symptoms, such as anxiety and sleep disturbances; it is also inexpensive and easy to implement.

Stress management programs have two drawbacks:

1. The beneficial effects on stress symptoms can be short lived.

2. Focusing on individual stress levels ignores important root causes of stress.

When the stress management program is administered by an EAP, a third drawback may come into play:

3. A lack of confidentiality about shared personal information can help corporations fight employee-initiated lawsuits (Rosch, 1993). For that reason, referral to off-site programs, nurse-led programs, or organizational change may be more optimal choices.

Many colleges, universities, adult education centers, and distance education providers offer stress reduction programs. Nurse leaders can develop a list of resources and suggest that staff participate in them.

Nurse leaders can also develop their own stress reduction programs for staff, ask a mental health clinical nurse specialist to design one, or hand out stress reduction information at staff meetings or shift reports.

Box 4-5 provides a relaxation/imagery exercise that nurse leaders can use and teach to supervisees.

BOX 4–5   RELAXATION/IMAGERY EXERCISE

1. Find a quiet place where you won't be disturbed.
2. Slip off your shoes, loosen tight clothing, and sit or lie down and get comfortable.
3. Close your eyes.
4. Focus on your breathing. Let your breath slowly move toward your center as you inhale and exhale. Just let it move naturally.
5. Begin to breathe in relaxing and healing energy with each inhale. See that relaxing healing energy as a color.
6. With each exhale, let go of any old thoughts, feelings, or situations that you don't need anymore. Perhaps view them as a different color. Just breathe out whatever it's time to be rid of. Inhale relaxing energy, and exhale what you're ready to let go of for a while until you feel relaxed.
7. When you're ready, scan your body, and exhale any remaining tension or ideas you don't need anymore.
8. Slowly open your eyes, feeling relaxed and refreshed. Take this relaxed and refreshed feeling with you throughout the day.

Not only is relaxation important to enhance mood and ward off exhaustion, it is more important than chewing is to the digestion of complex carbohydrates (Morse, Schacterle, Furst, Zaydenberg, & Pollack, 1989). (See the following section on nutrition for why relaxation is important.)

Another stress reduction measure includes using coping thoughts. Much of the internal dialogue people have with themselves consists of negative words and feelings. Coping thoughts counteract such negativity and provide a positive supportive voice for nurses to use. **Box 4-6** provides coping thoughts you can use yourself and teach to employees.

Nutrition

Stress is not just a mental or psychological issue; it has very real physical effects, including:

- Slowing digestion
- Releasing fats and sugars into the bloodstream

BOX 4-6   COPING THOUGHTS

Directions: Read through the list of positive thoughts that follow. Choose at least two to use to reduce your stress and enhance your coping ability. Say them often to yourself. Consider writing them down on index cards and carrying them with you or posting them on your mirror, your refrigerator, your desk, or your dashboard to remind you to be positive.

Preparatory Stage (Use these comments when preparing to enter a stressful situation)
- I can handle this.
- There's nothing to worry about.
- I'm picturing myself succeeding again and again until I believe it.
- I'll jump right in and be fine.
- It will be easier once we get started.
- Soon this will be over.

The Situation (Use these comments in the stressful situation)
- I refuse to let this situation upset me.
- Take a deep breath and relax.
- I can take this step-by-step.

- I can do this; I'm handling it now.
- I can keep my mind on the task at hand.
- It doesn't matter what others think; I will do this.
- Deep breathing really works.

Reinforcing Success (Use these comments after the stressful situation to enhance self-esteem)
- Situations don't have to overwhelm me anymore.
- I did it!
- I did well.
- I'm going to tell _____ about my success.
- By not thinking about being afraid, I wasn't afraid.
- By thinking about staying calm, I stayed calm.
- By picturing myself being successful, I was successful.

Source: Used with permission from *Wellness Practitioner, Concepts, Research, and Strategies,* by Carolyn Chambers Clark, New York: Springer Publishing Company, 1996.

- Increasing adrenaline production, which causes the body to step up its metabolism of proteins, fats, and carbohydrates to produce a quick source of energy
- Excreting amino acids, potassium, and phosphorus
- Depleting magnesium stored in muscle tissue
- Storing less calcium

The result is the body becomes deficient in many nutrients, and in chronic stress, it is unable to replace them adequately (Balch & Balch, 1997).

A diet of meat, white bread, coffee, and donuts was associated with an incidence of cancer, ischemic heart disease, and all-cause mortality in a study of 34,192 Californians (Fraser, 1999).

LEADERSHIP CHALLENGE Compare this study's findings to the third, fourth, and fifth stages of burnout described in Box 4-4.

Research shows the following connections between eating habits and health problems:

- *Meat.* Eating meat is correlated with cancer of the colon, rectum, stomach, pancreas, bladder, endometrium and ovaries, prostate, breast, and lung; heart disease; rheumatoid arthritis; type 2 diabetes; and Alzheimer's disease. These correlations indicate the presence of factors in red meat that damage biological components (Qi, van Dam, Rexrode, & Hu, 2007; Tappel, 2007).
- *White bread.* Bread that is not whole grain is correlated with breast cancer (Augustin et al., 2001), gastric cancer (De Stefani et al., 2004), prostate cancer (Walker et al., 2005), insulin resistance and type 2 diabetes (Villegas, Salim, Flynn, & Perry, 2004), and polycystic ovary syndrome (Douglas et al., 2006).
- *Coffee and caffeine.* Foods (like chocolate), drinks (like sodas, teas, coffee), and prescription drugs that contain caffeine are associated with stress. Caffeine can trigger a drop in blood sugar that results in fatigue and irritability (Rogers et al., 2005). Caffeine has been associated with increased cholesterol (Kleemola, Jousalahti, Pietinen, Vaatiacinen, & Tuomilehto, 2000), systolic blood pressure, and heart rate—all of which are markers of heart inflammation (Hamer, Williams, Vuonvirta, Gibson, & Steptoe, 2006). Caffeine has also been associated with increased risk of ovarian cancer (stage 5 of burnout). The chances of such health problems may be decreased by eating at least three cruciferous vegetables a week (Goodman, Tung, McDuffie, Wilkens, & Donlon, 2003).

(Cruciferous vegetables that protect against stress include arugula, bok choy, broccoli, brussels sprouts, cabbage, cauliflower, collard greens, daikon, horseradish, kale, kohlrabi, mizuna, mustard greens, napa or Chinese cabbage, radishes, rutabaga, tatsoi, turnip greens, turnips, and watercress.

Clinically, caffeine can often be directly traced to sleeping problems and sometimes to panic attacks, including heart palpitations. Caffeine also adds to nervousness and irritability in susceptible individuals.

Caffeine is an addictive substance that can cause 49 different symptoms during withdrawal, including headache, fatigue, muscle pain and stiffness, mild nausea, decreased energy, drowsiness, depressed mood, irritability, and decreased alertness (Juliano & Griffiths, 2004). To prevent withdrawal symptoms, it is best to taper off by drinking cups of half coffee and half a cereal beverage for a few days and gradually increasing the cereal beverage until no coffee remains. Chocolate can be substituted with carob products. Tea can be substituted with herbal teas.

- *Donuts and other simple sugars.* Donuts contain a large amount of sugar, which has been associated with the suppression of the immune system (Ichimura et al., 1990; Ringsdorf, Cheraskin, & Ramsey, 1976), mineral imbalances (Fields, Ferritti, Smith, & Reiser, 1983; Kozlovsky, Moser, Reiser, & Anderson, 1986; Lemann, 1976; Sears, 2006), increased risk of diabetes (Schulze et al., 2004), and various cancers (Cornee, 1995; De Stefani et al., 2004; Michaud, 2002). Sugar can also be addictive (Colantuoni et al., 2002).

Reducing the intake of simple sugars and increasing the ingestion of the nutrients that follow can decrease stress:

- *Vitamin C.* This nutrient can reduce the levels of stress hormones in the blood and reverse other typical indicators of physical and emotional stress, such as weight loss, enlargement of the adrenal glands, and reduction in the size of the thymus gland and spleen (American Chemical Society, 1999).

  Food sources of vitamin C include asparagus, beet greens, berries, broccoli, brussels sprouts, cantaloupe, citrus fruit, collard greens, dandelion greens, green peas, kale, mangos, mustard greens, onions, papayas, pineapple, radishes, spinach, sweet peppers, Swiss chard, tomatoes, turnip greens, and watercress (Balch & Balch, 1997).

- *Vitamin B.* The B-complex vitamins in combination with vitamin C are called the "stress vitamins" because they reduce stress. Vitamin B6 deficiency is especially linked to stress, probably because it is one of the building blocks for serotonin, which fights depression and stress. Without B6, even when taking into account coping style and amount of social support, individuals had significantly more psychological distress and anxiety. Research conducted at the University of Miami School of Medicine confirmed that inadequate levels of vitamin B6 were related to stress ("Researchers at UM School of Medicine Link Vitamin B6 Deficiency to Stress," 1995). Researchers there suggested beginning with vitamin B6 rather than antidepressant or antianxiety medication because the vitamin carries none of the harmful side effects associated with certain prescription drugs.

Food sources of vitamin B6 include avocado, bananas, blackstrap molasses, brewer's yeast, broccoli, brown rice, cabbage, cantaloupe, carrots, chicken, corn, eggs, fish, peas, potatoes, soybeans, spinach, sunflower seeds, tempeh, walnuts, and wheat germ.

- *Vitamin E.* Researchers found that taking 200 mg of vitamin C and 250 IU of vitamin E can protect against the negative effects of stress (Sahin & Kucuk, 2001).

  Food sources of vitamin E include brown rice, cornmeal, dark green leafy vegetables, eggs, kelp, legumes, nuts, oatmeal, organ meats, seeds, soybeans, sweet potatoes, watercress, wheat germ, and whole grains.

- *Selenium.* Diets deficient in selenium and vitamin E can lead to liver damage; a diet with sufficient selenium and vitamin E can protect against stress effects (South, Smith, Guidry, & Levander, 2006).

  Food sources of selenium include Brazil nuts, broccoli, brown rice, chicken, garlic, kelp, liver, molasses, onions, salmon, seafood, tuna, vegetables, wheat germ, and whole grain breads and cereals (Balch & Balch, 1997).

- *Magnesium.* Animal and human studies have shown that magnesium deficiency increases stress-induced hypertension, stroke, myocardial infarction, rhythm disturbances, and sudden death. Conversely, the administration of magnesium protects against cardiac and blood vessel damage and damage caused by the stress-related hormones adrenaline and noradrenaline. Other stress-related conditions—such as migraines, depression, bipolar disease, panic disorder, and epilepsy—may all respond to additional magnesium (Rosch, 1997).

  Food sources of magnesium include apples, apricots, avocados, bananas, black-eyed peas, blackstrap molasses, brown rice, cantaloupe, dark green leafy vegetables, figs, fish, garlic, grapefruit, lima beans, millet, nuts, peaches, seafood, sesame seeds, soybeans, tofu, watercress, and whole grains.

When it is not feasible to eat the required foods, it may be necessary to take a high-grade multivitamin and a high-grade multimineral.

LEADERSHIP CHALLENGE How would you use this nutritional information to help your staff reduce their stress?

In additional to individual strategies to reduce stress, there are organizational strategies.

Other Stress Reduction Ideas

There are many ways to reduce stress, depending on the situation and the person, including:

- *Putting job stress in perspective.* Jobs are temporary, but friends, families, and health aren't. If your employer can't or won't change, begin looking for a new job.
- *Modifying your work situation.* If you like your employer but the job is too stressful, ask about tailoring your work to your skills or making a lateral transfer.
- *Taking a break.* Walk away from a stressful situation that you feel unable to handle at the moment. Take a walk up a few flights of stairs or out in the sunshine, doing a meditation—such as counting "one, two" or saying "left, right"—as you walk. Have a cup of peppermint or chamomile tea (unless you're allergic to flowers), and let your stress melt as you sip.
- *Organizing your workspace.* Clutter and disorganization can increase a sense of loss of control.
- *Keeping track of accomplishments.* Keep a to-do list, and cross off each item as you complete it.
- *Rewarding yourself for your achievements.* Your boss may not notice, but you should. Take yourself (or a friend or two) out for a nice dinner or cook at home together, and present yourself with a certificate of achievement. Don't forget to hang it on your wall and take pictures to carry around to remind you of your accomplishment.
- *Using your support system.* Talk out your frustrations and stress with supportive others. Ask for suggestions, but carefully weigh putting them into action until you've thought them through.
- *Cultivating allies at work.* Make a pact that you'll support each other when you encounter stress.
- *Finding humor in the situation.* Share a joke or a funny story with friends or colleagues. Write a story, making your boss (or whoever is adding to your stress) the victim in a mystery plot or someone who is the target of a bully.
- *Stopping micromanaging.* No situation is perfect, and no person is, either. Change your motto from "Everything must be perfect" to "Everyone must perform at the highest level possible given the situation."
- *Avoiding negative people and situations.* Maintain a positive attitude by relaxing, using coping skills, and making good nutritional decisions. Don't allow negativism to suck the energy and motivation out of you (Hansen, 2007).
- *Distinguishing between stress you can change and stress you can't change.* Write down stressors affecting you and separate them into those you can change

and those you can't. Focus on those you can change. Prioritize this list, and get to work (Rosch, 1998c).

- *Following a healthy lifestyle.* Eat healthy foods (hint: keep only healthy foods in your cabinets and refrigerator in case you binge), exercise daily, and use relaxation and coping strategies.
- *Finding time to be alone.* Turn off cell phones, iPods, faxes, and other forms of technology. Put a "do not disturb" sign on your door. Defend your time alone ruthlessly.
- *Keeping a stress diary.* Note when you feel stressed, and begin to notice patterns so that you can intercept stress and reduce it.
- *Cutting back on commitments.* You're only human. Talk to your boss and family about making a workable solution to overscheduling.
- *Developing a hobby.* Make sure that whatever you choose is low stress and noncompetitive.
- *Spending time outdoors.* Nature is a natural de-stresser, and 15 minutes a day of sun on your arms and face can enhance your health. If you have a yard, start a garden. If you don't, grow flowers, plants, or herbs on your terrace or even on your windowsill (Borgatti, 2000).
- *Relaxing with a hot bath.* Fifteen or 20 minutes alone in a bath can restore a feeling of calm, invigorate you, or help you unwind.
- *Writing in a journal.* Keep a journal by your bedside, and write about your best moments that day.
- *Speaking with your nurse manager.* Talk about an overwhelming assignment, and ask for a smaller assignment.
- *Speaking to the unit educator.* Ask for help with prioritizing your workload.
- *Saying no selectively.* Learn to say no appropriately. Take an assertiveness course, if necessary.
- *Being empowered by what you do.* You're a nurse who helps people; keep that in focus (Knight, 2003).
- *Tuning in to your signs of body stress.* Headache, upset stomachache, and back pain all have a cause; often, it's stress. Beware of quick fixes such as aspirin, antacids, pain killers, and sleeping pills. If you have to use them, your body is telling you something, and it's important to listen.
- *Taking a break.* Set aside 3 minutes for stretching, enjoying a low-fat treat, teaching your colleagues a dance step, or telling a humorous work-related story.

Organizational Approaches to Job Stress

According to Mariano (2007), organizations have tried quick-fix solutions (higher salaries, housing, benefits, and flexible scheduling) to increase nurse retention. These actions hide the real problem and underlying causes. An organization must nourish and care for its staff, or it will become sick—and the staff will become sick, too (Wright & Sayre-Adams, 2000).

Recent studies of so-called healthy organizations suggest that policies benefiting worker health also enhance profits. A healthy organization is defined as one whose workforce has low rates of illness, injury, and disability *and* is itself competitive in the marketplace. Research from the National Institute for Occupational Safety and Health has associated healthy, low-stress work and high levels of productivity with organizations that:

- Recognize employees for performance
- Offer opportunities for career development
- Foster an organizational culture that values the individual worker
- Makes management decisions that are consistent with organizational values (Sauter et al., 1999)
- See **Box 4-7** for information about stress prevention and job performance from an organizational viewpoint.

Judkins, Reid, and Furlow (2006) say that organizations can cultivate hardiness by instituting policies that promote:

- Collaborative practice
- Self-scheduling
- Shared governance
- Staff education on coping with stress

Let's consider the opening Leadership in Action vignette again. A new nurse manager took over as leader of Roberta's unit. The new manager not only taught the staff stress reduction measures but also brought in a consultant to recommend ways to improve working conditions.

BOX 4-7 STRESS PREVENTION AND ORGANIZATIONAL CHANGE

St. Paul Fire and Marine Insurance Company conducted several studies on the effects of stress prevention programs in hospital settings that included:

- Employee and management education on job stress
- Changes in hospital policies and procedures to reduce organizational sources of stress
- Establishing employee assistance programs

As a result of these changes:

- Medication errors declined by 50% after prevention activities were implemented in one 700-bed hospital.
- Malpractice claims declined by 70% in 22 hospitals that implemented stress prevention activities.
- In a matched group of 22 hospitals where no stress prevention activities were implemented, no reduction in claims was found.

(Sauter et al., 1999)

Such a direct approach involves identifying stressful aspects of work, including excessive workload and conflicting expectations, and designing strategies to reduce or eliminate stressors. The advantage of this approach is that it deals with the roots causes of stress. Several of the nurses who had grown comfortable with work routines and schedules fought the suggested changes; they eventually left the unit. Although not everyone reported a large reduction in job stress, most staff did.

A combination of organizational change and stress management can be the most useful approach for preventing stress at work, especially when the organization is sick. In this case, nurses must tune in to their own stress and empower themselves with personal stress management procedures, including assertiveness skills. Empowerment can help nurses be more assertive and raise their voices regarding the dangers of the practice environment (Mariano, 2007). For suggestions on changing an organization to prevent job stress, see **Box 4-8**.

LEADERSHIP CHALLENGE   Brainstorm ways to incorporate the ideas for changing an organization to reduce stress. How can these principles be applied to the units you're familiar with? Give a rationale for your answer.

Implementing a Stress Prevention Program

At a minimum, preparation for a stress prevention program should include:

- Building general awareness about the causes, costs, and control of job stress
- Securing top management's commitment and support for the program

---

BOX 4-8   CHANGING THE ORGANIZATION TO REDUCE JOB STRESS

- Ensure the workload is in line with worker capabilities and resources.

- Design jobs to provide meaning, stimulation, and opportunities for workers to use their skills.

- Clearly define staff roles and responsibilities.

- Give employees opportunities to participate in decisions and actions that affect their job.

- Improve communications and reduce uncertainty about career development and future employment prospects. (See Chapter 7 for suggestions on improving communications.)

- Provide opportunities for social interaction among workers.

- Establish work schedules that are compatible with demands and responsibilities outside the job.

(Sauter et al., 1999)

- Incorporating employee input and involvement in all phases of the program
- Establishing the technical capacity to conduct the program, including specialized training for staff or the use of stress consultants (Sauter et al., 1999)

Box 4-9 provides details of a study of a hardiness program that could be used to reduce staff stress.

It may not always be clear that job stress is high. Sometimes employees are fearful of losing their jobs and hide the signs of stress. A lack of obvious signs is not a good reason to dismiss concerns about job stress. The National Institute for Occupational Safety and Health (Sauter et al., 1999) suggests a problem-solving approach to prevention.

Step 1: Identify the Problem

Ways to identify job stress include:

- Holding group discussions with employees
- Designing and administering an employee survey that measures perceptions of job conditions, stress, health, and satisfaction (Box 4-8 may provide ideas; using an anonymous survey may reap more information because participants will feel more comfortable participating)
- Collecting information about absenteeism, illness, and turnover rates or performance problems to gauge the scope of job stress
- Analyzing data to identify problems and stressful job conditions

BOX 4-9   EXPLORATORY STUDY OF HARDINESS AND STRESS

Judkins, Arris, and Keener (2005) conducted an exploratory study of hardiness and stress.

Purpose: To measure the effect of a hardiness program to reduce workplace stress.

Sample: A select group of graduate nursing administration students at the University of Texas–Arlington.

Measures: Participants completed the hardiness scale and perceived stress scale at the beginning and end of their program. Six to 12 months after graduation, each student participated in a telephone survey with items related to hardiness and the core competencies of the American Association of Colleges of Nursing and the American Organization of Nurse Executives.

Treatment: Participants received 6 weekly 2-hour sessions and 2-hour sessions at 5 and 8 months. Topics covered included hardiness, stress management, power, negotiation, communication, and problem and conflict management.

Findings: Mean scores for hardiness and stress improved after taking the program, and telephone interviews revealed that graduates were engaged in hardiness behaviors. The researchers concluded that such a problem could increase resiliency to workplace stresses.

Step 2: Design and Implement Interventions

Once information has been collected and analyzed, the stage is set for designing an intervention strategy. On small units, informal discussions may provide fruitful ideas for prevention. In larger organizations, a team may be asked to develop recommendations alone or in concert with outside experts.

Substeps to this step include:

- Targeting the sources of stress
- Proposing and prioritizing intervention strategies
- Communicating planned interventions to employees
- Implementing interventions

Step 3: Evaluate the Intervention

Short- and long-term time frames for evaluating interventions should be established. Evaluations should include objective measures, such as absenteeism and healthcare costs, and subjective measures, such as employee perceptions of job conditions, stress, health, and satisfaction.

LEADERSHIP IN ACTION

Roberta's new supervisor sensed an escalating level of tension and deteriorating morale among her staff. Headaches and absenteeism were on the rise. Roberta's supervisor held an all-hands meeting to explore her concerns. After reviewing a list of employee comments about their jobs, the supervisor asked one of the mental health clinical nurse specialists to conduct informal classes and hand out information about job stress causes, effects, and prevention. The supervisor also asked the clinical specialist to distribute and collect an anonymous survey about job satisfaction. Analysis of the survey data suggested that three conditions were linked to stress complaints: unrealistic deadlines, low levels of support from administration, and lack of worker involvement in decision making. The supervisor used the data to plan interventions, including greater staff participation in work scheduling and more frequent meetings between workers, managers, and administration to keep everyone updated on developing problems.

Nursing Research Needed on Job Stress and Health

McNeely (2005) evaluated studies on nurse job stress and found that even in Magnet hospitals, the focus is on healthy hospitals, not healthy nurses. Mason (2001) agreed and questions the agenda of many state-of-the-art hospitals. If they are truly places of healing, they ought to provide support groups for staff and other interventions to lessen the effects of traumatic stress. Nurses working in emergency, trauma, burn care, and psychiatry/behavioral health are especially at risk.

GUIDED LEADERSHIP TIP

JOB STRESS RESOURCE

You can reach the National Institute for Occupation Safety and Health (NIOSH) at 1-800-35-NIOSH. This federal agency provides information and publications about a wide range of occupational hazards, including job stress. Its "Stress at Work" Web page is http://www.cdc.gov/niosh/topics/stress.

McNeely (2005) stated that the following research regarding nurses' job stress is needed:

- *The relationship between nurses' work, chronic job stress, and career and health trajectories* (e.g., studying stress as a risk factor for disease and disability, physiological markers of stress linked with particular working conditions and health outcomes, nurses' health in the context of work and over the course of time, how nurses adjust to their daily work or their career trajectories because of disability, why hospital nurses are younger than nurses in other settings and why so many work part-time, and the relationship between symptoms of stress exposure)
- *How or if work can be reorganized to improve the nurses' health* (e.g., determining which nursing models are healthy or unhealthy for nurses)
- *The relationship between work and a productive, safe, and affordable healthcare system* (e.g., studying whether a nurse's health explains some of the variation in quality of care, establishing the affect of work conditions on nurses' disabilities, and determining nurses' true health status)

McNeely (2005) maintains that if we asked nurses about job stress, they would tell us how to improve their job conditions and, as a result, our healthcare systems.

Summary

This chapter introduced information about quantifying job stress and the sources of workplace stress. Burnout, hardiness theory, and Bandura's theory of self-efficacy provided ideas for reducing job stress, as did nutritional changes and other individual and organizational actions.

Key Term Review

- **Burnout** is a stage of exhaustion that can result from unrelieved work stress or from an erosion of the soul.
- **Focusing** helps individuals recognize body signals of stress.
- **Job strain** is the result of psychological demands of a job exceeding the worker's discretion in deciding how to do the job.
- **Job stress** is the result of a mismatch between a worker's capabilities, resources, or needs and the job's requirements.
- **Psychological hardiness** is composed of a commitment to self, work, family, and other important values; a sense of personal control over one's life; and the ability to see change in one's life as a challenge.
- The **social readjustment rating scale** ranks and rates 43 stressful life-change events.
- **Stages of burnout** include honeymoon, balancing act, chronic symptoms, crisis, and enmeshment.
- **Stress** is the feeling or perception of having little control.
- A **stressor** is a cause of stress.
- **Technostress** is the result of difficulties dealing with computer technologies or of an unusual attraction to them.
- Bandura's **theory of self-efficacy** focuses on the belief in one's ability to perform adequately.

Leadership Development Exercises

Leadership Development Exercise 4-1
Demonstrate three ways to use Bandura's self-efficacy theory to help at least three colleagues reduce stress.

Leadership Development Exercise 4-2
Try out information in Boxes 4-5 and 4-6. Report your findings to at least two colleagues.

Leadership Development Exercise 4-3
Teach at least two peers stress reduction measures, and analyze the results. Share your findings with the class or with at least two other learners.

Leadership Development Exercise 4-4
a. Choose at least one nutritional action to reduce job stress, and make it part of your daily regime.
b. Provide stress reduction nutrition information to at least two other people. Evaluate the results, and share them with the class or with two other learners.

■ **Leadership Development Exercise 4-5**

a. Observe a unit for signs of job stress.
b. Write down your findings.
c. Share them with the class or with two other learners.

■ **Leadership Development Exercise 4-6**

Design a job stress reduction plan for the unit you observed, and share your plan with the class or with two other learners.

■ **Leadership Development Exercise 4-7**

Share your job stress reduction plan with staff members or supervisors on the unit. If that's not possible, imagine a scenario of presenting your plan, identifying potential obstacles, and picturing yourself overcoming them.

Advanced Leadership Development Exercises

■ **Leadership Development Exercise 4-8**

a. Using McNeely's suggestions for research or other information in this chapter, develop a problem statement for some aspect of job stress reduction.
b. Ask for a critique from a more advanced nurse researcher; if that's not possible, ask the class or two other colleagues for one.
c. Revise your problem statement, if necessary, based on feedback.

■ **Leadership Development Exercise 4-9**

a. Develop a research design for your problem statement on job stress reduction.
b. Ask for a critique from a more advanced researcher, the class, or two other colleagues.
c. Revise your plan, if necessary.

References

Aiken, L. H., Clarke, S. P., Sloane, D. M., Sochalski, J., & Silber, J. H. (2002). Hospital nurse staffing and patient mortality, nurse burnout, and job dissatisfaction. *Journal of the American Medical Association, 288*(16), 1989–1993.

American Association of Critical-Care Nurses. (2005). *AACN standards for establishing and sustaining healthy work environments: A journey to excellence.* Retrieved March 1, 2006, from http://www.aacn.org/AACN/pubpolcy.nsf/vwdoc/workenv

American Chemical Society. (1999). *Vitamin C may alleviate the body's response to stress.* [Press release]. Retrieved February 18, 2007, from http://www.sciencedaily.com/releases/1999/08/990823072615.htm

American Nurses Association. (2001, September). *Nurses say health and safety concerns play a major role in employment decisions.* [Press release.] Washington, DC: Author.

American Nurses Association. (2005). *Survey of 76,000 nurses probes elements of job satis-faction, USA*. Retrieved February 16, 2007, from http://www.medicalnewstoday.com/medicalnews.php?newsid=21907

Augustin, L. S., Dal Maso, L., La Vecchia, C., Parpinel, M., Negri, E., Vaccarella, S., et al. (2001). Dietary glycemic index and glycemic load, and breast cancer risk: A case-control study. *Annals of Oncology, 12*(11), 1533–1538.

Balch, J. F., & Balch, P. A. (1997). *Prescription for nutritional healing*. Garden City Park, NY: Avery.

Bandura, A. (1977). *Social learning theory*. New York: General Learning Press.

Bandura, A. (1986). *Social foundation of thought and action: A social cognitive theory*. Englewood Cliffs, NJ: Prentice Hall.

Bandura, A. (1997). *Self-efficacy: The exercise of control*. New York: W. H. Freeman.

Bandura, A. (2001). Social cognitive theory: An agentic perspective. *Annual Review of Psychology, 52*, 1–26.

Bandura, A. (2004). The evolution of social cognitive theory. In K.G. Smith & M.A. Hitt (Eds.), *Great minds in management* (pp. 9–35). New York: Oxford University Press.

Biesalski, H. K., Jentzsch, A., & Kirschbaum, C. (1994, February). *Oxidative stress following acute mental stress*. Paper presented at the First World Congress on Stress, Montreux, Switzerland.

Borgatti, J. C. (2000). Stressed for success. *Nursing Spectrum Career Fitness Guide*. Hoffman Estates, IL: Nursing Spectrum.

Canadian Institute for Health Information & Health Canada. (2005). *National survey of the work and health of nurses, 2005*. Retrieved February 18, 2007, from http://secure.cihi.ca/cihiweb/dispPage.jsp?cs_page=hhr

Charles, C. L. (2001). *Why is everyone so cranky? The ten trends that are making us angry and how we can find peace of mind instead*. Burbank, CA: Hyperion.

Charles, J. (2003). Inspire yourself! *Meetings and Incentive Travel, 31*(3), 14.

Colantuoni, C., Rada, P., McCarthy, J., Patten, C., Avena, N. M., Chadeayne, A., et al. (2002). Evidence that intermittent excessive sugar intake causes endogenous opioid dependence. *Obesity Research, 10*(6), 478–488.

Cornee, J. (1995). A case-control study of gastric cancer and nutritional factors in Marseille, France. *European Journal of Epidemiology, 11*, 55–65.

Cox, T., & Griffiths, A. (1996). *Work-related stress in nursing: Controlling the risk to health*. Retrieved September 24, 2007, from http://www.ilo.org/public/english/protection/condtrav/pdf/wc-cgc-96.pdf

D'Anna, B. A. (2006). Advancing knowledge through collaboration: Nurses need rest, too! *Reflections on Nursing Leadership*. Retrieved February 15, 2007, from http://www.nursinghonor.org/RNL/2Q_2006/features/feature2.html

De Stefani, E., Correa, P., Boffetta, P., Deneo-Pellegrini, H., Ronco, A. L., & Mendilaharsu, M. (2004). Dietary patterns and risk of gastric cancer: A case-control study in Uruguay. *Gastric Cancer, 7*(4), 211–220.

Detmer, D. E., Steen, E. B., & Dick, R. S. (Eds.). (1997). *The computer-based patient record: An essential technology for health care*. Washington, DC: Institute of Medicine.

Douglas, C. C., Norris, L. E., Oster, R. A., Darnell, B. E., Azziz, R., & Gower, B. A. (2006). Differences in dietary intake between women with polycystic ovary syndrome and healthy controls. *Fertility and Sterility, 86*(2), 411–417.

Fields, M., Ferritti, R. M., Smith, J. C., Jr., & Reiser, L. (1983). Effect of copper deficiency on metabolism and mortality in rats fed sucrose or starch diets, *Journal of Clinical Nutrition, 113*, 1135–1345.

Fraser, G. E. (1999). Associations between diet and cancer, ischemic heart disease, and all-cause mortality in non-Hispanic white California Seventh-Day Adventists. *American Journal of Clinical Nutrition, 70*(Suppl. 3), 532S–538S.

Freudenberger, H., & Richelson, G. (1980). *Burnout: The high cost of high achievement.* Garden City, NY: Anchor Press.

Gendlin, E. T. (1978). *Focusing.* New York: Everest House.

Goodman, M. T., Tung, K. H., McDuffie, K., Wilkens, L. R., & Donlon, T. A. (2003). Association of caffeine intake and CYP1A2 genotype with ovarian cancer. *Nutrition in Cancer, 46*(1), 23–29.

Hamer, M., Williams, E. D., Vuonvirta, R., Gibson, E. L., & Steptoe, A. (2006). Association between coffee consumption and markers of inflammation and cardiovascular function during mental stress. *Journal of Hypertension, 24*(11), 2149–2151.

Hansen, R. S. (2007). *Managing job stress: 10 strategies for coping and thriving at work.* Retrieved September 24, 2007, from http://www.quintcareers.com/managing_job_stress.html

Holmes, T., & Rahe, R. (1967). Holmes-Rahe social readjustment rating scale. *Journal of Psychosomatic Research 2,* 213–248.

Ichimura, K., Sato, I, Qu, J., Shimojima, T., Fujihashi, H., & Ikeda. (1990). Relationship between development of periodontitis and macrophage's defensive power against infection in rats fed a high-sucrose diet. *Nippon Shishubyo Gakkai Kaishi, 32*(1), 175–188.

Judkins, S., Arris, L., & Keener, E. (2005). Program evaluation in graduate nursing education: Hardiness as a predictor of success among nursing administration students. *Journal of Professional Nursing, 21*(5), 314–321.

Judkins, S., Massey, C., & Huff, B. (2006). Hardiness, stress, and use of ill-time among nurse managers: Is there a connection? *Nursing Economics, 24*(4), 187–192.

Judkins, S., Reid, B, & Furlow, L. (2006). Hardiness training among nurse managers: Building a healthy workplace. *Journal of Continuing Education in Nursing, 37*(5), 202–207.

Juliano, L. M., & Griffiths, R. R. (2004). A critical review of caffeine withdrawal: Empirical validation of symptoms and signs, incidence, severity, and associated features. *Psychopharmacology, 176*(1), 1–29.

Kleemola, P., Jousalahti, P., Pietinen, P., Vaatiacinen, E., & Tuomilehto, J. (2000). Coffee consumption and the risk of coronary heart disease and death. *Archives Internal Medicine, 160:* 3393–3400.

Knight, K. A. (2003). Fired up or burned out? *Nursing Spectrum Career Fitness Guide.* New York: Nursing Spectrum.

Kobasa, S. O. (1984). How much stress can you survive? *American Health, 3*(7), 64–72.

Kohn, L., Corrigan, J., & Donaldson, M. (Eds.). (1999). *To err is human: Building a safer health system.* Washington, DC: National Academies Press.

Kozlovsky, A. S., Moser, P. B., Reiser, S., & Anderson, R. A. (1986). Effects of diets high in simple sugars on urinary chromium losses. *Metabolism, 35,* 515–518.

Leggiere, P. (2002). What happened to the leisure society? *Across the Board, 39*(4), 42.

Lemann, J. (1976). Evidence that glucose ingestion inhibits net renal tubular reabsorption of calcium and magnesium. *Journal of Clinical Nutrition, 70,* 236–245.

Maddi, S. R. (2006). Hardiness: The courage to grow from stresses. *The Journal of Positive Psychology, 1*(3), 160–168.

Mariano, C. (2007). The nursing shortages: Is stress management the answer? *Beginnings, 27*(1), 3, 18.

Maslach, C., & Leiter, M. (1997). *The truth about burnout.* San Francisco: Jossey-Bass.

Mason, D. J. (2001). Places of healing? With some state-of-the art hospitals, it's in question. [Editorial.] *American Journal of Nursing, 101(5)*, 7.

Mason, D. J., & Smith, T. (2006, November). *Who will care for me?* Paper presented to the New York Academy of Medicine, New York.

McNeely, E. (2005). The consequences of job stress for nurses' health: Time for a check-up. *Nursing Outlook, 53*, 291–299.

Michaud, D. (2002). Dietary sugar, glycemic load and pancreatic cancer risk, in a prospective study. *Journal of the National Cancer Institute, 94*, 1293–1300.

Montague, J. (1994). Averting burnout crucial to health of care-giver, hospital survival. *Hospital & Health Networks, 68*(15), 178.

Morse, D. R., Schacterle, G. R., Furst, L., Zaydenberg, M., & Pollack, R. L. (1989). Oral digestion of a complex-carbohydrate cereal: Effects of stress and relaxation on physiological and salivary measures. *American Journal of Clinical Nutrition, 49*, 97–105.

Qi, L., van Dam, R. M., Rexrode, K., & Hu, F. B. (2007). Heme iron from diet as a risk factor for coronary heart disease in women with type 2 diabetes. *Diabetes Care, 30*(1), 101–106.

Researchers at UM School of Medicine link vitamin B6 deficiency to stress. (1995, June 6). *Vital Signs*, 19.

Ringsdorf, W., Cheraskin, E., & Ramsey, R. (1976). Sucrose, neutrophilic phagocytosis and resistance to disease. *Dental Survey, 52*(12), 46–48.

Robinson, J. (2003). *Work to live*. Toronto, Canada: Perigee.

Rosch, P. (1993). A biopsychosocial approach to job stress. *Health and Stress, 8*, 4.

Rosch, P. (1997). Stress and magnesium. *Health and Stress, 5*, 6.

Rosch, P. (1998a). Can stress be quantified or qualified? *Health and Stress, 9*, 2.

Rosch, P. (1998b). Coping with college stress, a new job, or any change. *Health and Stress, 9*, 1–3.

Rosch, P. (1998c). Perception and sense of control. *Health and Stress, 9*, 3.

Rosch, P. (2000). Technostress due to information overload. *Health and Stress, 2*, 1–8.

Rogers, P. J., Heatherley, S. V., Hayward, R. C., Seers, H. E., Hill, J., & Kane, M. (2005). *Psychopharmacology, 179*, 742–752.

Sahin, K., & Kucuk, O. (2001). Effects of vitamin C and vitamin E on performance, digestion of nutrients and carcass characteristics of Japanese quails reared under chronic heat stress. *Journal of Animal Physiology and Animal Nutrition, 85*(11), 335–341.

Sauter, S., Murphy, L., Colligan, M., Swanson, N., Hurrell, J., Scharf, F., et al. (1999). *Stress . . . At work* (NIOSH Pub. No. 99–101). Retrieved September 24, 2007, from http://www.cdc.gov/niosh/stresswk.html

Schulze, M. B., Manson, J. E., Ludwig, D. S., Colditz, G. A., Stampfer, M. J., Willett, W. C., et al. (2004). Sugar-sweetened beverages, weight gain, and incidence of type 2 diabetes in young and middle-aged women. *Journal of the American Medical Association, 292*(8), 927–934.

Sears, R. (2006). *Best carbs*. Retrieved September 24, 2007, from http://www.askdrsears.com/html/4/T045000.asp

Selye, H. (1978). *The stress of life*. New York: McGraw-Hill.

Shimko, B. W., Meli, J. T., Restrypo, J. C., & Oehlers, P. F. (2000). Debunking the "lean and mean" myth and celebrating the rise of learning organizations. *The Learning Organization, 7(2)*, 99–109.

Shirey, M. R. (2006a). Authentic leaders creating healthy work environments for nursing practice. *American Journal of Critical Care, 15*, 256–268.

Shirey, M. R. (2006b). Stress and coping in nurse managers: Two decades of research. *Nursing Economics, 24*(4), 193–203, 211.

South, P., Smith, A., Guidry, C., & Levander, O. (2006). Effect of physical restraint on oxidative stress in mice fed a selenium and vitamin E deficient diet. *Biological Trace Element Research, 109*(3), 293–300.

Tappel, A. (2007). Heme of consumed red meat can act as a catalyst of oxidative damage and could initiate colon, breast and prostate cancers, heart disease and other diseases. *Medical Hypotheses, 68*(3), 562–564.

Veninga, R. L., & Spradley, U. P. (1981). *The work stress connection: How to cope with job burnout.* Boston: Little, Brown.

Villegas, R., Salim, A., Flynn, A., & Perry, I. J. (2004). Prudent diet and the risk of insulin resistance. *Nutrition and Metabolism in Cardiovascular Disease, 14*(6), 334–343.

Walker, M., Aronson, K. J., King, W., Wilson, J. W., Fan, W., Heaton, J. P., et al. (2005). Dietary patterns and risk of prostate cancer in Ontario Canada. *International Journal of Cancer, 116*(4), 592–598.

Wright, S.G., Sayre-Adams, J. (2000). Sacred space. *Australian Occupational Therapy Journal, 52*(1), 2–9.

Managing Time

CHAPTER OBJECTIVES

After reading this chapter, answering the leadership challenges, and participating in the leadership development exercises, you will be able to:

- Analyze one nurse leader's time management skills
- Assess whether you exhibit characteristics of hurry sickness and time urgency
- Identify inappropriate time management procedures and time traps
- Apply the steps of effective time management
- State two short-term and two long-term time management goals
- Develop two top-drawer and two bottom-drawer goals
- Break two long-term goals into manageable steps
- Apply approaches to overcoming procrastination
- Use at least four different ways to "make" time

Advanced nurses will be able to:

- Interview a nurse leader about time management
- Develop a time management program
- Role-play appropriate times to say no

Introduction

Although futurists predicted in 1960 that people would have more leisure time, the fact is, Americans now complain that there are not enough hours in the day to satisfy work and personal needs. Almost everything moves at a quickened pace. Eventually, this fast tempo pervades all activities and becomes a way of life. People think that they accomplish less and feel constantly hurried. Always being in a hurry and worrying whether you're accomplishing anything can be stressful.

This chapter explores hurry sickness and time management procedures and gives you a chance to develop a time management program for yourself or for a nurse leader. To begin, read about Audrey and her time management issues.

LEADERSHIP IN ACTION

Audrey, a new nurse manager, felt overwhelmed with the number of meetings, deadlines, and goals she faced. Each time someone invited her to attend a meeting or join a committee, she agreed. Her desk was soon piled high with reports, files, and books. She couldn't find anything in the piles and had no idea when her next appointment was. She considered throwing everything out the window but decided instead to consult with a mental health clinical nurse specialist with special time management skills.

LEADERSHIP CHALLENGE If you were the nurse consultant, how would you assess Audrey's time management skills? Give a rationale for your answer.

Hurry Sickness

KEY TERM

Hurry sickness or **time urgency** is the struggle to achieve as much as possible in the shortest period of time.

Hurry sickness or **time urgency** is the struggle to achieve as much as possible in the shortest period of time (Rosch, 2000a). It may be a reaction to the process of not managing time efficiently. Time urgency can manifest in different ways. Nurse leaders who tend to fall into all the categories that follow could be classified as having a time urgency problem:

- Having an abundance of nervous energy that leads to being on edge when sitting and waiting
- Rarely taking time to eat three meals in a slow, relaxed manner
- Being urged by others to slow down
- Trying to force events into a specific and arbitrarily allotted amount of time

- Becoming excessively annoyed in slow traffic or meetings that move slowly
- Walking faster than most other people

LEADERSHIP CHALLENGE Assess your tendency for hurry sickness and time urgency. The more items from the time-urgency problem list that describe you, the more likely you have hurry sickness and time urgency.

What Is Time Management?

Time management is the ability to use time effectively. Efficient time management is neither hurrying nor procrastinating, but using tried processes to make the most of the available hours. Rather than manage time, nurse leaders should manage themselves. Time is a constant that marches on despite what gets done.

Characteristics of Inappropriate Time Management

When nurse leaders find themselves well behind schedule, they could have a time management problem. People who have difficulty managing time often have similar characteristics (Rosch, 1998), such as a tendency to:

- Assume that they must do everything themselves, even when portions of the work could be delegated
- Procrastinate or put things off until the last moment
- Have difficulty saying no to requests that they know they do not have enough time to accomplish
- Be late for appointments
- Have difficulty making decisions or vacillate back and forth between options
- Be irritable and frustrated
- Have an aura of hurrying
- Be easily distracted
- Not be able to set realistic goals

Brumm (2003) added the following time traps that can lead people to feel that time is slipping away without them accomplishing anything:

- Trying to accomplish too much without planning ahead
- Not setting deadlines
- Stacking their desk with papers with no apparent organization
- Too much socializing
- Not asking questions about assignments, which leads to misunderstandings

LEADERSHIP CHALLENGE Identify which of the inappropriate time management procedures and time traps apply to you.

The perception of time is relative, but you can learn to use your time more efficiently. Effective time management can not only increase productivity but also improve quality of life.

Steps in Effective Time Management

According to Rosch (2000b), the important thing you can do is to establish goals. Effective time management can help minimize deadline anxiety, avoidance anxiety, and job fatigue (Davis, McKay, & Eshelman, 2003). It consists of a series of planned and focused steps, including:

- Exploring how time is currently being spent
- Setting short-term goals
- Setting long-term goals
- Prioritizing
- Breaking goals into manageable steps

Exploring How Time Is Currently Being Spent

An easy way to explore how you spend your time is to divide the day into three segments: waking through lunch, end of lunch through dinner, and end of dinner until bedtime. Carry a small notebook, logging in the number of minutes you spend on different activities. Keep this inventory for 3 days. At the end of that time, note the total amount of time you spent in each activity. **Table 5-1** shows the amount of time that Audrey, the nurse in the Leadership in Action vignette at the beginning of this chapter, spent on different activities during 1 day.

Over the week, Audrey noticed that she spent many hours attending or organizing unnecessary meetings. She vowed to stop going to such meetings; if she had to organize one, she would keep it as brief as possible (Hill, 2002).

Audrey found herself spending too much time on the phone and promised herself to keep future conversations to a minimum and to the point. She also realized that she skipped lunch sometimes, even though she knew it was important to take meal breaks because they would keep her energy level high (Hill, 2002). When Audrey found herself taking home a report she needed to read, she wondered whether her brain might be more focused the next day, after a good night's sleep.

TABLE 5-1 TIME MANAGEMENT ASSESSMENT			
Activity	**Time (minutes)**	**Activity**	**Time (minutes)**
Waking through Lunch		**After Lunch through Dinner**	
Lie in bed and plan day	20	Meeting	65
Shower	20	Daydream while staring at paperwork	20
Decide what to wear and dress	25	Meeting with assistant director	30
Cook breakfast	20	Phone call with colleague	30
Eat and read paper	30	Meeting with head nurse	40
Commute to work	30	Phone calls (which interrupted writing report)	20
Routine paperwork	30	Commute	30
Nonmandatory meeting	50	Shop	30
Mandatory report	45	Cook	40
Mandatory meeting	60	Eat and clean up kitchen	50
Lunch	40		
		End of Dinner until Bedtime	
		Phone calls	30
		Watch TV and procrastinate	70
		Read reports	60
		Prepare for bed and read novel	40

Setting Short-Term Goals

Based on a review of the information in Table 5-1, Audrey set the following short-term goals:

- Put out clothes for the next day before going to bed
- Get up at the alarm, and limit shower to 5 minutes
- Make breakfasts that don't require cooking, cut dinner preparation to 30 minutes, and enlist family to do food preparation and cleanup three days a week
- Take a late lunch to make the best use of the most productive work hours (9 a.m.–1 p.m.)
- Use thought stopping to limit daydreaming (see **Box 5-1** for directions)
- Stop attending nonmandatory, nonproductive meetings

LEADERSHIP CHALLENGE Set two short-term time management goals, and share them with two colleagues or the class.

BOX 5-1   THOUGHT STOPPING

Directions: Use when nagging thoughts interfere with your work. Practice for at least 3–7 days to extinguish unwanted thoughts.
- Start work.
- Interrupt unwanted thoughts with the verbal, thought, or pictured directive to stop.
- Return to work.
- If saying, thinking, or picturing the word *stop* doesn't work, use a loud noise, such as a buzzer or bell. If that's not effective, wear a rubber band around your wrist, and snap it when an unwanted thought occurs.

Setting Long-Term Goals

Audrey's next step was to set long-term goals. These goals were things she wanted to accomplish that she knew would require energy, planning, and time. She began by:

- Making a list of things she most wanted to accomplish in the near future without censoring any items
- Comparing her list to how she spent her time
- Visualizing herself being told she had 6 months to live
- Picturing how she could best spend the time

Audrey thought about going back to school for her doctorate, initiating a mentor program at work, writing a nurse management article, and teaching a continuing education course on stress management at the local community college.

LEADERSHIP CHALLENGE Set two long-term time management goals, and share them with two students or the class. Ask for feedback.

Prioritizing

Once Audrey had her lists, she separated her goals for the next day into those activities that had to be done that day and the items that could wait a day by using the top-drawer/bottom-drawer system for prioritizing.

KEY TERM

Top-drawer items must be accomplished today.

Top-drawer items were the items that she absolutely had to accomplish, such as those items that:

- Were due that day
- Would otherwise cause clients or their families distress
- Were needed by staff so they could do their job
- Presented a risk or hazard
- Were needed by her supervisor

LEADERSHIP CHALLENGE List two top-drawer items, and share them with two colleagues or the class. Ask for feedback.

Bottom-drawer items were items that could wait for a day or more before being completed:

KEY TERM

Bottom-drawer items can be accomplished at a later date.

- Items without a personal or work-related time frame
- Items that if left until later would not affect care on the unit

---

LEADERSHIP CHALLENGE List two bottom-drawer items, and share them with two students or the class. Ask for feedback.

Audrey then chose her bottom-drawer goals, categorizing them as lifetime goals, 1-year goals, and 1-month goals:

- Take an introductory nursing management course at the doctoral level (1-year goal)
- Write an article for the *Journal of Nursing Administration* (lifetime goal to contribute to the profession)
- Have dinner with husband and friends once a week (1-month goal to reduce stress)
- Start a mentor program at work (1-year goal)
- Complete report at work (1-month goal)

Breaking Goals into Manageable Steps

When Audrey took a look at her five goals, she felt overwhelmed. She decided to break each one down into manageable steps.

The steps for taking an introductory management course at the doctoral level included:

- Calling the university and finding out how to apply
- Filling out the application materials and mailing them in
- Finding out about any exams or courses that were needed to meet application criteria
- Making the appointment to take any necessary exams
- Finding out where any necessary courses could be taken
- Taking the exams
- Taking the courses

LEADERSHIP CHALLENGE List one long-term goal, and break the goal into manageable steps. Share your steps with at least two classmates, and ask for a critique.

RULES FOR MAKING TIME

- *Learn to say no.* Remind yourself that this is your life and your time to spend as best befits you. You should spend time on bottom-drawer items only when your boss asks you to. Be prepared to say, "I don't have the time." If necessary, take an assertiveness training course to help you.
- *Build time into your schedule for unforeseen events and interruptions.* Such occurrences will otherwise wreck havoc in your schedule.
- *Set aside several time periods during the day for structured relaxation.* Being relaxed will allow more efficient use of available time.
- *Keep a list of short 5-minute tasks.* You can do these anytime you are waiting or are between other tasks.
- *Learn to do two things at once.* Plan dinner while driving home, or organize an important letter or list while waiting in line at the grocery store.
- *Delegate bottom-drawer tasks to family or assistants.* You don't have to do everything yourself.
- *Get up 15 to 30 minutes earlier every day.* This extra time quickly adds up to hours of gained time.
- *Allow no more than 1 hour of television watching daily.* Use time in front of the TV as a reward for working on a top-drawer item.

Other Key Time Management Approaches

Audrey just stared at the list of steps. Even though they seemed manageable, she could not get herself to take action. She remembered a tip she read in an online article and developed a daily to-do list. She included the first step in her school goal in that list.

This approach helped Audrey with some of her goals, but she still had difficulties taking action until she discovered the rules for making time (Davis, McKay, & Eshelman, 2003), which appear in the leadership tip.

LEADERSHIP CHALLENGE Choose at least three ways from "Rules for Making Time," and plan how to add them into your daily regime. Share your plan with at least two other students, and ask for their critique.

Fighting Procrastination: The Great Time Robber

KEY TERM

Procrastination is the inability or lack of incentive to make a decision or take action.

Even with the tools Audrey developed, she still occasionally **procrastinated** and found it difficult to make a decision or take action. There are specific steps to take to overcome procrastination:

- *List the pros and cons of taking action.* Compare the unpleasantness of making a decision versus the unpleasantness that can accrue from putting it off. Analyze the costs and risks of delay.
- *Examine the payoffs of procrastination.* Possible payoffs include being protected against possible failure, having others rush in to take responsibility and help, and gaining attention.
- *Bolster your procrastination efforts.* Exaggerate and intensify whatever you are doing to put off the decision to act. Keep it up until you are bored and making the decision seems more attractive than whatever you are doing to procrastinate.
- *Take responsibility for delaying tactics.* Write down how long each delay took.
- *When you get stuck making unimportant decisions, resort to a predetermined action.* When you get lost in the car, for example, always choose south or east over north or west; or always take a left-hand turn over a right-hand turn. For other decisions, choose the closer option instead of the one farther away. Or when in doubt, take the option whose first letter is closest to the beginning of the alphabet.
- *Take small steps toward the decision to act.* Take out the materials for a report you need to write, and place them by you as a lead-in to taking action.
- *Avoid beginning a new task until you've completed a predecided segment of the current one.* Fully experience the reward of finishing something before moving on. This is one of the great payoffs of decision making. (Davis, McKay, & Eshelman, 2003)

Summary

This chapter presented information on managing time, including hurry sickness, the definition of time management, characteristics of inappropriate time management, and steps in effective time management.

Key Term Review

- **Bottom-drawer items** can be completed later.
- **Hurry sickness** or **time urgency** is the struggle to achieve as much as possible in the shortest period of time.
- **Procrastination** is the inability or lack of incentive to make a decision or take action.
- **Time management** is the ability to use time effectively.
- **Top-drawer items** must be accomplished today.

Leadership Development Exercises

■ Leadership Development Exercise 5-1

With at least two other colleagues, discuss ways to better manage time. Use the information in this chapter to assist you.

■ Leadership Development Exercise 5-2

Keep a monthly or weekly planner or a daily to-do list. Review it weekly with a trusted peer, and ask for feedback.

■ Leadership Development Exercise 5-3

Set goals to accomplish your assignments. Evaluate how well you accomplish goals. Ask for feedback and suggestions for meeting your goals from a trusted peer.

■ Leadership Development Exercise 5-4

Plan a hypothetical or real "day in the life" to make sure you accomplish the most difficult tasks first while you're the most energetic.

■ Leadership Development Exercise 5-5

Set up a "tickler file" to prompt you about important class assignments. Go over your file and the results with a trusted peer.

Optional: Report back your findings to the class or group.

■ Leadership Development Exercise 5-6

Pair off with a partner, and interview each other about how you manage time. Brainstorm new ways to handle your time better.

More advanced option: Interview a nurse leader about how he or she manages time. Consider writing up your interview and making it the basis of a publishable paper.

■ **Leadership Development Exercise 5-7**

Pair off and role-play a situation in which a nurse leader must say no to an invitation to join a committee or attend a meeting.

   a. Flip a coin or draw a role from a hat to determine which partner will play the nurse leader first.
   b. Role-play the situation.
   c. Ask for feedback on whether the nurse leader sounded firm.
   d. Keep role-playing the situation until the person playing the nurse leader sounds convincing.
   e. Switch roles.

■ **Leadership Development Exercise 5-8**

Develop a time management program for either a hypothetical nurse leader or yourself, if you are a nurse leader.

More Advanced Leadership Development

■ **Leadership Development Exercise 5-9**

Collaborate with a nurse leader to help set up a time management program for that person using concepts you learned in this chapter.

■ **Leadership Development Exercise 5-10**

Develop a research problem statement related to time management. Obtain at least three critiques from savvy nurse researchers and revise your statement as needed.

■ **Leadership Development Exercise 5-11**

Develop a research design that matches your problem statement. Obtain at least three critiques from more experienced nurse researchers and revise your design as needed.

References

Brumm, J. (2003). Time can be on your side. *Nursing Spectrum Career Fitness Guide.* New York: Nursing Spectrum.

Davis, D., McKay, M., & Eshelman, E. R. (2003). *The Relaxation and Stress Reduction Workbook* (4th ed.). Oakland, CA: New Harbinger.

Hill, B. (2002). Under pressure. *Nursing Standards, 16*(16), 59.

Rosch, P. (1998). Tips on how to manage time. *Health and Stress, 9,* 4.

Rosch, P. (2000a). Do you have "hurry sickness"? *Health and Stress, 3,* 6.

Rosch, P. (2000b). Tempus fugit. *Health and Stress, 3,* 7.

Critical Thinking

CHAPTER OBJECTIVES

After reading this chapter, answering the leadership challenges, and participating in the leadership development exercises, you will be able to:

- Explain what critical-thinking skills are
- Describe the relationship between critical-thinking skills, problem solving, and decision making
- Discuss the research on evaluating critical-thinking skills
- Choose appropriate action for two critical-thinking situations
- Identify the steps in the problem-solving process
- Develop three high-level critical-thinking questions
- Identify problem-solving assumptions
- Construct a design or system model
- Construct a structural or recipe model

Advanced nurses will be able to:

- Chart a group's decision-making process
- Use the Six Hats technique to enhance group decisions
- Use algorithmic methods to solve a problem

Introduction

As a nurse leader, you will use critical-thinking skills every day to assess, diagnose, plan, intervene, and evaluate. Merely acquiring information or possessing a particular skill set is not enough to qualify as critical thinking. This chapter focuses on what critical thinking is, how it's measured, and what you can do to enhance critical thinking in yourself and others. Ms. Jeffries provides an example of how critical thinking is important in nursing.

LEADERSHIP IN ACTION

Ms. Jeffries, a nurse manager, has been evaluating her staff. She has noticed that some nurses use poor judgment and/or biased thinking when providing nursing care, especially when determining what treatments to provide or which actions to take. Several of the nursing staff seemed to go on intuition alone when making decisions; some are obviously new to nursing and have been asking for advice on what to do next.

LEADERSHIP CHALLENGE What critical-thinking situations deserve a nurse manager's immediate attention?

KEY TERM

Critical thinking is the process of actively conceptualizing, applying, analyzing, synthesizing, and/or evaluating information to guide action.

Nurses and Critical Thinking

Critical thinking is the process of actively conceptualizing, applying, analyzing, synthesizing, and/or evaluating information to guide action.

Why is critical thinking so important in nursing? Nurses must not rely on biased, distorted, partial, uninformed, or prejudicial thinking in their approach. In addition, noncritical thinking is costly and affects quality of life. When action is taken without using appropriate guiding information, mistakes are easily made, helpful measures are overlooked, and client wellness is at risk.

Scriven and Paul (2004) propose that a critical thinker:

- Raises vital questions and problems in a clear and precise manner
- Gathers relevant information and comes to well-reasoned conclusions and solutions by testing them against relevant criteria and standards
- Assesses assumptions, implications, and practical consequences
- Communicates effectively with others to figure out solutions to complex problems

Measures of Critical Thinking

Two instruments for measuring critical-thinking skills are available. They were selected by the task force at one northeastern university because of their wide acceptance and use as sound psychometric measures (Walsh & Seldomridge, 2006). They focus on the ability to infer, recognize assumptions, deduce, interpret, and evaluate arguments; as a result, they allow for comparison across settings. Both are relatively inexpensive, can be scored by hand, and take less than an hour to administer.

The first instrument is the Watson-Glaser Critical Thinking Appraisal Form S (Watson & Glaser, 1994.) This instrument was selected for its ability to evaluate critical-thinking dispositions, such as open-mindedness, truth seeking, systematicness, confidence, analyticity, inquisitiveness, and maturity. The other instrument is the California Critical Thinking Dispositions Inventory (Facione, 1992).

Several researchers have used one instrument or the other in their work. Walsh and Seldomridge (2006) found only modest critical-thinking gains in their population of learners as those learners progressed through years of nursing studies. This led the authors to question their definition of critical thinking ("knowing what to believe or do") and the usefulness of standardized measuring instruments.

Because their research findings were inconsistent, Walsh and Seldomridge (2006) concluded that it is time to rethink the usefulness of standardized measurements.

Insights about Critical Thinking

The research on critical thinking may provide some answers for nurse leaders who want to help their staff develop and use critical-thinking skills.

Oral questioning shows promise as a way to teach learners critical thinking, but it's only effective if higher-level questions that use verbs such as *compare*, *contrast*, *analyze*, and *evaluate* are posed (Sellappah, Hussey, Blackmore, & McMurray, 1998). **Logic client concept maps and models** use a visual format (such as boxes and arrows to show the relation between resources, inputs, activities, outputs, and outcomes or goals) to develop an account of an illness or health issue, using inductive and deductive thinking to examine alternative actions that nurses should take. A qualitative analysis of learner reactions to logic models provided evidence that learners found them helpful in making decisions about client care, predicting outcomes of their interventions, and thinking critically (Ellermann, Kataoka-Yahiro, & Wong, 2006).

Many methods can promote learners' critical thinking, including:

> **KEY TERM**
>
> **Logic client concept maps and models** use a visual format to develop an account of illness or health issue.

- Written or simulated case studies (Baumberger-Henry, 2005; Ellermann, Kataoka-Yahiro, & Wong, 2006; Reising, 2004; Tomey, 2003)
- Concept mapping (Akinsanya & Williams, 2004; Luckowski, 2003; Staib, 2003)
- Journal reading (Ibarreta & McLeod, 2004; Wagner & Ash, 1998)
- Role-play and simulations (Cote-Arsenault, 2004; Jeffries, 2005; Phillips, 2005)

Stages of Critical Thinking in Nursing Practice

Benner (1984) studied stages of clinical competence in nurses. She found that nurses moved from being a novice or beginner to being an expert. The five stages she identified are:

Stage 1: Novice. These are nurses who have no experience and use rules to help them perform. Critical thinking at this stage is minimal. Beginners at this stage follow the motto "Just tell me what I need to do, and I'll do it."

Stage 2: Advanced beginner. As nurses gather experience, they formulate principles to guide their actions.

Stage 3: Competent. Nurses at this stage need conscious, deliberate planning and analysis to achieve efficiency and organization.

Stage 4: Proficient. Proficient nurses can perceive a situation as a whole and its meaning in terms of long-term goals.

Stage 5: Expert. At this stage, nurses no longer need analytic principles or rules; they now have an intuitive grasp of each situation and zero in on the problem without wasting time on considering alternative diagnoses and solutions.

LEADERSHIP CHALLENGE Using Benner's stages of nursing, which stages of clinical competence are exemplified by Ms. Jeffries at the beginning of this chapter? Give a rationale for your answer.

KEY TERM

Problem solving provides a format for critical thinking.

Problem Solving and Critical Thinking

Critical thinking requires a format. **Problem solving** can provide that format. In nursing, problem solving occurs in the contexts of client care, team leadership, client advocacy, and case management. **Box 6-1** provides a problem-solving format that you can use to enhance critical thinking.

BOX 6-1   PROBLEM-SOLVING FORMAT

1. **Definition of the problem**
   a. What is the nature of the problem?
      Questions to elicit answers include:
      "Tell me what the problem is."
      "What is the problem as you see it?"
      "Correct me if I'm wrong, but
         what I hear you saying is
         _____."
   b. How severe is the problem?
      "What effect is the problem having on you?"
      "How is the problem making it difficult for
         you to do your work?"
      "How often does this problem occur?"
      "Let me see if I have understood what you
         said. You told me _____
         _____. Is that
         correct?"
   c. When does the problem occur?
      "How long has this problem been going on?"
      "When does the problem usually come up?"
      "What else is going on when the problem
         comes up?"
2. **Determinants of the problem**
      "What makes the problem worse?
      "What else is going on when the problem
         occurs?
      "What improves the problem?
      "What have you tried to do that reduces
         the problem?"
      "What do you think is causing the
         problem?"
      "What evidence or facts do you have to
         support the problem?"
      "What brings the problem on?"
      "What sorts of things are going on when
         the problem surfaces?"
      "What do your colleagues do to help when
         the problem occurs?"

"What do your colleagues do to improve
   the problem?"
"What do your colleagues do to worsen
   the problem?"
"What feelings are you having about the
   effects of the problem?"
"How is this problem affecting your
   motivation?"
"In what ways does this problem create
   stress for you?"
"On one hand, I hear you saying
   _____. On the other hand, I
   hear you saying _____.
   I wonder how these two things go
   together."

3. **Possible solutions**
   "What do you think should be done to
      improve the situation?"
   "Looking back, how could you have reacted
      differently to the problem?"
   "What is the best way to decide what to
      do?"
   "What would be a good backup decision?"
   "What could you or I do to improve the
      chances of being successful?"
   "What can I do to help with the problem?"
   "What other information do you need to
      help solve the problem?"
   "What support do you need to help solve
      this problem?"
   "Let's consider how we might find out
      more about the problem together."
   "We've covered a lot of ground. Is there
      anything I've said that was confusing
      or troubling?"

Source: Copyright, 2007, Carolyn Chambers Clark. Used with
permission from *Holistic Assertiveness Skills for Nurses.* New
York: Springer Publishing Company.

Creative Problem Solving

Creative problem solving involves identifying assumptions, using multiple techniques to approach a problem (including visualization, modeling, and using metaphors), and asking for criticism and suggestions (Harris, 2002).

Identifying Assumptions

A frequently overlooked step in problem solving is identifying assumptions that you make. An unidentified assumption can prevent you from developing a solution. Assumptions may be hidden or unidentified and still affect the problem-solving process. Some areas where assumptions may lie hidden include:

- *Time.* What assumptions are being made about how long the solution will take?
- *Money.* What assumptions are being made about the availability of money?
- *Cooperation.* What assumptions are being made about who will support the solution?
- *Law.* Can a law be changed or reinterpreted to permit the solution?
- *Energy.* What assumptions are being made about the amount of energy necessary to find a solution? Is it better to expend more energy now than later?
- *Information.* What assumptions are being made about the available information, and has it been triple-checked for accuracy?
- *Cultural binds.* How are attitudes about the culture interfering with thinking and limiting solutions? (Harris, 2002)

LEADERSHIP IN ACTION

Anna leads a nursing unit where clients and visitors complain that noise interferes with their sleep. Her problem is this: how can we reduce noise on this unit? Phrased this way, Anna realized certain solutions would be more likely, such as putting silencers or mufflers on the PA system and noisy monitors, soundproofing some rooms or hallways, installing sound-absorbing panels, and so forth. None of these seemed plausible, so Anna decided to check her assumptions and found that she was assuming that the unit really was noisy and that noise was interfering with sleep. From there, she decided to obtain information about the number of hours clients were sleeping on the unit to find out just how much of a problem noise was.

Techniques for Approaching a Problem

There are a number of techniques to approaching a problem, including examining the problem carefully, formulating the problem statement carefully, breaking the problem into small parts, choosing a different entry point, visualizing the problem, using models, trying metaphors, and using searching techniques. Explore a wide range of ideas and solutions to find the best fit for you and your problem (Harris, 2002).

Examine the Problem Carefully

You should examine the problem carefully before looking for a solution. Part of examining the problem is recognizing that something can always be done to solve it and that a problem is not a punishment. Denying a problem only perpetuates it.

   Make sure that the problem you think exists does exist. Once a problem has been identified, use the opportunity to demonstrate the power of leadership and to increase happiness in the workplace. Before jumping into action, take enough time to examine and explore the problem thoroughly. Understanding the problem often solves it (Harris, 2002).

Formulate the Problem Statement Carefully

You should formulate problem statements carefully and with the knowledge that the questions you ask will determine the range of choices and the answers that you will receive. Make sure that you are not approaching a problem with a preconceived solution and that you are focusing on the problem itself, not just on the symptoms of a problem or on a problem that someone else thinks exists (Harris, 2002).

Break the Problem into Small Parts

Problems can be solved more easily when they are broken into smaller parts or goals. Each subproblem or subgoal can then be solved.

Choose a Different Entry Point

Most people attack problems in a linear way at the front end, as Anna did, but you can start at the solution and work backward. This is especially useful when the goal is clear but the present situation is ambiguous (Harris, 2002).

LEADERSHIP IN ACTION

Todd hadn't been able to improve relationships with his supervisees by asking them what was wrong or by trying to figure out what was going wrong between them. As soon as he gave up trying to understand the problem and envisioned how he wanted the relationships to change, he worked backward to find the problem that had been hampering him. He wrote himself a note to remember that whenever the goal is clearer than the problem, he should start at the solution and work backward.

   Entry points could just as well be in the middle. For example:

LEADERSHIP IN ACTION

Rebecca was in charge of planning a new nursing center. The task was overwhelming, and the deadline for ideas seemed so close. She decided to attack the middle of the problem, pretending as if the funding and planning had already been done, and to begin with the construction and design phase. From there, she moved in both directions, working backward toward planning where the unit would attach to the current building and how to get funding, and forward toward arranging for clients to move into the center. Split that way, she felt less pressured, and the project moved along to completion.

LEADERSHIP CHALLENGE **What kind of note should Rebecca make to herself about when to start a solution in the middle instead of at the beginning? Give a rationale for your answer.**

Visualize the Problem

Before attempting a solution or taking action, it may be helpful to practice or picture the solution mentally. Once you can visualize the problem and its solution, it will be easier to solve. Imaging being someone else who is involved in either the solution or the problem may also be helpful (Harris, 2002).

LEADERSHIP IN ACTION

Cara was having difficulty with one staff nurse who argued with her about everything. When Cara imagined herself as the staff nurse, she began to get some insight into what made the staff nurse act that way, what might improve their relationship, and what the nuances of the staff nurse's personality were.

Another way is to use visualization to imagine being an expert or mentor who can solve the problem with special knowledge.

KEY TERM

A **model** is a simplified, concrete, visual, or symbolic representation of reality.

Use Models

A **model** is a representation or pattern of an idea or problem. Models can make an idea more concrete, especially when they use a picture or symbol. A drawing can simplify and show a relationship or connection more quickly than words alone.

Models serve several purposes, including to:

- *Make an idea concrete.* A picture, drawing, symbol, map, box, or circle can show relationships, connections, hierarchy, and more in a dramatic way that enhances understanding by converting an idea into something that stimulates the senses.

- *Reveal relationships between ideas.* Models can have profound effects on perception and conceptualization. They can help viewers think about the relationships between parts and the associated possibilities. Multiple models allow viewers to think about the same concept in different ways without the controlling influences that a single model might present.
- *Simplify the complex.* All models make complex concepts manageable or understandable. When using models, it is important not to eliminate important aspects of a prime concept. (Harris, 2002)

Several types of models exist. **Conceptual models** concretize an idea and aid memory. **Structural models** concretize physical structures, such as nursing centers or nursing units.

A model is created before all large construction projects. Models can be visual (a door, a machine, a bathroom); physical (a blueprint for a nursing unit); or mathematical (a decision matrix can help a nurse leader decide whom among many applicants to hire).

There are many paradigms to use when creating models:

- *System model.* A **system model** is a collection of interacting elements that work together to accomplish a specific goal.

  Example: Improving relationships on a clinical unit
  Input: Words, actions
  Processing: Reactions
  Output: Mutual support/dissatisfaction
  Feedback: Communication through words and actions
  Control: Processing is changed to positive reactions, actions, and output
- *Design model.* A **design model** is used to plan an overall pattern.
- *Construction model.* A **construction model** emphasizes the parts in a sequential manner. It can be used for a year-end report, for ordering information, or for building a clinical unit.
- *Recipe model.* The **recipe model** emphasizes proportions and ingredients. Spice or flavor can be added to a recipe. Toolkits can be used, along with formulas for success. (Harris, 2002)

KEY TERM

Conceptual models concretize an idea and aid memory.

KEY TERM

Structural models concretize physical structures.

KEY TERM

A **system model** is a collection of interacting elements that work together to accomplish a specific goal.

KEY TERM

A **design model** can be used to plan an overall pattern.

KEY TERM

A **construction model** emphasizes the parts in a sequential manner.

KEY TERM

A **recipe model** emphasizes proportions and ingredients.

Try Metaphors to Solve Problems

When using a model to solve problems, it is often helpful to incorporate metaphors. For example, ask yourself:

- How is this problem or its solution like a garden? Clue: Consider words like *vegetative*, *growing*, *expansive*, and *infested*.
- How is this problem or its solution like a machine? Clue: Consider concepts like energy input, the driving force, work output, and how the parts work together.
- How is this problem or its solution like a symphony? Clue: Consider factors like the conductor, soloists, the type of music, harmony, and the orchestration of various parts.
- How is this problem or its solution like the human body? Clue: Consider the functions of hands, feet, mouth, eyes, and ears.
- How is the problem or its solution like a vehicle? Clue: Consider the kind of vehicle, what powers it, its passengers, where it's going, and what propels it.

Use Searching Approaches

Searching techniques can help with problem solving and decision making. Some common searching techniques are:

KEY TERM

A systematic **trial-and-error method** includes searching for a solution with a plan in mind and keeping a record of attempts and failures.

KEY TERM

Algorithmic methods use computer programs and math formulas such as the maze and split-half method.

KEY TERM

A **public solution** helps workers take responsibility for others' problems and fosters problem-solving and decision-making skills by posting the problem and asking for suggestions.

- *Trial-and-error method.* Make this method more efficient by keeping a record of attempts and failures so that ineffective solutions are discarded and not retried.
- *Algorithmic methods.* Algorithms use computer programs and math formulas. A maze algorithm follows a maze or intricate passageway. The split-half method involves going to the halfway point and seeing whether the problem appears there (e.g., somewhere in the process of feeding clients, they aren't being fed; where is the problem occurring?). This method can be used with many leadership situations, including bathing clients, completing intake interviews, and transmitting data from staff to the nurse leader (and vice versa).
- *Public solution.* Post the problem on a bulletin board, in a newsletter, in an e-mail, or in a memo. This can work well with employee absenteeism or dissatisfaction, budgets, and reward systems. This kind of approach develops interest and discussion about the problem, helps workers take responsibility for others' problems, and fosters problem-solving and decision-making skills in all members of the work group. Be aware that people will work to implement their own ideas and solutions more energetically than they will work to implement yours (Harris, 2002).

Asking for Criticism and Suggestions

It is always wise to accept criticism and suggestions when problem solving. Nurse leaders must be careful not to get so involved in an idea that they are unwilling to alter it once they discover a better way of viewing the problem or the solution. Other people—even those not knowledgeable on the subject—including children who are especially open to giving honest feedback—can provide valuable insights. Suggested ways to frame a request for feedback include:

- I'm asking you to help me improve on my idea to _____ _____. Can you give me some feedback on it?
- I'm working on the problem of _____. Do you have any ideas about a solution? Take a look at what I've come up with so far, and tell me your reactions. Can you think of anything I'm missing? Is there anything wrong with this? Is there anything you can improve on?

Group Decision Making

Group decision making is a key component to the functioning of an organization. Whenever a decision could impact employees, it is helpful to involve them in making that decision (Burke, 1994; Sandifer, 2005; Winch, 1995).

Learning about Group Decision Making

Decision making and problem solving are often the same process in groups. The best way to learn about the decision-making process is to sit in on a task group that is going to make a decision or to lead a group and help its members come to a decision. If you're leading a group, your role may include:

- *Initiating.* Keep the group moving by suggesting an action step ("Let's poll the group"); pointing out a goal ("As I remember, our goal is to make this decision today"); proposing a procedure ("Let's role-play to see whether that helps us"); or identifying potential obstacles ("I'm wondering whether pushing too hard to come to consensus has become an obstacle for us").
- *Regulating.* Summarize what's happened so far ("So far, we've listed some alternative solutions"); point out time limits ("We have 10 minutes left today"); and restate the agreed-upon goals ("We agreed to set priorities in the next 15 minutes").
- *Informing.* Bring information or opinions to the group ("I brought these summaries of possible solutions based on what we discussed last time").
- *Supporting.* Create an emotional climate that makes it easy for group members to get along, stay calm, and voice their feelings ("Let's try a relaxation exercise to keep us calm" and "It's OK to share your feelings").

- *Evaluating.* Help the group evaluate its decisions by noting a group process that either helps or hinders decision making and by testing for a consensus ("I'm wondering if polling the group so soon has prevented us from considering alternatives" and "Are we ready to test for a consensus?"). (Clark, 2003)

Using the Six Hats Method

KEY TERM

Lateral thinking uses a set of systematic techniques, not just one, to change concepts and perceptions and to generate new ones.

Six Hats is a structured process for introducing lateral thinking into problem solving, especially group problem solving. **Lateral thinking** is a set of systematic techniques used to change concepts and perceptions and to generate new ones. Lateral thinking allows the user to explore multiple possibilities and approaches instead of pursuing only one.

Each hat in the Six Hats method represents a different perspective or way of thinking. Participants can put on or take off these metaphorical hats to indicate the kind of thinking they are using. Sometimes, groups are asked to put on the different hats in a particular sequence to facilitate the problem-solving process. According to de Bono (1995), the hats are:

- *The white hat.* When group members put on the white hat, they ignore arguments and proposals. They examine facts, figures, and information and identify needed information and how it can be obtained.
- *The red hat.* This hat means that it is time to focus on feelings, hunches, and intuition. The red hat gives the wearer permission to share his or her feelings without explaining them, justifying them, or apologizing for them.
- *The black hat.* This is the hat of caution and critical judgment, and it is the one most often used, even though it can kill creative ideas with its negativity and it makes references to rules, policies, and procedures, which can make progress impossible.
- *The yellow hat.* This hat signifies optimism and a positive view of the situation. When wearing the yellow hat, a person observes how something can be accomplished and the benefit of a particular solution.
- *The green hat.* Creative thinking, new ideas, and additional alternatives are associated with the green hat. When a group wears the green hat, creative effort is encouraged, and people have permission to ask, "Could we do this in a different way, or could there be another explanation?"
- *The blue hat.* The last hat helps set the agenda for thinking, suggests the next step for thinking, and asks for conclusions, decisions, and summaries.

The Six Hats technique is a cooperative technique to get a group back on track when participants get bogged down in arguments or take positions and defend them to death. The Six Hats method challenges participants to see all sides of a problem or decision (de Bono, 1995).

Dilemmas Related to Enhancing Critical Thinking

Because critical thinking has not been adequately defined to date, it may be wise for nurse leaders to decide which kinds of critical thinking to promote and then define and operationalize them for various learner levels. For example:

- **Problem solving** allows the transfer of theory into practice
- **Decision making** anticipates potential problems
- **Diagnostic reasoning** helps settle on a client's condition by ruling out improbable conclusions or diagnoses (Walsh & Seldomridge, 2006)

KEY TERM

Problem solving provides a format for critical thinking.

KEY TERM

Decision making anticipates potential problems.

LEADERSHIP CHALLENGE Decide on one kind of critical thinking, and suggest ways to operationalize a program for that aspect.

KEY TERM

Diagnostic reasoning helps settle on a client's condition by ruling out improbable conclusions.

Summary

This chapter presented information on critical thinking, including measures of critical thinking, insights gained about critical thinking, stages of critical thinking in nursing practice, problem solving in critical thinking, creative problem solving, group decision making. and suggested ways to operationalize a critical thinking skills program.

Key Term Review

- **Algorithmic methods** use computer programs and math formulas such as the maze and split-half method.
- **Conceptual models** concretize an idea and aid memory.
- **Construction models** emphasize the parts in a sequential manner and can be used for a year-end report, for ordering information, or for building a clinical unit.
- **Creative problem solving** involves identifying assumptions, using multiple techniques to approach a problem (including visualization, modeling, and using metaphors), and asking for criticism and suggestions.
- **Critical thinking** is the process of actively conceptualizing, applying, analyzing, synthesizing, and/or evaluating information to guide action.
- **Decision making** anticipates potential problems.
- **Design models** are used to plan an overall pattern; if harmony is the goal, all the components of achieving a harmonious whole are presented.
- **Diagnostic reasoning** helps settle on a client's condition by ruling out improbable conclusions.
- **Lateral thinking** uses a set of systematic techniques, not just one technique, to change concepts and perceptions and to generate new ones.
- **Logic client concept maps and models** use a visual format to develop an account of illness or health issue.
- A **model** is a simplified, concrete, visual, or symbolic representation of reality.
- **Problem solving** provides a format for critical thinking.
- A **public solution** helps workers take responsibility for others' problems and fosters problem-solving and decision-making skills by posting the problem and asking for suggestions.
- **Recipe models** emphasize proportions and ingredients; spice or flavor can be added to give a recipe a twist; toolkits can be used, along with formulas for success.
- **Structural models** concretize physical structures.
- **System models** portray a collection of interacting elements that work together to accomplish a specific goal.
- A **systematic trial-and-error method** includes searching for a solution with a plan in mind and keeping a record of attempts and failures.

Leadership Development Exercises

Leadership Development Exercise 6-1

Develop three high-level critical-thinking questions, using verbs such as *compare*, *contrast*, *analyze*, and/or *evaluate*. Share them with at least three colleagues, and obtain feedback.

■ **Leadership Development Exercise 6-2**

Pick a problem that needs to be solved. Identify any assumptions that could prevent a solution. (See the "Identifying Assumptions" section in this chapter for ideas, p. 118.)

■ **Leadership Development Exercise 6-3**

Construct a design or system model.

■ **Leadership Development Exercise 6-4**

Construct a structural or recipe model.

Advanced Leadership Development Exercises

■ **Leadership Development Exercise 6-5**

Sit in on a task group (or join with your classmates who agree to portray a task group), and use the decision steps that follow to chart the group's process to making a decision.

Steps in the Decision	**Examples**
a. Stating the problem/decision	
b. Clarifying and elaborating	
c. Developing alternative solutions	
d. Keeping the discussion relevant	
e. Testing the group's commitment to the emerging decision	
f. Summarizing	
g. Agreeing to the decision	
h. Testing the consequences of solutions	

■ **Leadership Development Exercise 6-6**

Use the Six Hats method to enhance group decision making. Choose a common nursing leadership situation from the following list or develop your own and use the Six Hats method to solve the problem or keep the group from getting bogged down in argument.

- ■ Staffing
- ■ Role transition
- ■ Conflict management

■ **Leadership Development Exercise 6-7**

Teach critical thinking techniques to a group of nursing students or staff members.

■ **Leadership Development Exercise 6-8**

Develop a research problem statement for some aspect of critical thinking. Obtain critiques from at least two nurses with advanced research skills.

■ **Leadership Development Exercise 6-9**

Develop a research design to test one problem statement. Obtain feedback from at least two nurses with advanced research skills.

References

Akinsanya, C., & Williams, M. (2004). Concept mapping for meaningful learning. *Nurse Education Today, 24*(1), 41–46.

Baumberger-Henry, M. (2005). Cooperative learning and case study: Does the combination improve learners' perception of problem-solving and decision making skills? *Nurse Education Today, 25,* 238–246.

Benner, P. (1984). *From novice to expert: Excellence and power in clinical nursing practice.* Menlo Park, CA: Addison Wesley.

Burke, W. W. (1994). Diagnostic models for organizational development. In A. Howard, *Diagnosis for organizational change: Methods and models* (pp. 53–84). New York: Guilford Press.

Clark, C. C. (2003). *Group leadership skills* (4th ed.). New York: Springer.

Cote-Arsenault, D. (2004). Planning for a new baby: A creative approach to learning, *Nurse Educator, 29*(1), 6–9.

de Bono, E. (1995). Serious creativity. *Journal for Quality and Participation, 18*(5), 12–18.

Ellermann, C. R., Kataoka-Yahiro, M. R., & Wong, L. C. (2006). Logic models used to enhance critical thinking. *Journal of Nursing Education, 45*(6), 220–227.

Facione, P. A. (1992). *The California critical thinking dispositions inventory* (2nd ed.). [Test manual.] Millbrae, CA: California Academic Press.

Harris, R. A. (2002). *Creative problem solving: A step-by-step approach.* Los Angeles: Pyrczak.

Ibarreta, G. I., & McLeod, L. (2004). Thinking aloud on paper: An experience in journal writing. *Journal of Nursing Education, 43,* 134–137.

Jeffries, P. (2005). A framework for designing, implementing, and evaluating: Simulations used as teaching strategies in nursing. *Nursing Education Perspectives, 26*, 96–103.

Luckowski, A. (2003). Concept mapping as a critical thinking tool for nurse educators. *Journal for Nurses in Staff Development, 19*, 225–230.

Phillips, J. M. (2005). Chat role play as an online learning strategy. *Journal of Nursing Education, 44, 43*.

Reising, D. L. (2004). The outcome-present state-testing model applied to classroom settings. *Journal of Nursing Education, 43*, 431–432.

Sandifer, L. (2005). *Group decisionmaking with the organization*. Retrieved March 25, 2007, from http://www.worldteams.unt.edu/listerature/paper-rlahti.html

Scriven, M., & Paul, R. (2004). *Defining critical thinking*. Retrieved September 14, 2006, from http://www.criticalthinking.org/aboutCT/definingCR.shtml

Sellappah, S., Hussey, T., Blackmore, A. M., & McMurray, A. (1998). The use of questioning strategies by clinical teachers. *Journal of Advanced Nursing, 28*, 142–144.

Staib, S. (2003). Teaching and measuring critical thinking. *Journal of Nursing Education, 42*, 498–508.

Tomey, A. M. (2003). Learning with cases. *Journal of Continuing Education in Nursing, 34*(1), 34–38.

Wagner, P. S., & Ash, K. L. (1998). Creating the teachable moment. *Journal of Nursing Education, 27*, 278–280.

Walsh, C. M., & Seldomridge, L. A. (2006). Critical thinking: Back to square two. *Journal of Nursing Education, 45*(6), 212–218.

Watson, G. B., & Glaser, E. M. (1994). *Watson-Glaser critical thinking appraisal form S manual*. San Antonio, TX: Harcourt Brace.

Winch, G. W. (1995). Developing consensus: Reflections on a model-supported decision process. *Management Decision, 33*(6), 22–31.

Communicating Effectively

CHAPTER OBJECTIVES

After reading this chapter, answering the leadership challenges, and participating in the leadership development exercises, you will be able to:

- List ingredients of effective interpersonal communication
- Identify ways to use emotional intelligence to communicate with others
- Discuss three ways to enhance support during nurses' intershift reports
- Describe strategies that are effective for communicating with various generations in the workforce
- Identify ways to enhance collaborative communication with physicians
- Describe group communication methods

Advanced nurses will be able to:

- Develop a problem statement to study aspects of leader communication
- Teach communication skills to novice leaders
- Complete a small research project related to leader communication

Introduction

Clear communication is crucial to being an effective nurse leader. Both verbal and nonverbal aspects of communication are important. This chapter explores theories that can help you communicate effectively with individuals and groups, including social cognitive theory, language expectancy theory, contagion theory, and cognitive dissonance theory. Interventions that show promise include emotional intelligence, assertiveness, and positive feedback. But first read about Hilda T.'s communication dilemma.

LEADERSHIP IN ACTION

Hilda T., a nurse leader, wanted to open up communication on her unit. Physicians were grumpy and disrespectful to nurses, who, in turn, were indirectly hostile (passive-aggressive). When Hilda observed nursing shift reports, she noted little supportive communication from the head nurse to staff nurses. When she thought about the staff, she realized that they spanned at least four generations of workers. Hilda also noticed that staff from different cultural or ethnic groups sometimes didn't get along. When she asked staff members what she could do to help, she got little information.

LEADERSHIP CHALLENGE   **What would you suggest Hilda do to improve communication on her unit?**

KEY TERM

An **effective communication** is easily understood and accepted.

The Importance of Communication

Humans are social creatures. We require information and feedback to feel good about ourselves. **Effective communication** is a message that is easily understood and accepted.

Communication has been cited as a critical skill for all aspects of nursing (Hays, 2002). Without clear and effective communication, employees feel isolated and dissatisfied. Effective interpersonal relationships are part of being a competent nurse leader (Nurse Leadership Institute, 2002).

KEY TERM

Human communication is **multimodal**, which means that more than one piece of information is interpreted to convey meaning, and includes verbal and nonverbal aspects.

Types of Human Communication

Human communication is **multimodal**, which means that more than one piece of information is interpreted to convey meaning (Baber & Mellor, 2001). Verbal communication is only one aspect of total communication. Nonverbal communication provides the major message. Often, people react to unspoken **elements of communication** more than they do to words, so it is important for you to know just what you are conveying.

Misunderstandings can often be clarified when the people involved observe and comment on nonverbal communication (Blatner, 2002).

Blatner (2002) developed one system of classification that includes 13 categories of nonverbal communication:

1. *Personal space* includes the comfortable or uncomfortable distance between people. People from parts of Latin America or the Middle East may prefer standing closer to each other than persons of northern European descent. Different distances are appropriate for coworkers, friends, people dining at a restaurant, and people in intimate relationships.

2. *Eye contact* includes glancing, gazing, staring, or not looking at another person. Limiting eye contact can lessen the discomfort of close personal space in elevators and other tight spaces. Modern management and business culture values a fair degree of eye contact; looking away may be interpreted as avoidance or deviance, but some cultures raise their children to minimize eye contact with authority figures for fear of appearing uppity or arrogant. Others may misinterpret this respectful looking away as passive aggressiveness.

3. *Position* includes sitting, standing behind, facing, being in front of, or standing opposite.

4. *Posture* includes slouching, stiffening, slumping, twisting, cringing, towering, crouching, angling, tilting the pelvis down and forward (swagger), or tilting the buttocks to the rear (mincing steps).

5. *Paralanguage* includes vocal inflection, such as rising, falling, rapid, slow, measured, changing, choppy, loud, soft, breathy, nasal, operatic, growling, wheedling, whining, high, medium, low, meaningful pauses, disorganized pauses, shy pauses, or hesitant pauses.

6. *Facial expression* includes using the face to express being pensive, amused, sad, barely tolerant, cautious, angry, pouting, anxious, sexually attracted, startled, confused, sleepy, or intoxicated.

7. *Gesture* includes clenching a fist, shaking a finger, pointing, biting fingernails, tugging at hair, squirming, rubbing chin, smoothing hair, folding arms, raising eyebrows, pursing lips, narrowing eyes, scratching head, looking away, hands on hips, hands behind head, rubbing nose, rocking, sticking out tongue, tugging earlobe, and waving.

8. *Touch* includes gentle, firm, hurrying, coercive, overly friendly, and respectful touches, as well as gripping a hand in a permission-giving way,

holding onto the arm or upper back, pushing, tugging, patting, rubbing, and grabbing.

9. *Locomotion* includes styles of moving, such as strolling, shuffling, hurrying, running, jogging, springing, tiptoeing, marching, crawling, tottering, walking, and swinging.

10. *Pacing* refers to how action is taken—for example, jerky, pressured, gradual, graceful, nervous, tense, easy, fatigued, deliberate, clumsy, shaky, or deliberate.

11. *Latency of response* refers to the time it takes to react to questions or interact in conversations.

12. *Context* refers to the amount and source of light, color of lighting, props, size of the room, colors of the walls and furniture, seating arrangement, number of people present, sounds, smells, temperature of the room, and people's proximity to each other.

13. *Physiological response* refers to signs of emotion—for example, flaring nostrils, trembling chin, sweating, cold or clammy skin, flushing, moisture in eyes, blushing, swallowing, blinking, breathing heavily, and blanching.

LEADERSHIP CHALLENGE How could Hilda use Blatner's categories to help examine communication on her unit?

Communication Theories

There are many communication theories. Some of these theories that are more relevant to nursing are discussed here, including social cognitive, language expectancy, contagion, and cognitive dissonance.

Social Cognitive Theory

KEY TERM

Social cognitive theory posits that if people are to perform a behavior, it is important to communicate what the behavior is and how to achieve it, to support the behavior, to model or observe the behavior, and to build confidence that the behavior will appear.

Social cognitive theory is relevant to health communication because it deals with the cognitive, emotional, and behavioral aspects of change. This theory, developed by Bandura (2001), explains how people acquire and maintain a certain behavioral pattern, which includes communication with others.

Concepts of social cognitive theory, including the following, can be applied to nursing leadership:

- *Behavioral capability.* If a person is to perform a behavior, it is important to communicate what the behavior is and how to achieve it. If nurse leaders expect staff to perform professionally, they must communicate the necessary behaviors clearly and explain how those behaviors can be achieved.

- *Expectations.* By anticipating and modeling positive outcomes of a behavior, success is more likely. Nurse leaders should suggest to staff that they will have a positive outcome, and then nurse leaders should model the behavior.
- *Observational learning.* Behavioral acquisition occurs by watching people's actions and observing the reinforcements they receive for performing the behavior. Nurse leaders can ask staff members to observe skilled staff members who perform the required task and then are rewarded with verbal praise or by some other mechanism.
- *Self-efficacy.* The more confidence people have in performing a particular behavior, the more successful they will be. Nurse leaders enhance staff self-confidence by rewarding and praising their successes.
- *Expectancies.* The greater value a person places on a given outcome, the more likely that outcome will occur. When nurse leaders verbalize the value of a given behavior, it encourages staff to produce the behavior.

LEADERSHIP CHALLENGE How could Hilda use social cognitive theory with her staff?

Language Expectancy Theory

Language expectancy theory is a formalized model about message strategies and attitude and behavior change. The theory, developed by Burgoon and Burgoon (2001), holds that language is a rule-governed system and that people develop expectations about the message strategies that others employ in their attempts to persuade. These expectations are a function of cultural and social norms and preferences.

> **KEY TERM**
>
> **Language expectancy theory** holds that language is a rule-governed system and that people develop expectations about message strategies that others employ in their attempts to persuade. It explains how speakers vary language intensity to make their messages more persuasive.

Buller et al. (2000) tested this theory by carefully adjusting features of a message about safety. The researchers knew that people do not always comply with prevention advice, and they predicted that messages with high language intensity and a deductive argument style would improve compliance with prevention recommendations. They presented newsletters, brochures, and tip cards that varied in language intensity and style of logic. These researches found that by carefully adjusting messages, they received a more favorable response—especially when advice was aimed at expectations about reducing personal risk. They found that people who received messages with high-intensity language were more apt to comply with safety recommendations.

LEADERSHIP CHALLENGE How could Hilda use language expectancy theory with her staff?

KEY TERM

Contagion theories explain how networks of people spread "infectious" attitudes and behavior.

KEY TERM

Contagion by cohesion refers to the influence of those with a tendency toward direct communication on those with a tendency toward indirect communication.

KEY TERM

Contagion by structural equivalence refers to the mutual influence of those who have similar communication patterns.

KEY TERM

Cognitive dissonance theory holds that when individuals are presented with information that is inconsistent with their beliefs, they will strive to reachieve balance.

Contagion Theories

Contagion theories seek to explain how networks of people spread "infectious" attitudes and behavior. **Contagion by cohesion** refers to the influence of those with a tendency toward direct communication on those with a tendency toward indirect communication. **Contagion by structural equivalence** refers to the mutual influence of those who have similar communication patterns (Contractor & Eisenberg, 1990).

Rice and Aydin (1991) tested contagion theory and found that hospital employees who communicated with one another or who had supervisory-subordinate relationships were more apt to share similar attitudes about recently introduced information technology (contagion by cohesion). Burkhardt (1994) examined individual attitudes about a recently implemented distributed data-processing computer network and found that they were significantly influenced by the attitudes and use of others in their communication network (contagion by structural equivalence).

Cognitive Dissonance Theory

In 1957 Leon Festinger synthesized a set of studies and distilled his **cognitive dissonance theory,** which examined the social influences of communication. *Cognitive* means the theory has to do with thinking, and *dissonance* indicates an inconsistency or conflict. Cognitive dissonance is the uncomfortable feeling that results when someone holds two or more incompatible beliefs at the same time. The theory views individuals as purposeful decision makers who strive to balance their beliefs. When presented with decisions or information that creates dissonance, they try to regain equilibrium, especially if the dissonance affects their self-esteem. Dissonance can be reduced by altering behavior or seeking information that is consonant with behavior. This theory is especially relevant when you make a decision or solve a problem. By presenting new or challenging information, you can create dissonance and, thus, an effort to regain equilibrium, solve problems, or make decisions.

LEADERSHIP CHALLENGE How can Hilda use cognitive dissonance theory with her staff?

GUIDED LEADERSHIP TIP

WAYS TO FIND OUT WHAT STAFF THINK

Finding out what staff think may not be easy. They may fear being fired or labeled as "trouble-makers" if they share information. It you want to obtain information, you may have to ask for feedback numerous times in groups and in one-to-one meetings.

It is important to inform staff why information is needed (e.g., "I need to be tapped into what is going on here to do my job well"). Once staff begin to share information, it's important to listen and interrupt only to clarify. Employees' suggestions should always be met with encouraging words (e.g., "That's helpful," "That's important to know," or "I understand"). Avoid using comments such as "That's interesting," which can be interpreted as though you don't really care or understand their suggestion.

Whistle-blowers who uncover the source of problems should be promptly rewarded. The reward can be made publicly (if that is appropriate) or with a personal handwritten note of thanks (Tanouye, 1990).

Providing staff with a survey and asking for feedback on unit problems can also work if answers are anonymous. Being visibly present on the unit and talking to staff can also elicit useful information. When staff bring up a problem, ask that they discuss the worst-case scenarios, potential pitfalls, and alternative actions. This will help them learn problem-solving skills, help them own the problem, and help them grow (Tanouye, 1990).

Effective One-on-One Communication

The Nursing Leadership Institute (2002) identified the following competencies for interpersonal effectiveness:

- Listens attentively to others' ideas and concerns
- Invites contact and is approachable
- Treats employees with respect
- Develops collaborative relationships within the organization
- Builds and sustains positive relations in the organization
- Shares information readily with staff
- Recognizes and uses the staff's ideas
- Articulates ideas effectively both verbally and in writing
- Succinctly communicates viewpoints
- Involves staff in building consensus on issues
- Models health communication and promotes cooperative behaviors

Effective nurse leaders use persuasive communication. They impart inspiration and vision to others in an exciting and motivating way (Stordahl, 1995).

LEADERSHIP CHALLENGE How could Hilda begin to share her vision with staff in an exciting and motivating way?

Emotional Intelligence

Rager (1998) underscored the importance of setting a positive tone in the work setting. Developing a high degree of emotional intelligence may be the most important ingredient in effective leadership, more important than having an MBA, an advanced nursing degree, or even vast leadership experience. Managing emotions and relating to others in a positive way can have the most influential results (Weisinger, 1998). **Box 7-1** lists characteristics of leaders with high emotional intelligence.

Weisinger (1998) offers advice for leaders and staff members about using and developing their emotional intelligence:

- Listen to and thank others for positive criticism: it is a vote of confidence that can lead to success. "Thank you for your critique. I'm going to think hard about what you said."
- Carry around an image of an inspiring person, and use it to picture how to handle a particular situation.
- Trust your feelings and behavior.
- Use constructive inner dialogue as a guideline. "I can handle this. I'm already handling it."
- Learn to manage fear and anger by saying or thinking positive coping messages, such as "I can stay calm so I can listen and help this person" and "I refuse to let this person upset me."

BOX 7-1   QUALITIES OF LEADERS WITH DEVELOPED EMOTIONAL INTELLIGENCE

Emotional intelligence includes the ability to:
- Perceive and identify emotions in others' faces, tone of voice, and body language and the ability to name one's own feelings, discuss emotions, and communicate clearly and directly
- Analyze, reason, solve problems, make decisions, and guide what is important to think about

- Understand how emotions, thoughts, and behavior affect each other and how feelings can lead to behavior
- Take responsibility for one's own emotions and happiness, to turn negative emotions into positive learning and growing opportunities, and to help others identify and benefit from their emotions

Source: Adapted from Steve Hein. (2005). *Emotional intelligence.* Retrieved April 15, 2007, from http://eqi.org

- Appreciate differing viewpoints by telling others, "I appreciate your viewpoint; let's see if we can come to a consensus on this."
- Avoid mind reading; check out intuitions or conclusions by asking for verification. "I heard you say _____; is this what you meant?"
- Keep things in perspective; don't overplay the significance of one bad encounter.
- Remember that emotions are contagious, so use positive messages. "We were in a difficult situation; we got through it, and I'm positive we can learn from it."
- Tune in to the emotional context within which words occur, and read between the lines. Always phrase findings as hunches, not verified facts. "I'm wondering whether you're feeling angry about the changes. Are you?"
- Remember past emotional experiences, and use them to be empathic with others.
- Invite disagreement; it will lead to learning on both sides. Make comments like "Let's hear some opposing viewpoints; we need to get everyone's ideas."

Bobulski (2002) added the following suggestion:

- Focus on the circumstances and how they can change, not on the negative characteristics of the person or situation; this will take the heat and emotion of the situation and transform it into a learning opportunity. "Let's look at the situation and what we can learn from it."

LEADERSHIP CHALLENGE Apply Weisinger's and Bobulski's principles to the situation that follows. Choose a response, and give a rationale for your choice.

Situation: A team member has handled a client situation poorly. Your supervisor has said that such behavior is bad for the hospital and that it is up to the nurse leader to handle the situation.

Response 1: "What you did was irresponsible and cannot be tolerated. I will be writing up an incident report about the matter."

Response 2: "Good afternoon. May I speak to you alone, Mr. Justin? (Move the conversation to a private area.) "I noticed you spoke with Mrs. Emerson this morning and it didn't turn out well. Let's take a look at what happened and see if we can come up with an alternate way to deal with the situation."

Assertive Communication

Assertive talk—such as communicating clearly with staff, allowing them to be autonomous, and supporting group cohesion—can increase job satisfaction. By seeking out and valuing contributions from staff, you can promote a climate in which information is shared, decisions at the staff nurse level are supported, and the coordination of work helps retain staff and decrease job stress (Boyle, Bott, Hanse, Woods, & Taunton, 1999).

Clear and open communication is a crucial skill for leaders to model and support. If nurse leaders cannot confront verbally abusive physicians or clients, how will staff members learn? Although all nurses receive some education in communication skills, only psychiatric/mental health nurses tend to master this aspect of their work, and even they may not zero in on assertive skills.

Box 7-2 provides ideas for being assertive in planned meetings.

Even nurse leaders who believe that they possess good communication skills could benefit from attending assertiveness workshops. By demonstrating their willingness to learn new skills, such leaders are more likely to convince staff members that it is not only safe but also useful to attend an assertiveness workshop.

Enhancing Supportive Communication during Shift Reports

The majority of a nurse leader's time is spent communicating with other nursing personnel. Staff interaction is key to nursing outcomes, satisfaction levels, and retention (Hays, 2002).

Curtin and Flaherty (1982) have called for nurses to improve their relationship with one another and suggested that educators need to teach nurses how to give and receive criticism, support, direction, and guidance.

Supportive behaviors are believed to result when two persons verbally and nonverbally influence each other to ease doubt and anxiety about themselves, the situation, and their relationship, leading to an increased sense of personal control over an otherwise unpredictable and confusing situation (Albrecht & Adelman, 1987). Supportive behaviors also occur when leaders listen and reassure, and reframe and redefine, situations (Albrecht & Halsey, 1991; Peterson, Halsey, Albrecht, & McGough, 1995).

This kind of supportive behavior can even occur during shift reports, which are an important and recurrent example of leader-follower communication (Hays, 2002). Although Wolf's (1998) 12-month study of a hospital unit found that shift reports served as a forum where "negative criticism prevailed, not praise for work well done," interaction during shift reports can affect staff retention and quality of client care because of the intensity of the exchange of information and the potential for reducing anxiety and increasing confidence (Hays, 2002).

Using Hersey and Blanchard's situational leadership theory (see Chapter 1) as the guiding framework for a repeated-measures single-case study, Hays (2002) set out to videotape 16 nurse leader-follower dyads (i.e., the off-going shift RN nurse leader and the oncoming RN) during shift reports in a hospital setting.

BOX 7-2   HOW TO BE ASSERTIVE IN PLANNED MEETINGS

- **Set up an appointment well in advance whenever possible, and prime the other person.** For the purpose of an upcoming interview or meeting, speak to the person, or send a memo or e-mail, stating the objective for the meeting and any requests (like that the appointment not be interrupted). A written reminder is preferable because it stands as a permanent record of the purpose of the meeting.
- **Role-play upcoming anxiety-provoking situations with a friend or colleague.** Anticipate intimidating or unclear comments, and practice responding to them before the actual meeting or interview.
- **Write down important points or statements on an index card, and bring it with you to the meeting.** If necessary, read them aloud to the other person, saying something like "I've written this down because it's very important, and I don't want to forget anything." Reading your points aloud is preferable to stumbling or forgetting to stay on the topic.
- **When the meeting begins, structure the discussion environment for clear and open communication.** Move chairs to face one another (without desks in between), use direct eye contact, and stick to the topic.
- **Restate the purpose of the meeting.** For example, say, "I'm here to clarify . . ." or "I want to talk with you about . . ." or "I'd like us to work together to solve the problem of . . ."
- **Avoid getting sidetracked by irrelevant issues.** Keep the discussion on the identified issues with such comments as "Before you go on, I'd like to clarify . . ." or "I'd like to finish discussing . . ."
- **Concentrate on the words the other person says.** This is especially important if the other person's tone of voice, facial expressions, or nervous movements intimidate you.
- **Use relaxation exercises and deep-breathing techniques to remain calm.** Write a reminder like "Breathe in your abdomen" or "Picture peace and serenity" on your index card.
- **Determine what motivates the other person, and use that information to support your argument or purpose.** If the other person is motivated by budgetary concerns, use that to support your argument. For example, say, "Not only will this program help employees be more effective, but it will also save money because participants will have learned to be more efficient in their communication and everyday work."
- **Keep time limitations in mind.** Move the meeting along. If necessary, make such comments as "We have 10 minutes left, and I'd like to come to an agreement on . . ." or "If I don't hear from you about this by Thursday, I'll call you."

Source: Adapted from *Holistic Assertiveness Skills for Nurses*, by Carolyn Chambers Clark, 2003, New York: Springer. Copyright 2003 by Carolyn Chambers Clark. Used with permission.

Hays used the target behavior instrument, an investigator-developed research tool based on Hersey and Keilty's interaction influence analysis, to identify individual and dyad communication. Interrater reliability was 100% when the behaviors were analyzed in a 2-day period (Hays, 2002).

GUIDED LEADERSHIP TIP

ASSERTIVENESS OPPORTUNITIES FOR NURSE LEADERS

- Implement a plan so staff have more influence and input in their work assignments. Describe your plan:

    Date to implement:
    Date to monitor program effectiveness:

- Devise a plan to ensure ongoing monitoring of head nurses (e.g., supervisors, assistant directors of nursing, clinical nurse leaders) so they provide verbal and visible support for those they supervise.
    Date to implement:

- Ensure that all employees attend an assertiveness training class or a 2-day assertiveness workshop.
    Date to implement:
    Dates to monitor program effectiveness and plan follow-up consultations:

- Start an employee suggestion box that is regularly read and implemented.
    Date to implement:
    Dates to monitor program effectiveness:

- Open up communication so that it flows up, down, and across all organizational levels. Start with a newsletter that shares information from all levels, including anticipated organizational changes, achievements, and rewards.
    Date to implement:
    Dates to monitor program effectiveness:

Source: Clark (2003).

The findings included:

- Few supportive behaviors were observed, and none were observed among the leaders.
- The supporting behaviors exhibited by both men and women were all non-verbal head nods.
- Neither the nurse leaders nor the staff nurses used verbal statements of praise or acknowledgment.
- RN followers who demonstrated supporting behaviors were younger but had longer current employment.

- Education level appeared not to relate to supporting behaviors. In this study, nurse leaders with master's degrees exhibited no supportive behaviors.

Based on her findings, Hays made the following recommendations for shift reports:

- *Develop an in-service nursing leadership course to elevate self-esteem among nurses by promoting a sense of value and respect of others.* Value clarification exercises can help nurses assess their values and learn to recognize and appreciate others. A planned brief socialization period before or after a report could enhance feelings of belonging and approval among nursing leadership and staff.
- *Review the selection process of the current leaders.* It is vital to select, educate, and retain staff who share similar values and goals.
- *Explore the significance of various dyads.* Female-male dyads, cross-cultural dyads, and other groupings may lead to rejection, negativity, and other signs of nonsupport.
- *Link the shift report process to performance appraisals.* Such an action acknowledges that this act of exchanging information is significant and part of the unit's reward system.

See **Boxes 7-3** and **7-4** for value clarification exercises that could bring staff to a greater understanding and acceptance of their differences.

Communicating with Different Generations

Today's nursing workforce is composed of staff and nurse leaders from as many as four different generations. Their differences in attitudes, beliefs, work habits, and expectations can be viewed as potential strengths. Communicating with nurses from different generations can be a challenge. As a nurse leader, you will be responsible for helping bridge gaps between generations and create unique solutions that appeal to different belief and operating systems (Sherman, 2006).

Some communication suggestions follow:

- *Veteran nurses, born 1925–1945.* Nurses in this generation are most comfortable with inclusive communication systems that build trust. Face-to-face or written communication may be more effective than communication that involves technology, but query individual nurses about which communication channels they're most comfortable with (Duchscher & Cowin, 2004).
- *Baby boomers, born 1946–1962.* This generation prefers communication that is open, direct, and less formal. Boomers enjoy processing information as a group and value staff meetings that provide an opportunity for discussion. They prefer face-to-face or telephone communication but will use e-mail (Duchscher & Cowin, 2004).

BOX 7-3   CONTROVERSIAL ISSUES EXERCISE

Objective:
To communicate feelings about a controversial issue and to allow others to communicate theirs.

Directions:
- Read the controversial issue statement below.
- Without signing your name, make one comment illustrating how you feel about the statement or issue (Part A).
- Route this paper around the group. Each person reads every other person's comment without judging it. The idea is to communicate your feelings and allow others to do the same.
- Reroute the paper, read other people's reactions to the exercise, and decide whether you feel the same or different about the issue now. Give a rationale for your response (Part B).
- If you wish, record your reactions to the exercise itself (Part C).

Controversial issue statement:
Whenever a doctor writes, "Do not call code 99" for a client, the nurse should not call the cardiac arrest team for that person.

Part A: My reaction to this statement is:

Part B: Now that I have read others' reactions, I feel the following way about the issue (give a rationale for your reaction):

Part C: My reactions to this exercise are:

- *Generation X, born 1963–1979.* This is the first generation that experienced technology as a part of daily life. Gen Xers may become bored with meetings that include considerable discussion (Karp, Fuller, & Sirias, 2002).
- *Millennials, born 1980–2000.* This generation grew up with instant messaging and cellular phones. Millennials prefer immediate feedback and may become frustrated if they do not get it. They appreciate team meetings and use them as a forum for communication. They read less than other groups, so limit the distribution of lengthy policies and procedures to them. Chat rooms and e-mails are good ways to provide communication updates (Sherman, 2006).

BOX 7-4   UNDERSTANDING OTHER VIEWPOINTS

Objective:
To share values with others and understand their viewpoints.

Directions:
- Using the list below, all participants choose a topic of interest about which they have a strong point of view.
- They share their point of view regarding that topic with all other participants either in writing or verbally.
- Each participant reads or listens to value statements from others without commenting and tries to understand their point of view.
- In one month, all participants examine their point of view on the topics that were discussed.

Topics:

Health	Physical appearance
Aging	Abortion
Sex	Family relationships
Handicapped people	Friendship
Rules	Euthanasia
Salary	Drugs
Lifestyles	Learning
Work	Institutions
Leisure	

I choose the following topic:

My position on this topic is:

I have come to this position based on:

Other people or situations that have influenced my position are:

Follow-up: It is now one month later; my evaluation of my position on the topics discussed is:

Enhancing Collaborative Communication with Physicians

Collaborative communication is associated with positive client, nurse, and physician outcomes (Boyle, 2004). When nurses are dissatisfied, angry, or anxious during their interactions with physicians, nursing care can suffer. Collaborative communication can also increase client survival, shorten hospital stays, improve the staff's ability to meet family needs, and enhance professional relationships (Boyle, 2004).

Research Box 7-1 provides information about one study that improved collaborative communication between nurses and physicians.

Communicating with Groups

Is there a difference between face-to-face communication and virtual communication in terms of staff satisfaction? A study by Hoyt (2003) examined this question in a laboratory experiment.

Transformational and Transactional Leadership in Virtual and Physical Environments

Crystal Hoyt of the University of Richmond and Jim Blascovich of the University of California, Santa Barbara, examined the effect of leadership style (transformational or transactional) and group setting (face-to-face, immersion in virtual environment, or intercom) on three-person ad hoc work groups.

Results indicated that, compared to transactional leadership, transformational leadership was associated with decreases in quantity of performance but increases in quality of performance, leadership satisfaction, and group cohesiveness. Trust appeared to play an important role, but group performance and cohesiveness were similar across group settings and group members were most satisfied with their leader when the leader interacted with them face to face.

RESEARCH BOX 7-1   STUDY OF COMMUNICATION BETWEEN NURSES AND PHYSICIANS

Collaborative communication is associated with positive client, nurse, and physician outcomes. Using a pretest-posttest repeated-measures design incorporating baseline data collection, implementation of the intervention over 8 months, and immediate and 6-month post-data collection, Boyle (2004) tested an intervention to enhance collaborative communication among nurse and physician leaders (e.g., nurse manager, medical director, clinical nurse specialist) in two diverse ICUs.

Seven nurse (all women) and three physician (two men, one woman) leaders participated in the intervention, which consisted of six core development dimensions modules: leadership, core skills for communication, guiding conflict resolution, helping others adapt to change, teams, and trust. Collaborative skills included agreeing and focusing on the goal, checking for understanding, agreeing on a plan of action, acknowledging good ideas, and following through; relationship skills included the key principles of esteem, empathy, involvement, sharing, and support.

Each intervention incorporated multiple learning activities, small-group skill practice and problem-solving sessions, feedback and reinforcement of newly learned skills, a planning assignment for on-the-job application, and assessment and feedback after the intervention. Total training time was 23.5 hours, and participants received continuing education credit for each module they attended and a certificate upon completion of the intervention. All participants participated in a collaboration skills simulation vignette of seven sequenced situations that included all elements of the interaction process and tested participants' collaborative skills. Repeated-measures of multivariate analysis of variance were used to analyze data.

Findings provided evidence that nurse-physician collaborative communication can be improved, specifically:

- Communication skills of ICU nurse and physician leaders improved significantly.
- Leaders reported increased satisfaction with their own communication and leadership skills.
- Staff nurses reported lower personal stress (e.g., more respect from coworkers, physicians, and managers), even though they perceived significantly more situation stress (e.g., fewer staff members and less time).

Communicating about Being a Leader

Being a manager does not automatically mean staff or clients will view you as a leader. To boost others' perception of you as a leader, it is important to communicate like a leader. Follow the advice of Hodson (1998). To be viewed as a nurse leader:

- *Be visible as a leader.* Give a short presentation, or plan an event, letting staff or clients know about it in advance.
- *Give 60-second informationals.* Talk about successes and how they've benefited your unit or institution.

- *Invite staff or clients to help with a project.* Organizing an event makes others perceive you as a leader.
- *Provide sincere praise.* Address important staff behavior—saying, for example, "Your comment was very helpful to me."
- *Validate opinions.* Comment on what you have in common—saying, for example, "That's a wonderful idea. I had a similar situation a few months ago."
- *Resolve problems.* Come up with solutions, and ask people to participate in them. For example, instead of reprimanding two feuding staff members, invite them to come to your office and state their side of the story. Even better, ask feuding staff to meet with you and come up with suggestions for how to solve the problem between them. When staff are involved in decision making, they own the solutions and are more apt to follow their own advice.

Communicating by Involving Others

Whether communicating with a boss, a supervisee, or a client, it is important to remember the 90-20-8 rule.

According to Pike (1998), adults can either listen for 90 minutes and understand what they hear or listen for 20 minutes and retain content. To maintain interest, they need to be involved in the presentation every 8 minutes.

Long-winded leaders can lose listeners after 8 minutes. To keep their interest, ask a question to provide a dialogue at least once every 8 minutes.

Determining How Often to Communicate as a Nurse Leader

Many meetings are unnecessary, yet groups continue to meet. Sometimes, it is just out of habit. Use the following guidelines to make meetings more effective:

- *Huddle spontaneously* for no more than 15 minutes to brainstorm, give vital updates, boost enthusiasm, and renew collaboration.
- *Meet daily* for no longer than 30 minutes when you must direct team activities, discuss emerging changes, or make announcements that everyone needs to know to complete work that day.
- *Meet weekly* for less than an hour to check progress on reports or projects and to review employee, staff, or client concerns.
- *Meet monthly or quarterly* for less than 90 minutes to review long-term program progress, assess group or team progress, or analyze performance patterns. (Humphrey & Stokes, 1998)

Communicating in the Managed Care Environment

Hospital nurses must cope with the changing healthcare environment. They must deal with radically redefined roles that include collaboration and coordination with others (Miller & Apker, 2002). As a nurse leader, it will be your responsibility to help nurses and nurse assistants adapt to their roles. Steps you can take to improve communication include the following:

- Directly communicate to staff nurses about how client-centered environments are designed to heighten collaborative decision making. Strengthen this message by holding regular brown-bag lunches for nurses and establishing central nursing lounges for RNs to gather and communicate informally. These strategies can replace vital relational resources that may be depleted in the move to client-centered hospitals.
- Communicate to staff nurses that they are change agents and can successfully transition to different work situations and be positive role models for clients and caregivers. These messages can be disseminated through organizational newsletters and town hall meetings, giving staff nurses a greater voice in the changes occurring in their work environments.
- Few workers can adequately anticipate the extent to which their roles might change in response to managed care. The more information that you can provide, the more apt nurses and others will be able to adjust. (Miller & Apker, 2002)

Communicating by Empowering Staff

Although the competencies identified by the Nursing Leadership Institute (2002) are certainly ideals to strive for, the reality for many work environments is that they have limited resources and their clients are very ill. This can lead to increased stress and pressure to complete a seemingly endless list of assignments, which, in turn, can result in anxiety and blame.

Elizabeth Tonkin, a chief nursing officer at Westside Regional Medical Center in Plantation, Florida, contends that it is still possible to be a positive communicator. According to Tonkin (1995), the greatest gift a leader can offer staff who blame other shifts for leaving them too much work is to shift from being a controller of behavior to being a facilitator of empowerment.

A suggested intervention is to call a series of staff meetings that overlap shifts, explain how blaming wastes energy, and ask employees to identify and correct the root of the problem. By enlisting two staff members from each shift to serve on a task force or quality circle to resolve issues, and by establishing a cooperative relationship that puts clients first, blame can be eliminated or at least reduced. With this intervention, it is important to provide guidelines for the group because not all solutions may be feasible in the work setting (Tonkin, 1995).

It may seem easier to dictate an expected outcome, but Tonkin reminds nurse leaders to "trust the process" of letting staff members take leadership of their own destinies. In her experience, all empowered staff flourish.

Using Positive Feedback

Praise can reinforce positive behaviors and inspire hard work. Sometimes, praise can backfire if it makes employees or clients complacent and encourages them to slack off. Nelson (1998) suggests taking the following actions to reduce that possibility:

- Link praise to results.
- Find another way to provide inspiration if verbal praise disrupts work.
- Ask employees or clients what type of praise they value most. Verbal praise, written notes or memos, certificates, approving special requests, and occasional perks are all possible positive feedback actions.
- Use praise to build up other performance areas that need growth. For example, say, "That was well done. Excellent work. What about complimenting your clients once in a while to show them you respect their work, too?"

Giving and Accepting Criticism

Criticism is one of the most important forms of communication, yet it can carry a hurtful sting if not presented in a respectful way. One way to criticize painlessly is to:

- *Begin with two positive statements.* "You really have presented some very good ideas, and I like working with you."
- *State the criticism.* "I'd like us to stay on topic and not stray off it."
- *Add another positive statement and a ray of hope.* "You've shown the ability to work on complex goals, and I believe we'll get this accomplished by tomorrow."

Receiving criticism can be difficult especially if you catastrophize, obsess over the comment, or allow negative self-talk. It is important to recognize criticism as a problem-solving tool. When you heed reasonable criticism, you can avoid greater conflict.

When receiving criticism, it is useful to:

- *Avoid catastrophizing.* For example, do not assume that one criticism is tantamount to being fired.
- *Acknowledge the criticism.* "You're right, I did . . ." (If the criticism is true.)
- *Use assertiveness techniques to counter unfair criticism.* See **Box 7-5** for suggestions.
- *Vow to learn from the mistake.* Bemoaning what should have been done will not help. Instead, focus on what you can do in the future to prevent criticism. When you're successful, vow to repeat the successful behavior.

BOX 7–5   ASSERTIVENESS TECHNIQUES WHEN BEING CRITICIZED

- **Fogging/negative assertion.** Fogging means that you offer no resistance yet are persistent and independent, admitting errors while refusing to be manipulated. One way to do this is to agree with any truth in the other person's statement—for example, "That's right, I am 5 minutes late," "You're right, I haven't finished the report," or "I guess I did make an error."

- **Negative inquiry.** Negative inquiry can help you desensitize yourself to negative criticism so that you can listen to what you are being told, decrease others' repetitive criticism, and reduce the idea that there is a strict right or wrong method of interaction. Negative inquiry is a method of clarifying the other person's point of view. Examples include "I don't understand; what are you basing that on?" or "What exactly do you think I didn't do?"

- **Assertive probing.** Assertive probing can help you decide whether criticism is constructive or manipulative. The aim of assertive probing is to clarify unclear comments. Examples include "What is it about my work that bothers you?" and "What is it that you are displeased about?"

- **Broken record.** When others won't listen to your viewpoint, sometimes continuing to repeat your opinion works. A short, specific statement that is repeated again and again may eventually be heard. This technique is like saying no except that the objective is to get the other person to accept your criticism or comment. Examples include repeating the same statement no matter how the other person tries to make you feel guilty, appeal to your sense of fairness, order you to do something, or whatever—for example, repeat, "I can't, I have other priority items to complete" until the other person runs out of options.

- **Content–to–process shift.** When the focus of conversation drifts away from the original topic, because of strong feeling or some other reason, a content-to-process shift can help move you back on course. Examples include "Let's get back to what we were discussing," "I really don't want to argue about this," and "You seem upset; do you want to talk about it?"

- **Momentary delay.** Take your time. You don't have to answer right away. Take a moment to think of your answer and reply.

- **Time out.** When you or the other person is angry, it's always wise to call for a time out to cool down. A day or more is preferable.

- **Deflection.** Changing the topic can deflect or redirect an attack. For example, saying, "Is that a new suit?" can help you take the criticism less seriously and free you from stress.

- **Joining the attacker.** When you join with the attacker, you agree with the other person's right to experience a feeling.

- **Parley.** This approach is most effective when you are involved in no-win situation. Use comments such as "Let's try to work out a compromise," or "Let's see if we can iron out the problem."

- **Fighting back.** When there is no other option, when it is a question of life or death, or the problem has a high priority, express your anger directly and stand up to insults with comments such as, "I'm angry about what you said, and I'd like to talk about it," or "I feel insulted. Please don't talk to me like that. I deserve respect."

- **Multiple attack.** It can feel quite intimidating when you are attacked by several people at once. Keep one of your attackers between you and the other by asking one of the group what he or she sees as the main problem, and then practice deep breathing and listening skills.

Source: Adapted from *Holistic Assertiveness Skills for Nurses,* by Carolyn Chambers Clark, 2003, New York: Springer. Copyright 2003 by Carolyn Chambers Clark. Used with permission.

- *Use positive self-talk.* Everyone talks to themselves about situations. Talking about how having an error pointed out can benefit you, how learning and change can occur, and how everyone makes mistakes or grows can go a long way. Examples are such comments as "I can handle this" and "This isn't so bad," or "focus on your positive points."
- *Count to 10.* When emotion wells up, count to 10 to provide time to sort out thoughts and feelings. If the criticism turns into a harangue, ask the person to take a moment so they might state their complaint more clearly.
- *Seek support.* Reach out to support persons for help in clarifying reactions to the criticism and in recognizing that it isn't the end of the world.
- *Acknowledge truth.* Think through the criticism, and look for a grain of truth. If you don't find one, communicate that the criticism seems inaccurate, and allow time for additional discussion.
- *Recognize that time heals.* The sting of criticism will fade as days pass. Carry on with your daily activities, and focus on your goals.

Communicating with Supervisors

Everyone has a supervisor, someone they report to. It is important to have a positive relationship not only with peers and supervisees but also with your supervisor. Krieff (1996) provides the following strategies:

- *Learn about your supervisor's goals, and align with them.* If you help supervisors achieve their goals, you will be viewed as a valuable resource.
- *Anticipate problems.* Avoid waiting until a problem occurs by addressing issues as they surface and reporting actions to supervisors.
- *Close gaps.* Tackle tasks that your supervisor cannot or does not want to deal with.
- *Keep your supervisors informed.* Provide them with needed information.
- *Use positive reinforcement.* Avoid emphasizing your supervisor's bothersome behavior; instead, comment on the times when he or she models effective behavior. For example, if your supervisor allows phone calls and other interruptions to prevent work from getting done, say things like "It's amazing how much we accomplished by ourselves" or "Thank you for giving me the chance to finish the project with just you and me working on it."

Disagreeing with Supervisors

All nurse leaders eventually have a supervisor who asks that they do something unreasonable or unethical. In these cases, it is important to ask yourself, "Isn't it my responsibility to speak up when I see something wrong?"

GUIDED LEADERSHIP TIP

Some ways to disagree in a positive way include:

- Having a positive attitude and always communicating a willingness to cooperate and be helpful.
- Presenting ideas in the form of a question. For example, you could say, "I wonder if Sarah might be helpful with this; she's dealt with it quite a bit."
- Agreeing to disagree and offering to help with some of the work. You might say, "I'll get right on it, but Dan does this kind of thing a lot. He's already established a protocol and could probably get faster results. Do you mind if I call him and ask him to make the calls?"
- Offering to begin the work and then consulting with or passing the task onto a more experienced person. Novice nurse leaders can say, "I'll get started, but do you mind if I take this to Esther? She's much more qualified and experienced in this kind of action."
- Asking for clarification on the goal. Say, "Help me understand why we're doing it this way." Once you understand the goal, you may be able to say, "I think this will work quite well if we just change _____. What do you think?"
- Explaining your personal ethics in advance. When hired or shortly thereafter, state, "I notice it is common practice here to _____. I have a personal ethic that won't allow me to do that. I just wanted to let you know that up front so you won't unknowingly put me into a position where I can't follow your directive." (McDonald, 1988)

McDonald (1988) states that although it is important to obey a directive, it is also important to provide supervisors with information that could help them make better decisions.

Things to avoid when disagreeing with a supervisor include:

- Assuming you are right and your boss is wrong
- Implying you refuse to do what has been ordered
- Saying the action is not in your job description
- Implying the directive won't work
- Claiming the action is unethical (even if it is)

Avoiding Communication Mistakes

The pressure of day-to-day activities can lead people to ignore the importance and power of good manners. To improve morale and serve as a positive role model, it is important to:

- *Greet everyone.* Saying "good morning" or "good afternoon" sets a tone of openness, warmth, and caring.

- *Avoid misusing beepers and cell phones.* Turn off beepers and/or cell phones during meetings. On the rare occasions when you must stay in touch, set your beeper or cell phone to vibrate.
- *Take invitations seriously.* Accepting an invitation and then not showing up or showing up late is rude and gives the impression that you're disinterested or disorganized. Invitations must be replied to within a week. If you accept, you should attend. Unless the invitation specifies bringing a guest, it is not wise to bring one.
- *Return phone calls and e-mails.* Set aside a certain time during the day to return phone calls and e-mail. Not doing so may convey an air of self-importance. And even a seemingly unimportant message could be a vital one.
- *Apologize after a mistake.* After making a verbal or nonverbal gaffe, it is important to apologize in person and then follow it up with a phone call apology. For serious mistakes, a small thoughtful gift accompanied by a note of apology is in order.
- *Listen carefully.* Avoid getting caught up in personal agendas. When someone needs to talk with you, listen. Do not forget that important information may be transmitted during even a short communication. If there is an emergency, set a time to talk with the person later, and then follow through and be available as agreed.
- *Say no.* Learn to say no to unreasonable demands or invitations that do not support nurse leader priorities. (Baldrige, 1994)

Summary

This chapter defined communication, described communication theories and research findings, provided ways to communicate with staff and supervisors, and suggested assertive ways to give and take criticism.

Key Term Review

- **Cognitive dissonance theory** holds that when individuals are presented with information that is inconsistent with their beliefs, they will strive to reachieve balance.
- **Contagion theories** explain how networks of people spread "infectious" attitudes and behavior.
- **Contagion by cohesion** refers to the influence of those with a tendency toward direct communication on those with a tendency toward indirect communication.
- **Contagion by structural equivalence** refers to the mutual influence of those who have similar communication patterns.
- **Effective communication** is a message that is easily understood and accepted.
- **Elements of communication** include words, gestures, movement, posture, eye contact/gaze, adornment and other artifacts, rate of speech, pauses, facial expression, silences, touch, sound effects, intonation, and proxemics or use of space.
- **Language expectancy theory** holds that language is a rule-governed system and that people develop expectations about message strategies that others employ in their attempts to persuade. It explains how speakers vary language intensity to make their messages more persuasive.
- Human communication is **multimodal,** which means that more than one piece of information is interpreted to convey meaning, and includes verbal and nonverbal aspects.
- **Social cognitive theory** posits that if people are to perform a behavior, it is important to communicate what the behavior is and how to achieve it, to support the behavior, to model or observe the behavior, and to build confidence that the behavior will appear.

Leadership Development Exercises

Leadership Development Exercise 7-1

Identify which of the characteristics in Box 7-1 (p. 138) match up with your leadership style. Devise a plan to incorporate at least three characteristics into your work relationships in the next 3 months, and then monitor your progress and share your findings with three classmates or colleagues.

Leadership Development Exercise 7-2

Examine the goals in the section on assertive communication, pages 139–142. Make three recommendations for involving the nursing staff in the implementation of three goals. Present your findings to three classmates or colleagues.

■ Leadership Development Exercise 7-3

From the list of ingredients of effective interpersonal communication (see Effective One-on-One Communication, pages 137–141) select one and identify at least one personal goal to take action on. Write up a plan, and set an implementation date. Share your findings with three other learners.

■ Leadership Development Exercise 7-4

Identify at least two ways to use emotional intelligence to communicate with others, and draw up a plan for using this concept with staff. Monitor your results, and share your findings with three other learners.

■ Leadership Development Exercise 7-5

Sit in on four or more nurses' intershift reports. Summarize your findings, and share them with three others learners. If you observed problems, identify a solution, and discuss your suggestion with one head nurse, if possible.

■ Leadership Development Exercise 7-6

Describe communication strategies for various generations in the workforce. Identify a plan for enhancing communication between generations, and try it out. Write up your results, and share them with three other learners.

■ Leadership Development Exercise 7-7

Identify ways to enhance collaborative communication with physicians by rereading pages 146–147. Decide on a plan for enhancing communication between nurses and physicians. Discuss your ideas with three other learners. Together, find a way to try out or participate in an action that enhances nurse-physician communication.

■ Leadership Development Exercise 7-8

Sit in on a staff meeting. Describe the group communication that you observe. Share your findings with three other learners. Brainstorm together, and come up with at least four possible solutions for enhancing group communication.

Advanced Leadership Development Exercises

■ Leadership Development Exercise 7-9

Develop a problem statement to study one aspect of leader communication.

■ Leadership Development Exercise 7-10

Teach communication skills to novice leaders. Write up your experience, and share it with three other learners.

■ **Leadership Development Exercise 7-11**

Plan and complete a small research project related to leader communication. Write up your findings, and share them with three other learners.

Optional: Submit an article based on your findings to an appropriate journal.

References

Albrecht, T. L., & Adelman, M. B. (1987). Communicating social support: A theoretical perspective. In T. L. Albrecht, M. B. Adelman, & Associates, *Communicating Social Support* (pp. 18–29). Newbury Park, CA: Sage.

Albrecht, T. L., & Halsey, J. (1991). Supporting the staff nurse under stress. *Nursing Management, 22*(7), 60–61.

Baber, C., & Mellor, B. (2001). Using critical path analysis to model multimodal human-computer interactions. *International Journal of Human Computer Studies, 54*, 613–636.

Baldrige, L. (1994, March 1). 10 mistakes in manners that executives make over and over again. *Bottom Line Personal*, 10–11.

Bandura, A. (2001). Social cognitive theory: An agentive perspective. *Annual Review of Psychology, 52*, 1–26.

Blatner, A. (2002). *About nonverbal communication: General considerations*. Retrieved April, 10, 2007, from http://www.blatner.com/adam/level2/nverb1-htm

Bobulski, E. D. (2002, August 26). A message for managers: Care, teach, connect. *Nursing Spectrum*, 9.

Boyle, D. K., Bott, M. J., Hanse, H. E., Woods, C. Q., & Taunton, R. L. (1999). Managers' leadership and critical care nurses' intent to stay. *American Journal of Critical Care, 8*, 361–371.

Boyle, D. K. (2004). Enhancing collaborative communication of nurse and physician leadership in two intensive care units. *Journal of Nursing Administration, 34*(2), 60–70.

Buller, D. B., Burgoon, M., Hall, J. R., Levine, N., Taylor, A. M., Beach, B. H., et al. (2000). Using language intensity to increase the success of a family intervention to protect children from ultraviolet radiation: Predictions from language expectancy theory. *Preventive Medicine, 30*, 103–114.

Burgoon, J. K., & Burgoon, M. (2001). Expectancy theories. In W. P. Robinson & H. Giles (Eds.), *The new handbook of language and social psychology* (2nd ed.). Sussex, UK: Wiley.

Burkhardt, M. E. (1994). Social interaction effects following a technological change: A longitudinal investigation. *Academy of Management Journal, 37*, 868–896.

Clark, C. C. (2003). *Group leadership skills*. New York: Springer.

Contractor, N. S., & Eisenberg, E. M. (1990). Communication networks and new media in organizations. In J. Fulk & C. W. Steinfield (Eds.), *Organizations and communication technology*. Newbury Park, CA: Sage.

Curtin, L., & Flaherty, M. J. (1982). *Nursing ethics: Theories and pragmatics*. Bowie, MD: Robert J. Brady.

Duchscher, J. E., & Cowin, L. (2004). Multigenerational nurses in the workplace. *Journal of Nursing Administration, 34*(11), 493–501.

Festinger, L. (1957). *A theory of cognitive dissonance*. Stanford, CA: Stanford University Press.

Hays, M. M. (2002). An exploratory study of supportive communication during shift report. *Southern Online Journal of Nursing Research, 3*(3). Retrieved November 15, 2007, from http://www.snrs.org/publications/SOJNR_articles/Iss03vol03.htm

Hein, S. (2005). *Emotional intelligence*. Retrieved April 15, 2007, from http://eqi.org /history.htm

Hodson, D. (1998). Learn to lead with these steps [Preview Issue]. *Manager's Edge*, 4.

Hoyt, C. L. (2003). Transformational and transactional leadership in virtual and physical environments. *Small Group Research*, *34*(6), 678–715.

Humphrey, B., & Stokes, J. (1998). How often should you meet? [Preview Issue]. *Manager's Edge*, 1.

Karp, H., Fuller, C., & Sirias, D. (2002). *Bridging the boomer-Xer gap*. Palo Alto, CA: Davies-Black.

Krieff, A. (1996). *Manager's survival guide*. Paramus, NJ: Prentice Hall.

McDonald, D. M. (1988, December). How to tell your boss he's wrong. *Management Solutions*, 3–9.

Miller, K. I., & Apker, J. (2002). On the front lines of managed care: Professional changes and communicative dilemmas of hospital nurses. *Nursing Outlook*, *50*(4), 154–159.

Nelson, B. (1998). Giving feedback . . . How to deliver useful recognition [Preview Issue]. *Manager's Edge*, 6.

Nursing Leadership Institute. (2002). *The nursing leadership institute competency model*. Retrieved March 27, 2007, from http://www.fau.edu/nli/model2.pdf

Peterson, L. W., Halsey, J., Albrecht, T. L., & McGough, K. (1995). Communicating with staff nurses: Support or hostility? *Nursing Management*, *26*(6), 36–38.

Pike, B. (1998). Involve the audience to make your point. *Manager's Edge*, Preview Issue, 1.

Rager, P. (1998, March 9). Emotional intelligence and the management edge. *Nursing Spectrum*, 3.

Rice, R. E., & Aydin, C. (1991). Attitudes toward new organizational technology: Network proximity as a mechanism for social information processing. *Administrative Science Quarterly*, *9*, 219–244.

Sherman, R. O. (2006). Leading a multigenerational nursing workforce: Issues, challenges and strategies. *Online Journal of Issues in Nursing, 11*(2), 1–8.

Stordahl, N. (1995, April 11). Effective leadership, *Vital Signs*, 16.

Tanouye, E. T. (1990, April). What is your staff afraid to tell you? *Working Woman*, 35–38.

Tonkin, E. (1995, February 21). Management perspectives: Hall of blame. *Nursing Spectrum*, 5.

Weisinger, H. (1998). *Emotional intelligence at work*. San Francisco: Jossey-Bass.

Wolf, Z. R. (1988). *Nurses' work, the sacred and the profane*. Philadelphia: University of Pennsylvania Press.

Resources

Avtgis, T. A. (2000). Unwillingness to communicate and satisfaction in organizational relationships. *Psychological Reports*, *87*(1), 82–84.

Johnson, R. S. (1993). Difficult people. *TQM: Leadership for the quality transformation*. Milwaukee, WI: ASQC Quality Press.

Sego, S. (2005, November). Overcoming staff hostility. *Clinical Advisor*, 72.

Weiss, D. H. (1988, February). How to handle difficult people. *Management Solutions*, 33–38.

Williams, R. T. (1985). *The power of criticism*. Madison, WI: The Wisconsin Clearinghouse.

Managing Conflict

CHAPTER OBJECTIVES

After reading this chapter, answering the leadership challenges, and participating in the leadership development exercises, you will be able to:

- Define conflict
- Compare and contrast conflict resolution models
- Analyze one example of nursing conflict
- Examine the concept of conflict in nursing work environments
- Identify sources of generational conflict
- Assess your conflict resolution skills
- Facilitate the development of conflict resolution skills in your staff

Advanced nurses will be able to:

- Teach conflict resolution skills to two clients, staff on a nursing unit, or a group of colleagues
- Formulate a problem statement for a nursing project related to conflict
- Design a research project related to conflict

Introduction

In many nursing settings, conflict between nurses is a significant factor in job dissatisfaction. It occurs in every work environment because of differences in people's goals, needs, desires, responsibilities, perceptions, and ideas. Unresolved conflict can result in job dissatisfaction, absenteeism, and turnover, whereas resolved conflict can lead to better relationships. Resolving issues leaves staff feeling more integrated, adjusted, powerful, and competent (Almost, 2006).

For these reasons, you need conflict resolution skills based on a strong conceptual framework. This chapter focuses on helping you learn both skills and the theories behind them.

LEADERSHIP IN ACTION

Rose L., a nurse leader on a busy medical-surgical unit, noticed signs of unrest among nurses when the unit moved from a total patient care delivery model to a team nursing model, and she feared that she'd done something wrong to disturb the peacefulness she usually experienced at work. Individual nurses complained about changes in their workloads, and arguments broke out between staff. Some nurses refused to help colleagues. Many were bitter and angry, and their feelings carried into their relationships with clients.

LEADERSHIP CHALLENGE What concept is being enacted by the nurses?

KEY TERM

Conflict is a normal occurrence and a multidimensional construct whose antecedents are individual, interpersonal, and/or organizational. Conflict can be either beneficial or detrimental, and either internal or external.

Conflict Defined

Conflict is a normal phenomenon in nursing (Stroeder, Znaniecki, & Brennerman, 2006) and part of the ebb and flow in any human relationship (Lederach, 2003). Conflict is a multidimensional construct whose antecedents are individual, interpersonal, and/or organizational (Almost, 2006). Conflict can be either beneficial or detrimental, and either internal or external. It develops when values or beliefs clash, and when leaders use conflict to increase communication within a healthcare team, it can be turned into a learning event.

Intrapersonal conflict can occur when you (or someone else) have two opposing goals. When you are not sure whether to uphold unit policy or support individual nurse's attempts to be creative with client care, you can experience conflicting feelings. When you are not sure whether to confront a staff member who never completes an assignment or to overlook it because confronting him or

her intimidates you, intrapersonal conflict can arise. Intrapersonal conflict is even more likely to occur when staff begin to
complain about how little work their peers do.

Interpersonal conflict can occur when you are involved
with one or more staff members and one of you perceives
opposition from the other. If you are modeling a leadership
behavior that clashes with another learner's, client's, or staff
member's values, conflict can occur.

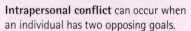

KEY TERM

Intrapersonal conflict can occur when
an individual has two opposing goals.

KEY TERM

Interpersonal conflict can occur when
two or more individuals are involved
and one perceives opposition from the
other.

Conflict can also occur in groups, such as staff meetings,
nursing reports, or other group gatherings. Group conflict is
caused by opposing forces within the work group and can be experienced by an
individual member, by subgroups, or by the entire group. Conflict may be dis-
guised and covered up at first, but it can soon burgeon into hostility or out-and-
out warfare if not subdued or resolved. Subgroups may appear as one or more
group members vie for control of the group, but subgroups can also be a sign of
group growth (Clark, 2003).

Other authors have viewed conflict as positive. As early as 1964, Blake and Mouton
claimed that complete resolution of conflict might stifle growth and creativity.

LEADERSHIP CHALLENGE What kind of conflict was Rose identifying? Give
a rationale for your answer.

Before attempting to manage, resolve, or transform conflict, it is a good idea to
understand the context within which it developed. Theory and models can assist you.

Conflict Theory and Models

We'll examine several models and theories of conflict and conflict management,
including Almost's model of antecedents and consequences of conflict, Kupperschmidt's model of multigenerational conflict, the human needs theory of conflict, Wehr's model for conflict mapping, Lambourne's model of reconciliation,
and Lederach's theory of conflict transformation.

Almost's Model of Antecedents and Consequences of Conflict

Almost (2006) developed her model for conflict within nursing work environments by using concept analysis. The model provides a thorough understanding
of the sources and outcomes of conflict and could enable preventive action.

Almost's model includes the following parts:

- Conflict antecedents (including individual characteristics, interpersonal factors, and organizational factors)

- Perceived conflict
- Conflict consequences

See **Figure 8-1** for a more in-depth look at Almost's model.

LEADERSHIP CHALLENGE How might Almost's model of conflict help Rose identify what to do on her unit. Give a rationale for your answer.

Kupperschmidt's Model of Multigenerational Conflict

Today, four generations of RNs often work side by side in nursing situations. Because they bring different values and cultures to the work environment, conflict is common.

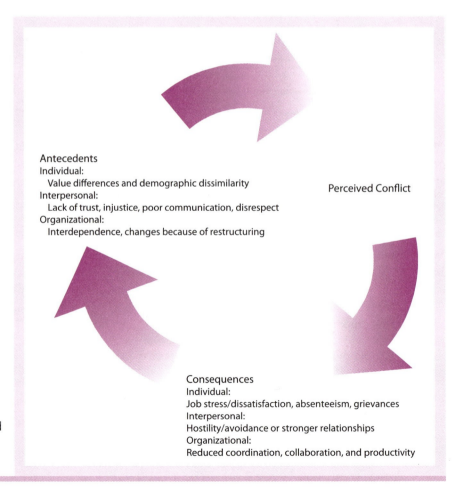

Antecedents
Individual:
    Value differences and demographic dissimilarity
Interpersonal:
    Lack of trust, injustice, poor communication, disrespect
Organizational:
    Interdependence, changes because of restructuring

Perceived Conflict

Consequences
Individual:
Job stress/dissatisfaction, absenteeism, grievances
Interpersonal:
Hostility/avoidance or stronger relationships
Organizational:
Reduced coordination, collaboration, and productivity

Figure 8-1
Antecedents, Perceived Conflict, and Consequences in Almost's Model

Kupperschmidt (2006) developed a model to address multigenerational conflict in nursing, and that model provides an explanation for the recent exodus of nurses from the profession. The **Kupperschmidt model of multigenerational conflict** describes four generations—from traditional professionals to Net generation professionals—and explains how differing values may cause conflict:

> **KEY TERM**
>
> The **Kupperschmidt model of multigenerational conflict** explains the challenges faced by nurses who work side by side with colleagues from a variety of generational cohorts and value systems.

- *Traditional RNs* were born before 1944; they value hard work, respect authority, and may tell younger nurses to "do it because I say so."
- *Baby boomer RNs* were born between 1944 and 1960; they value teamwork and like to reach consensus.
- *Generation X RNs* were born between 1961 and 1980 and value self-reliance; they might say that they will do the job themselves.
- *Net generation RNs* were born between 1981 and 2000; they value achievement and might not care who does the job as long as it gets done.

LEADERSHIP CHALLENGE How could Rose use these generational differences to understand conflict on her unit? Give a rationale for your answer.

The Human Needs Theory of Conflict

The **human needs theory of conflict** is based on the writings of psychologist Abraham Maslow (1998). He theorized that all people are driven to fulfill fundamental human needs for safety, security, love, a sense of belonging to a group, self-esteem, and attaining their goals.

> **KEY TERM**
>
> The **human needs theory of conflict** suggests that people are driven to fulfill fundamental human needs for safety, security, love, a sense of belonging to a group, self-esteem, and attaining their goals.

A group of conflict theorists—among them, Herbert Kelman (1997)—adapted Maslow's ideas to conflict theory, suggesting that these needs underlie many deep-rooted conflicts. When needs are denied, conflict can continue indefinitely.

If this theory is true, it explains why needs conflicts can be so intractable—a person's needs or a group's needs do not run out. But providing security, safety, or a sense of belonging to one individual or one group does not deny them to others. In fact, needs are often mutually reinforcing. If one individual or group stops threatening, the opposition will also stop because the mutual reinforcement ends (Maiese, 2003).

LEADERSHIP CHALLENGE Which needs may have been denied, leading to conflict, on Rose's unit? Give a rationale for your answer.

Wehr's Model for Conflict Mapping

Conflict has many elements. Wehr (1979) theorized that if mediators or those involved in a conflict could produce a road map, it would be easier to understand the dynamics of specific conflicts, enabling participants to solicit cooperation from their opponents.

Important elements identified by **Wehr's model for conflict mapping** include the context of the conflict, parties involved, causes and consequences of the conflict, values and beliefs, goals and interests, dynamics, functions, and any regulations or rules that affect the conflict. For more specifics on how to identify and use these elements, see the section "Conflict Assessment" on pages 166–167.

LEADERSHIP CHALLENGE How could Wehr's model for conflict mapping help Rose?

Lambourne's Model of Reconciliation

Lambourne (2004) developed a model of reconciliation that may be helpful. The model includes five elements:

1. *Truth.* This element includes an acknowledgment of past injustices and wrongs committed, a validation of pain and suffering, and an apology for harm caused.
2. *Mercy.* This element includes forgetting and letting go to end the cycle of revenge, releasing pain and identifying pain in the other, and engaging in rituals of healing and joint sorrow.
3. *Justice.* This element includes sharing power, responsibility, or resources.
4. *Identity.* This element includes replacing animosity with mutual acceptance and respect and accepting the other's autonomy.
5. *Recommitment.* This element includes a commitment to risk, trust, and change; the assurance that hurtful actions will not be repeated; and an anticipation of mutual security.

LEADERSHIP CHALLENGE Which elements of Lambourne's model of reconciliation could Rose use on her unit?

Lederach's Theory of Conflict Transformation

John Paul Lederach's theory of conflict transformation may help you understand what happened on Rose's unit. Lederach advocated the pursuit of conflict transformation, as opposed to conflict resolution or conflict management. He asserted that conflict resolution implies that all conflict is bad and should be ended and that, while conflict management correctly assumes that conflicts are long-term processes that cannot be quickly solved, the notion of management suggests that people can be directed or controlled as though they were objects (Lederach, 1995, 2003).

Conflict transformation goes beyond eliminating or controlling conflict and recognizes and works with conflict's interactive nature. Once conflict appears, it transforms the people and events involved, altering relationships, communication patterns, social organization, and people's images of themselves and others (Lederach, 1995, 2003).

Conflict transformation takes place at both the individual and organizational levels. At the individual level, conflict transformation includes the pursuit of awareness, growth, and commitment to change that occurs once a person identifies his or her fear, anger, grief, or bitterness. At the organizational level, justice and equality in the social system as a whole is pursued. This may involve eliminating oppression, improving the sharing of resources, and resolving conflict between groups in nonviolent ways. Key to both kinds of transformation are identifying the truth about what happened, righting any wrongs, extending forgiveness, empowering people to right wrongs, and establishing interdependence.

Lederach (1995, 2003) also counsels that the process of how conflict is resolved is more important than the outcome. During times of heated conflict, too little attention is often paid to the conflict resolution process, including how the issues are approached, discussed, and decided, and when discipline must be used to create an adequate and clear process for achieving an acceptable result.

KEY TERM

Conflict transformation theory suggests that people, events, and relationships are altered by a conflict but that destructive consequences can be prevented by transforming perceptions of issues, action, and other people or groups to improve mutual understanding.

LEADERSHIP TIP

Conflict can have destructive consequences that can be prevented by transforming perceptions of issues, action, and other people or groups to improve mutual understanding. Even when interests, values, and needs differ, progress can be made by gaining a relatively accurate understanding of each other.

LEADERSHIP CHALLENGE How could Rose use conflict transformation theory with staff on her unit?

Conflict Assessment

Wehr's (1979) conflict map provides a systematic way to plot out the origins, nature, dynamics, and possibilities for conflict resolution. Categories to consider include:

- *Conflict context.* Gather information about the history of the conflict and its physical and organizational settings. Use geographic boundaries, political structures, relationships, communication networks and patterns, and any legal jurisdictions. Look for conflicts nested within conflicts. For example, an ongoing conflict between medicine and nursing at the highest levels can be played out at the unit level.
- *Parties.* Individuals involved in the conflict can be primary (the ones who oppose another's values and goals and who have a direct stake in the outcome), secondary (those who have an indirect stake in the outcome), or third parties (mediators or peacekeepers who facilitate resolution). All these individuals have some stake in the conflict's outcome.
- *Causes and consequences.* Causes and consequences may blend; for example, hostility may be a consequence of one phase of a conflict and the cause of another. A basic cause of social conflict is incompatible goals and interests. Cultural differences, especially language, can create separateness and cause a group to become defensive.
- *Contrasting beliefs and values.* This category includes such things as one side's negative images of its opponents, opinions about a Supreme Being, the need to argue or fight, and a low capacity or priority for cooperation.
- *Goals and interests.* Goals are specific positions or demands made by one party or the other. Interests are what motivates those involved: security, recognition, respect, justice, and so on. Mapping can help opposing parties distinguish their positions from their needs and bring them as close to unity as possible.
- *Dynamics.* Conflicts can change. Mapping changes in escalation and polarization can make dynamics more visible. Other dynamics to map include precipitating events that led to the dispute, escalatory and de-escalatory spirals (during which time participants can be carried away from cooperative resolution and toward greater hostility). Stereotyping opponents only reinforces these runaway responses.
- *Functions.* Conflicts can have positive consequences for those involved, such as the release of tension or aggression. A conflict has a purpose for those involved and new alliances may be formed. The group may even become more unified as it defends itself against unfair accusations. Studying the consequences of these functions can help understand ways to move the conflict toward resolution.

- *Regulation potential.* Each conflict contains its own conflict-limiting elements, such as the wish to maintain the relationship, laws or policy, or a higher authority.

Now that you've learned about conflict theories and models, including Wehr's conflict assessment, read **Box 8-1.**

LEADERSHIP CHALLENGE How could Rose use this conflict assessment? What other information would she need to understand the conflict?

Conflict Approaches

"Clients can sense immediately when nurses are not working as a team," says Terri Irwin, an RN and college practice consultant (Stroeder, Znaniecki, & Brennerman, 2006, p. 14). As a nurse leader, it is important for you to "recognize, manage and deal with conflict before it becomes an issue that affects client care" (Stroeder et al., 2006, p. 14).

Once you have assessed the conflict and have sufficient information, you will need to choose a conflict approach. Conflict approaches include using Weiss's model of conflict patterns, managing strong emotions, using "I" statements,

---

BOX 8-1   ASSESSING MY CONFLICT RESOLUTION SKILLS

Directions: Answer yes or no for each statement.
- I know how to assess conflict by using Wehr's conflict assessment.
- I have filled out Wehr's conflict assessment for at least one conflict situation.
- I can identify Almost's antecedents and consequences of conflict.
- I can describe Kupperschmidt's four generations.
- I can identify elements for each of Kupperschmidt's generations that could lead to conflict.
- I can describe how Maslow's theory of fundamental human needs relate to conflict.
- I can identify the five areas of Lambourne's model of reconciliation.
- I can describe Lederach's conflict transformation theory.
- I have chosen a conflict resolution model or theory to resolve a conflict.
- I can describe five approaches to conflict resolution, management, or transformation.
- I have tried out at least two approaches to conflict resolution, management, or transformation.

Reread the items that you've answered no to, and complete the related leadership development exercises at that end of this chapter.

Source: Adapted from Almost (2006).

dealing with needs conflicts and reconciliation, conflict resolution programs, problem-solving workshops, analytical problem solving, transformative mediation, and fostering dialogue.

Weiss's Model of Conflict Patterns

One model that may be helpful for choosing a conflict approach is Weiss's (1988) model of three basic patterns of reaction:

1. *In control and unresponsive.* An example of this pattern is an individual who is aggressive with other people, which easily sets up conflict. When confronted in a group, this individual can either become more aggressive or ignore the confrontation. Taking this person aside and asking what he or she thinks could resolve the conflict. Unresponsive behavior can change when the individual gets credit for solving the conflict.

2. *Not in control and responsive.* An example of this pattern is a demanding individual who starts conflicts by promising to complete work tasks but then doesn't fulfill those promises.

3. *Not in control and unresponsive.* An example of this pattern is an individual who stammers, trembles, and cannot speak.

Weiss (1988) also discussed conflict-ridden patterns of game playing that can add havoc and stress to a work setting. Some patterns of game playing include:

- *Gotcha.* This game includes blaming other people, using exaggerated sarcasm, and enjoying watching other people's discomfort.
- *Woe is me.* This game includes constant whining or complaining without taking appropriate problem-solving steps for the purpose of winning sympathy.
- *Let's fight.* This game involves starting arguments for the purpose of fighting or winning a fight.
- *How about you two fight?* This game involves instigating fights between other people, usually over trivial or petty matters, for the purpose of watching other people fight.
- *Why don't you . . . ?* This game includes offering unsolicited advice (often to "woe as me" players) for the purpose of appearing to be helpful while really wishing to control the other person.

LEADERSHIP CHALLENGE Which of these games, if any, might Rose have to deal with? What advice would you give her?

No matter how difficult a conflict is, there's a specific method of taking action:

1. Find a private room, and engage the involved individuals in a discussion.
2. State the purpose of the meeting in nonthreatening terms, accepting responsibility for working on the problem by using "we" statements rather than "you" statements.
3. Ask the other persons to express their opinions and solutions first; then express yours.
4. Resolve any disagreements by returning to step 2.
5. Design an action plan for ending the difficulty, including deadlines and progress review dates. (Weiss, 1988)

That action plan contains the following items:

- Describe the way that the involved individuals act.
- Decide what exact action to take when the identified behaviors occur.
- Write out and rehearse the plan.
- Carry out the plan at the first opportunity.
- Evaluate the outcome.
- Revise the plan as necessary. (Johnson, 1993)

Managing Strong Emotions

Strong emotions can be the cause and effect of conflict. These emotions can mask the issues in dispute, so they must be dealt with. Some strategies to use include:

- *Use symbolic gestures to express respect and defuse negative emotions.* These include apologies, sympathetic notes, shared meals, or handshakes.
- *Help participants identify their emotions.* Are they angry or just excited?
- *Model how to express feelings.* For example, say, "I feel angry because I don't like to be shouted at" or "I'm confused about what's happening on the unit," rather than "You made me angry."
- *Acknowledge that everybody's feelings are legitimate.* Allowing feelings to be expressed and recognized often defuses them.
- *Avoid retaliating to outbursts with anger.* If you feel as if you're losing control, step out of the room for a new perspective, and take some deep breaths. Leaving the scene gives you a chance to calm down and plan an effective response rather than reacting automatically, which can escalate the situation. A useful response is to acknowledge the outburst with active listening and to paraphrase what you hear; this shows that you understand the strength of the speaker's feelings.

Using "I" Statements

"You" statements, such as "You aren't really listening to me," are intrusive, blaming, or attacking. They can be manipulative or coercive because they seek to change another person's behavior, and they can provoke a defensive reaction, counterattack, or withdrawal and escalate a destructive communication cycle. These aggressive statements often mask insecurities.

"I" statements, such as "I feel as if I'm not being understood," disclose your feelings without attacking others, invalidating their feelings, or criticizing them. "I" statements can halt defensive and hostile escalation because they tend to invoke trust and create space for the parties to explore their unacknowledged feelings. Such communication has the potential to transform situations. "Personal growth is largely a function of our capacity to be with feelings in an accepting, sensitive manner" (Amodeo & Wentworth, 1995, p. 210). By risking honest self-expression and taking responsibility for your feelings, you can encourage others to change their behavior.

LEADERSHIP CHALLENGE How could Rose use "I" statements with her staff? Give some examples of what she might say.

Needs Conflicts and Reconciliation

When conflict is a result of the denial of one or more essential needs, fighting can go on until those needs are filled (Marker, 2003). As a nurse leader, it is important for you to identify the legitimate needs of all staff and begin to meet those needs. If safety or security needs have top priority, then they should be the focus. If staff do not feel part of the work group, then that should be the priority. When self-esteem is low, make attempts to raise self-esteem. by praising staff attempts and pointing out staff strengths.

Conflict Resolution Programs

Conflict resolution programs use negotiation to settle conflicts. Negotiation can be distributive or integrative. **Distributive negotiation** is focused on each party winning as many concessions as possible; this can result in a win-lose situation. **Integrative negotiation** is focused on parties discovering solutions that embody mutual self-interest; this can result in a win-win situation.

The face-to-face conversations involved in direct negotiation can influence people to act in the group's interest. Talking with the opposition sends the message that both parties are committed to positive resolution and tends to be integrative (Kagan & Gall, 1998).

Conflict resolution skills overlap with social competence skills and include:

- Awareness of others
- Awareness of the distinctions between self and others
- Listening skills (see chapter 11)
- Awareness of and ability to express one's own thoughts and feelings
- Ability to respond to others' thoughts and feelings

LEADERSHIP CHALLENGE If you were a nurse leader on a unit where staff did not possess these skills, what could you do to ensure that they are learned?

Problem-Solving Workshops

Problem-solving workshops have been shown to contribute to transforming the relationship between conflicting parties. Interacting in this type of workshop promotes and models a new kind of relationship between the parties, one that is based on equality and reciprocity.

During the workshop process, a facilitator encourages participants to gain an understanding of the other side's needs, fears, and constraints. As a result, group members try to shape solutions that respond to the fundamental concerns of both sides. The group searches for ways to provide mutual reassurance. Such ideas emerge from acknowledgments participants make to each other while interacting. Empathy for the other side begins to develop, and trust grows. Workshop participants then return to their community or workplace and teach their respective colleagues not only ideas about transforming relationships but also the results of their workshop experience. They can testify that a mutually enhancing relationship is possible because they participated in one (Kelman, 1997).

LEADERSHIP CHALLENGE What could Rose take from that information on problem–solving workshops to use on her unit?

Analytical Problem Solving

Analytical problem solving is a social-psychological approach to dealing with protracted conflicts that is based on the human needs theory of conflict. During

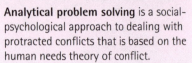

Analytical problem solving is a social-psychological approach to dealing with protracted conflicts that is based on the human needs theory of conflict.

this process, a great deal of emphasis is put on identifying and examining both parties' perspectives on the problem, including their values, interests, prejudices, hopes, fears, and needs. Emotions are not avoided; they are dealt with directly. Much emphasis is placed on recognizing each other's needs and empowering parties to approach their mutual problem in new ways. Although long-term conflict resolution is a primary goal, the short-term goal is increasing mutual understanding. This can be achieved in a workshop (Burgess & Burgess, 1997).

Some questions that such a workshop process could raise include:

- What are your interests, hopes, fears, and needs related to this situation?
- What feelings has this conflict brought forth that you are comfortable sharing?
- What do you believe are the other party's needs?
- How are these interests, hopes, fears, and needs similar to yours?

LEADERSHIP CHALLENGE   How could Rose use analytical problem solving with her staff? What if she couldn't bring her staff together in one place at the same time? In what other ways could she promote this kind of problem solving?

Transformative Mediation

Transformative approaches do not seek resolution of the immediate problem. They seek the empowerment and mutual recognition of the parties involved (H. Burgess, 1997).

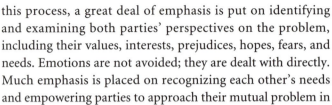

Empowerment means increasing the skills of all involved to make better decisions for themselves by learning how to clarify their goals, to find out about resources and options, and to choose their preferences.

Empowerment means increasing the skills of all involved to make better decisions for themselves by learning how to clarify their goals, to find out about resources and options, and to choose their preferences (Bush & Folger, 1996).

Transformative mediators help disputing parties deal with issues by providing a forum for discussion with a neutral third party present. This process can help clarify the nature of the problem from both parties' points of view and develop a range of options. In this approach, the involved parties are believed to be the experts who have the motivation and capacity to solve their own problems with minimum help (such as encouraging the expression of emotion and examining the past as a way of persuading the parties to recognize each other's accomplishments and discuss important issues even if such issues are not easily negotiable). The transformative mediator lets parties set goals, direct the process, and design the ground rules.

You can implement transformative mediation by using the information in the Guided Leadership Tip "Helping Combatants Resolve Their Difficulties."

LEADERSHIP CHALLENGE **What problems might Rose anticipate using conflict transformation, and how could she overcome those obstacles?**

Fostering Dialogue

In dialogue, participants speak as individuals, not as representatives of groups or positions. Parties speak directly to one another, and facilitators strive to create a safe atmosphere for discussion and to promote respectful exchanges.

Facilitators encourage participants to question the dominant public view and to express fundamental needs that may or may not be reflected in formal workplace directives. Three approaches foster dialogue:

1. Collaborating with participants
2. Refusing to take the role of expert
3. Acknowledging the parties are the best experts in their own experiences and wishes (Chasin et al., 1996)

Extensive preliminary work may be necessary with individual participants. Setting ground rules for conducting the sessions will help facilitators prevent each side from reenacting old patterns of interaction. Common ground roles include:

- Participants can decline to answer a question without explanation.
- Respectful language must be used.

GUIDED LEADERSHIP TIP

HELPING COMBATANTS RESOLVE THEIR DIFFICULTIES

Comments to help combatants include:

- "What ground rules do you want to use?"
- "Your goals are legitimate and should be considered seriously. You might want to clarify them. How you do that is up to you."
- "These resources are available to you to help you make informed choices" or "It's important to find out what resources you need to make an informed choice. How you do that is up to you."
- "Here is a list of your options for you to examine the relative costs and benefits of each."
- "It's important to reflect and deliberate on your preferences so you can make a conscious decision based on the strengths and weaknesses, advantages and disadvantages, of both sides. How you do that is up to you."
- "It's up to you how much you recognize the views of ____[name of opponent]____."

- Attempts to persuade others or use rhetorical questions are forbidden.
- No one is to share the specifics of the sessions outside the meetings. (Chasin et al., 1996)

Four tactics that help foster new patterns of communication are:

1. Making sure that the parties speak as individuals, not as representatives of their position
2. Exploring ideas and experiences that are usually dismissed or ignored by the mainstream discussion
3. Discovering new differences by asking sincere questions about unclear points
4. Using de-stereotyping exercises to break down polarization (Chasin et al., 1996)

Roth (1994) made the following additional suggestions for constructive dialogue:

- Address participants as coinvestigators in finding a solution.
- Request that participants avoid interrupting each other, pass if they don't want to speak (no questions asked), and keep their replies to 2 minutes.
- Begin by asking participants to talk about their life experiences in relation to the issue.
- Ask, "We would like to hear a little about your beliefs and perspectives about this issue. What is at the heart of the matter for you as an individual?"
- Then ask, "What dilemmas, struggles, and conflicts do you have about your prevailing view of this issue? Include any mixed feelings that you wish to share."

LEADERSHIP CHALLENGE **If Rose decides to foster dialogue on her unit, what specific actions must she take to ensure that staff follow the tactics that help foster new patterns of communication?**

Establishing an Environment of Care

Generational conflict and lack of respect can lead nurses to be abusive to other nurses. Kupperschmidt (2006) pointed out that nurses should respect each other and that when a nurse is disrespected, he or she should adopt an assertive attitude, not fall into silent withdrawal. An environment that's conducive to caring for colleagues needs to be established in the workplace. Failing to confront disrespect is "not kindness; rather it is a form of lying" (Augsburger, 1973, p. 25).

An article in *Nursing Management* (Sanford, 2005) described a toxic work environment that was allowed to continue for 14 years because nursing staff and managers refused to confront the disrespectful behavior of one RN. Allowing the RN's behavior to continue gave other nurses permission to be disrespectful. The article stressed that nurse leaders and staff nurses should learn confrontation skills to set the expectation of mutual respect.

Some ways to do that include using honest communication that confronts and addresses disrespectful behavior, such as:

- "I want and deserve to be treated with respect."
- "You and I have an ethical imperative to treat each other with respect." (See Chapter 10.)

When nurse leaders provide access to information, support and resources, and an opportunity for development, nurses perceive that they are being treated with respect (Laschinger & Finegan, 2005).

> **LEADERSHIP TIP**
>
> As a nurse leader, you can ask for cultural diversity education to address issues of generational diversity, and you can teach ways to confront disrespectful behavior.

Other Conflict Approaches

Other ways to deal with conflict and even prevent it are:

- Acknowledge conflict so it can be resolved before it escalates.
- Develop conflict prevention and management guidelines so staff can refer to them.
- Focus on behavior that contributes to the conflict, not on the person.
- Identify conflicting values or beliefs that may be fueling conflict.
- Avoid postponing dealing with conflict.
- Use open body language, and display a respectful attitude.
- Develop efficient reporting systems to help nurses manage conflict before it escalates.
- Allow concerns to be raised at team meetings.
- If you're a manager, adopt an open-door policy, and take actions to make a fair workplace environment (Stroeder, Znaniecki, & Brennerman, 2006).
- When you're at fault, give the other persons what they want or request.
- Strive to understand the problem from all viewpoints.
- Work with other parties to create a solution that meets everyone's needs.
- Work toward a win-win solution for all involved, or at least achieve a middle ground where everyone involved gives and gets a little.
- Always use tactful messages—for example, "I have a problem, can you help me?" "I need your help with . . ." "I feel this way about . . ." (Johnson, 1993).

Specific suggestions for dealing with difficult situations appear in **Box 8-2**.

BOX 8-2 SUGGESTIONS FOR DEALING WITH DIFFICULT SITUATIONS

Verbally Abusive Individuals

- Encourage a more relaxed situation by asking those involved to sit down and discuss the problem.
- Encourage people to vent their emotions by using open-ended questions ("Tell me what you're upset about"), but set rules ("No swearing, cursing, or attacking, please").
- Stand up for yourself ("I've listened to your views; now please listen to mine").
- Maintain eye contact, and hold your ground; bullies often back down and become friends when someone stands up to them.
- Focus on solving a problem, not the person's behavior ("What do you hope to accomplish; what are your goals?" or, in a group, "Does anyone else feel the way _____ does?").
- Avoid getting in between the aggressive person and a third party, and avoid counterattacking. Stay focused on solving the problem, not on group dynamics.
- Relay your perceptions of people's behavior and its effect on others in a neutral, nonjudgmental way.
- Empathize with others' needs ("I hear what you're saying and what you're asking for").
- When you understand an inkling of the other person's motivations, voice them ("I wonder if you're upset about . . ." or "Do you think _____ is affecting you?").
- State your objections to the other person's behavior, and request that he or she stop ("I don't like verbal abuse; please stop it").
- Never remain silent on an issue you disagree with; at least say, "I disagree with that last statement."

Naysayers

- State the worst possible thing that could happen, and ask, "What would you do if that happened?" (This demonstrates that even the worst-case scenario is controllable.)
- Respond positively to any valid reservations.
- Identify the rewards that naysayers will miss out on if they don't come on board.
- Be prepared to replace these team members if they still refuse.

Those Who Speak without Data to Back Them Up

- State the correct facts.
- Provide alternative opinions and perceptions ("Here's a new survey that shows . . ." or "A new study shows that . . .").
- Have individual meetings; without an audience, this behavior often ends.
- Never suggest that you may be wrong, but be sure that you have your facts right.
- Request proof for assertions and allegations that you believe are false.

Procrastinators

- Help procrastinators get started by having a task for them to work on.
- Develop solid reporting and follow-up procedures to track progress.
- Identify omissions, misinformation, and clues of problem areas.
- Never accept excuses.
- Follow up on any performance difficulties until work is back on track.

For All Problem Situations

- Reward high achievers by letting them mentor low achievers.

Source: Based on the ideas of Bramson (1981); Johnson (1993); and Keating (1984).

Summary

This chapter has focused on conflict in the workplace and the nurse leader's role. There is no appropriate or inappropriate strategy to deal with conflict, but detecting symptoms of conflict and adopting the most effective behavior to that specific situation is essential in nursing units (Vivar, 2006).

Key Term Review

- **Analytical problem solving** is a social-psychological approach to dealing with protracted conflicts that is based on the human needs theory of conflict.
- **Conflict** is a normal occurrence and a multidimensional construct whose antecedents are individual, interpersonal, and/or organizational. Conflict can be either beneficial or detrimental, and either internal or external.
- **Conflict transformation** theory suggests that people, events, and relationships are altered by a conflict but that destructive consequences can be prevented by transforming perceptions of issues, action, and other people or groups to improve mutual understanding.
- **Distributive negotiation** is focused on each party winning as many concessions as possible; this can result in a win-lose situation.
- **Empowerment** means increasing the skills of all involved to make better decisions for themselves by learning how to clarify their goals, to find out about resources and options, and to choose their preferences.
- The **human needs theory of conflict** suggests that people are driven to fulfill fundamental human needs for safety, security, love, a sense of belonging to a group, self-esteem, and attaining their goals.
- **Integrative negotiation** is focused on parties discovering solutions that embody mutual self-interest; this can result in a win-win situation.
- **Interpersonal conflict** can occur when two or more individuals are involved and one perceives opposition from the other.
- **Intrapersonal conflict** can occur when an individual has two opposing goals.
- **"I" statements** can halt defensive and hostile escalation because they tend to invoke trust and create space for the parties to explore their unacknowledged feelings.
- The **Kupperschmidt model of multigenerational conflict** explains the challenges faced by nurses who work side by side with colleagues from a variety of generational cohorts and value systems.
- **Wehr's model for conflict mapping** includes the context of the conflict, parties involved, causes and consequences of the conflict, values and beliefs, goals and interests, dynamics, functions, and any regulations or rules that affect the conflict.
- **"You" statements,** such as "You aren't really listening to me," are intrusive, blaming, or attacking.

Leadership Development Exercises

- **Leadership Development Exercise 8-1**

Use Wehr's conflict assessment for at least one real or hypothetical situation.

■ Leadership Development Exercise 8-2
Identify Almost's antecedents and consequences of conflict for at least one real or hypothetical situation.

■ Leadership Development Exercise 8-3
Observe staff members at work, and determine which of Kupperschmidt's four generations each belongs to and possible areas of conflict. Give a rationale for your findings.

■ Leadership Development Exercise 8-4
Pick a real or hypothetical conflict situation, and describe how Maslow's theory of fundamental human needs relates to it.

■ Leadership Development Exercise 8-5
Identify the five areas of Lambourne's model of reconciliation, and explain how you could use them to end a conflict.

■ Leadership Development Exercise 8-6
Describe a real or hypothetical situation and how you'd apply Lederach's transformation theory to it.

■ Leadership Development Exercise 8-7
Choose a real or hypothetical conflict situation, and try out at least two approaches to conflict resolution, management, or transformation with a classmate, staff member, or friend. Write up your findings, and share them with the class.

Advanced Leadership Development Exercises

■ Leadership Development Exercise 8-8
Teach conflict resolution skills to two clients, staff on a nursing unit, or a group of colleagues using at least two of the methods presented in this chapter.

■ Leadership Development Exercise 8-9
Write up your findings from teaching conflict resolution skills, and make them the basis for a class assignment.

Alternate exercise: Use your findings to prepare a paper suitable for submission for publication.

■ Leadership Development Exercise 8-10
Formulate a problem statement for a nursing project related to some aspect of conflict.

■ **Leadership Development Exercise 8-11**

Design a research project related to some aspect of conflict.

References

Almost, J. (2006). Conflict within nursing work environments: Concept analysis. *Journal of Advanced Nursing, 53*(4), 444–453.

Amodeo, J., & Wentworth, J. (1995). Self-revealing communication: A vital bridge between two worlds. In J. Steward (Ed.), *Bridges not walls* (6th ed.). New York: McGraw-Hill.

Augsburger, D. (1973). *Caring enough to confront.* Glendale, CA: Regal Books.

Blake, R. R., & Mouton, J. S. (1964). *The managerial grid.* Houston, TX: Gulf.

Bramson, R. M. (1981). *Coping with difficult people.* New York: Dell.

Burgess, G., & Burgess, H. (1997). Analytic problem-solving. *Conflict Information Consortium.* Retrieved September 19, 2007, from http://www.colorado.edu/conflict /transform/apsall.htm

Burgess, H. (1997).Transformative mediation. *Conflict Information Consortium.* Retrieved September 19, 2007, from http://www.colorado.edu/conflict/transform/tmall.htm

Bush, R. A. B., & Folger, J. P. (1996). *The promise of mediation.* San Francisco: Jossey-Bass.

Chasin, R., Herzig, M., Roth, S., Chasin, L., Becker, C., & Stains, R. J. (1996). From diatribe to dialogue on divisive public issues. *Mediation Quarterly, 13*(4), 323–344.

Clark, C. C. (2003). *Group leadership skills.* New York: Springer.

Johnson, R. S. (1993). *ASQC total quality management series: Vol. 1. TQM: Leadership for the quality transformation.* Milwaukee, WI: ASQC Quality Press.

Kagan, J., & Gall, S. B. (1998). *Encyclopedia of childhood & adolescence.* Farmington Hills, MI: Thomas Gale.

Keating, C. J. (1984). *Dealing with difficult people.* New York: Paulist Press.

Kelman, H. C. (1997). Group processes in the resolution of international conflicts. *American Psychologist, 52*(3), 212–220.

Kupperschmidt, B. R. (2006). Addressing multigenerational conflict: Mutual respect and carefronting as strategy. *Online Journal of Issues in Nursing, 11*(2). Retrieved April 24, 2007, from http://www.medscape.com/viewarticle/536481

Lambourne, W. (2004). Post-conflict peace-building: Meeting human needs for justice and reconciliation. *Peace, Conflict and Development, 4,* 1–23.

Laschinger, H., & Finegan, J. (2005). Using empowerment to build trust and respect in the workplace: A strategy for addressing the nursing shortage. *Nursing Economic$, 23,* 6–13.

Lederach, J. P. (1995). *Preparing for peace: Conflict transformation across cultures.* Syracuse, NY: Syracuse University Press.

Lederach, J. P. (2003). *The little book of conflict transformation.* Woodacre, CA: Good Books.

Lederach, J. P., & Maiese, M. (2003). *Underlying causes of intractable conflict.* Retrieved November 15, 2007, from http://www.beyondintractability.org/essay/transformation/

Marker, S. (2003). *Unmet human needs.* Retrieved November 15, 2007, from http://www .beyondintractability.org/essay/human_needs

Maslow, A. (1998). *Maslow on management.* New York: Wiley.

Roth, S. (1994). *Constructive conversation in the abortion debate: Use of the dialogue process.* Retrieved November 15, 2007, from http://www.colorado.edu/conflict/full_text_ search/AllCRCDocs/94-9.htm

Sanford, K. (2005). Becoming competent in confrontation. *Nursing Management, 36*, 14.

Stroeder, M. H., Znaniecki, K., & Brennerman, A. (2006). Learn through conflict. *The Standard, 31*(4), 12–16.

Vivar, C. G. (2006). Putting conflict management into practice: A nursing case study. *Journal of Nursing Management, 14*, 201–206.

Wehr, P. (1979). *Conflict regulation.* Boulder, CO: Westview Press.

Weiss, D. H. (1988, February). How to handle difficult people. *Management Solutions,* 33–38.

Delegating

CHAPTER OBJECTIVES

After reading this chapter, answering the leadership challenges, and participating in the leadership development exercises, you will be able to:

- Define delegation
- Discuss changes in healthcare delivery that make task delegation important
- Identify the essential elements of effective delegation
- Determine whether state law and facility policies permit the delegation of a specific task
- Decide when delegation is appropriate
- Discuss the procedure for delegating tasks to assistive personnel
- Analyze nursing delegation actions

Advanced nurses will be able to:

- Teach delegation skills to student nurses in an undergraduate leadership course
- Formulate a problem statement for a nursing project related to delegation
- Design a research project related to delegation

Introduction

According to an American Hospital Association survey, nearly all hospitals (97%) now employ unlicensed assistive personnel (**UAPs**), who carry titles like "nursing assistants," "nurse extenders," and "care partners." So no matter where you work, the use of this kind of worker is apt to increase as hospitals act to preserve their profits (Parkman, 1996). As a result, you will need to know how to delegate tasks effectively.

You may want to do all client care yourself, but the reality of the situation in many facilities is that delegation is a necessity. Because delegating is an expected professional nursing activity, begin to think about the many benefits of assigning appropriate tasks to UAPs. Effective delegation can free you to do what nurses do—make judgments about clients and coordinate their care (Anderson, Twibell, & Siela, 2006). This chapter will provide you with the information you need to practice safely while delegating tasks to UAPs.

To prepare you to delegate tasks to UAPs before you face the situation on a hospital unit, read the Leadership in Action vignette that follows, answer the questions you'll find throughout this chapter, and complete the leadership development exercises at the end of the chapter.

LEADERSHIP IN ACTION

It's a busy evening, and you're assigned to care for eight clients. Because your unit is short staffed, Ray, a nursing assistant, has been floated from another department to help you. Although you've worked with Ray before, you still feel uneasy delegating tasks to him because you're not sure that he has the skills and theory to make decisions about any of your clients. You're not sure which of the eight clients to delegate to Ray and how often you need to check on his progress. You're not even sure what the legal ramifications are if he makes a mistake and harms one of the clients. You wish there were more nurses on the unit so you could double-check your delegation decisions with them. As a result, you do most of the care for all eight clients yourself.

LEADERSHIP CHALLENGE   How would you evaluate your decision to do most of the care for all eight clients yourself?

The American Nurses Association (ANA, 1995) defines **delegation** as "transferring responsibility for the performance of an activity . . . while retaining accountability for the outcome." Accountability means being able to explain your actions and results. Responsibility means completing the task at an acceptable level.

Healthcare Changes and Delegation

According to the National Council of State Boards of Nursing (NCSBN) and the ANA, the escalating shortage of nurses, the greater acuity of clients, technological advances, and the increased complexity of therapies all contribute to changes in the healthcare environment. Because of these changes, RNs will be expected to work with assistive personnel and be able to delegate, assign, and supervise them (NCSBN & ANA, 2006).

> **KEY TERM**
>
> **Delegation** is "transferring responsibility for the performance of an activity . . . while retaining accountability for the outcome (ANA, 1995).

Both the NCSBN and the ANA believe that mastering the skill and art of delegation is a "critical step on the pathway to nursing excellence and, when used appropriately, can result in safe and effective nursing care" (NCSBN & ANA, 2006).

Some of the problems you may face when attempting to delegate tasks are because of the changes that have occurred in work settings. Since fewer full-time RNs may be on the unit and part-time nursing personnel are often hired, continuity of care may be compromised. As a new and inexperienced nurse, your care may focus on the details of procedures while working within a small number of paradigms. Mentors may not be available because clinical nurse specialists and more-senior nurses have been downsized. Even more experienced nurses may be confronted with delegation problems because they may assume that UAPs make the same complex assumptions about clients as they do (Boucher, 1998).

LEADERSHIP CHALLENGE Now that you know what the ANA and NCSBN think about delegating tasks, go back and reevaluate your choice in the Leadership in Action vignette to do most or all of the nursing tasks yourself.

Guidelines for Delegation

The ANA (2005) provided guidelines for delegation, recommending that nurses engage in a critical-thinking process before delegating care responsibilities to assistive personnel. Questions you will need to answer before delegating a task include:

- Will the client receive quality nursing care if the task is delegated?
- Should the task be delegated?
- How much supervision will the person doing the task require?
- Is the person to whom the task is being delegated competent to do the task?
- Is the person functionally able to perform the task based on other assignments?
- Can the person perform the task without an adverse client occurrence?

LEADERSHIP CHALLENGE Which of these questions can you answer about Ray, the nursing assistant in the Leadership in Action vignette at the beginning of the chapter?

Conceptual Models for Delegation

When you delegate a task, you give someone else the authority to carry it out, but you remain accountable. Because you're ultimately accountable, you need a conceptual model to guide your decisions to delegate.

One conceptual model for delegation is called "the rights of delegation." These rights are:

- *The right task.* You must be sure that the task is one that can be delegated and does not fall within the nurse's scope of practice.
- *The right person.* You must be sure that you delegate only to a person who is qualified and competent to do the job.
- *The right circumstances.* Some of the information you need to make this decision are that the task frequently recurs in the daily care of a client and that there is an established sequence of steps and a predictable outcome.
- *The right communication.* When working with assistive personnel, make sure that you are communicating clearly and concisely about the task, the objective, your expectations for the task (including any unique client requirements and characteristics), and your willingness to be available to guide and provide support. And verify that the assistant accepts the delegation and accompanying responsibility. See **Box 9-1** for ideas.
- *The right feedback/evaluation.* You must consider the healthcare status of the client, the predictability of responses and risks, the complexity of the task, and the required supervision and support (and then you need to provide that supervision and support). While the task is being completed, provide the worker with comments. The final step is to evaluate the outcome and to problem-solve about future delegation processes. Part of that evaluation includes asking the assistant whether the task was performed correctly, whether the client outcome was achieved at a satisfactory level, whether communication from you was timely and effective, what went well and what presented challenges, what the assistant learned, and whether the assistant received appropriate feedback from you (Center for American Nurses, 2006; Parkman, 1996).

LEADERSHIP CHALLENGE Use the rights of delegation and Box 9-1 to help you identify some ways to evaluate and approach the situation with Ray.

BOX 9-1   SUPERVISING UAPS AND MAINTAINING NURSING PRESENCE

When supervising UAPs, think like a UAP, and then communicate the needed information. and be sure to maintain a nursing presence. Steps to take include:

- Anticipate clinical problems that could be encountered by a UAP.
- Think of these problems as cues to help you organize your communication. For example, if you plan to delegate ambulation, what client cues does the UAP need to watch for? Postural hypotension might be one. In a diabetic client, signs of hypoglycemia or shock might be important. Signs of postoperative bleeding would be important for postoperative clients, and so on.
- Develop a clear statement of what the task entails and what outcome you expect from the UAP. You could even write this down on an index card (including important observations that the UAP needs to make) and hand it to the UAP as a reminder of what to watch for.
- Clarify what you expect. Use a tone of voice that says, "This is important, and I expect you to follow through." (You can read from the card if you like.) Be specific in your communication. Say, "Please take Mrs. Albert's temperature right away so we can get packed red cells from the blood bank"—not just, "Please take Mrs. Albert's temperature." Say, "Let me know if Mr. George's blood glucose is above 240"—not just, "Let me know if Mr. George's blood glucose is too high." By specifying the why of your request, you will teach the reason behind the nursing action and more likely receive a positive response.
- Ask UAPs to sign a specific assignment sheet, and/or ask them to repeat back to you what you've just assigned them to do.

- Give a specific time that you will be checking back to evaluate the UAP's performance; make sure that you check back at the agreed-upon time.
- When you check back, find out exactly what has not been accomplished. Provide praise and direction as needed, and always thank the UAP. If the job was not accomplished well, talk to the UAP in private to identify whether inadequate training, a lack of preparation, or an inability to prioritize tasks may be the reason why the UAP did not accomplish the task well. Reiterate why the task is done in a certain way and the benefit for the client. Work out a plan with the UAP for the assignment to be completed.
- Listen carefully to what UAPs say about clients; ask specific questions to learn what you need to know. Your questions will train UAPs to watch for what is important.
- To maintain a nursing presence and build trust, take minireports throughout a shift, and make frequent rounds. Such actions allow you to make your own observations, to supervise UAPs, and to provide a supportive presence for them. Be consistent in word and action; it is the hallmark of trust building.
- Document carefully when you run into problems with a UAP. This will protect you from being sued if a client is harmed by an assistant's actions.
- Remember: Being a leader includes teaching management skills to others so they can learn to be effective.

Source: Adapted from Boucher (1998); Clark (2003); and Parkman (1996).

Another conceptual model for delegation is the nursing process. Delegation shares some common facets with the nursing process, such as assessing, planning, implementing, and evaluating care. After assessing the client and planning care, identify which tasks someone else can perform, and assign and supervise the performance of these tasks. Once the care has been implemented by the nursing assistant, evaluate whether the assistant performed the task properly and whether he or she achieved the planned outcome (Parkman, 1996).

While models can help you understand the delegation process, only your state's nurse practice act and other policies can provide the information you need about what to delegate.

Determining Legal and Facility Delegation Policies

Before delegating a task, you must be familiar with your state laws and hospital policies. In the section defining nursing practice, you will find aspects of care, such as physical assessment and care planning, that belong only to the nurse. Other, more-specific skills, such as wound care, are not delegable. Most states may also identify the RN's actions in providing indirect care by delegating tasks and supervising their completion.

You can also consult your state board of nursing rulings. It can often tell you what can be legally delegated and what cannot. It may also provide job descriptions. According to Parkman (1996), state regulations and nursing board rules dictate that a nursing assistant or other UAP cannot be directly assigned to a group of clients, even though assignment sheets or boards may do so.

Legally, nurses who delegated tasks appropriately based on hospital policy and who followed up and evaluated the UAP's work correctly were not found liable when lawsuits arose (Anderson, Twibell, & Siela, 2006).

Job descriptions for UAPs should be available at your institution. These descriptions usually provide specifics of what UAPs can and cannot do (e.g., take vital signs, position clients, or even gather supplies for a dressing change). UAPs may not always be familiar with what they can do in your setting, so do not assume they are. Parkman (1996) also suggests reviewing policies and procedure skill requirements for specific treatments, the supervision needed, and the protocol for reporting problems or incidents. Also be familiar with standards of care for client safety, including infection control.

Typically, a task that you can delegate is one that does not require nursing judgment (e.g., measuring urine output or vital signs). But even that is not set in stone. UAPs may be assigned to take vital signs on someone who is recovering well from elective surgery, but you may want to take vital signs on a critically ill client because you are more apt to detect a downturn in that client's condition (Parkman, 1996).

Never delegate tasks that require monitoring chest pain or other complex procedures. Even if your hospital allows you to delegate ambulating a client, only you can decide whether a specific UAP can ambulate a specific client.

Your nurse practice act probably prohibits you from delegating initial assessments, discharge planning, health education, care planning, triage, and the interpretation of assessment data (Anderson, Twibell, & Siela, 2006).

Remember that UAPs are not trained to see a client within a specific context and know the significance of what they observe. They do not possess the critical-thinking ability that you do. They receive training for only a few weeks to a few months. They report observations; they cannot analyze the meaning of what they report. For example, they can record and report the amount of urinary output but not grasp the significance of decreased output (Boucher, 1998).

> **LEADERSHIP TIP**
>
> A general rule for delegation: do not delegate the assessment, planning, and evaluation steps of the nursing process.

Learning how to keep a nursing presence with clients while delegating simple and repetitive tasks to UAPs will require creative thinking and will be an ongoing challenge. The more you practice, the better you will become at delegation.

Determining When Delegation Is Appropriate

Delegation may be appropriate under the following two conditions:

1. You have assessed the client and have assured yourself that the task you wish to delegate does not require skilled nursing care. Only you can look at a client and use your critical-thinking skills to judge spiritual needs, emotional state, cognitive function, clinical condition, and physiological status.

2. You have assessed the UAP's ability to perform. The more stable the client, the more likely you can delegate aspects of care. There are specific questions that you can ask UAPs to determine their ability, including:

   - Have you been trained to do this task?
   - Have you ever performed this task with a client?
   - Have you ever completed this task unsupervised?

- How confident are you about performing this task correctly?
- What problems have you encountered when completing this task in the past? (Anderson, Twibell, & Siela, 2006)

If you are still not sure, you can demonstrate the procedure and request that the UAP does a demonstration. You can also consult with a senior nurse or your immediate supervisor. Be assertive about obtaining a consultation if you are unsure. Take notes on the conversation, including the date and time of consultation. Be sure to keep a copy.

If you're new to the idea of delegating or prefer to remain in charge of client care, see **Box 9-2.**

BOX 9-2   SIGNS OF DIFFICULTY IN DELEGATING TASKS

If you notice any of these signs in yourself, you may have difficulty delegating tasks:
- Always being very busy
- Needing to be three places at once
- Rushing from crisis to crisis
- Difficulty making and scheduling appointments with others
- Believing you're the only one who can do the task correctly

If you're not the designated leader, you may notice the above signs in the unit leader, and additionally:
- Team breakdown (the team falls apart when the leader is not there)
- Statements from the leader such as, "I'm so busy, I don't have time to do what I need to do."

Source: Adapted with permission from *Group Leadership Skills*, 2003, by C.C. Clark, New York: Springer Publishing Company.

LEADERSHIP CHALLENGE For what procedures could you set up a demonstration for a UAP? Where would you conduct the demonstration? Give a rationale for your answer.

Preparing UAPs

Preparation of UAPs varies widely by state. Competency-based training programs with checklist evaluations have shown positive results. Using a checklist can not only verify what UAPs are capable of doing but also bolster your confidence in a UAP's skill (Lugo, 2007).

Some suggestions for delegating duties to UAPs include:

- Assess client needs and UAP knowledge and skill level.
- Identify tasks that can safely be delegated.
- Prioritize tasks, and provide a time frame for completion.
- Communicate with UAPs, and encourage them to ask questions.
- Evaluate progress toward goals, and give feedback.
- Revise plans as client needs change. (Lugo, 2007)

Explaining Assistive Personnel's Role to Clients

Clients and their families need information about their care and who will be working with them. They also need to know who is a nurse and who is not. You are responsible for naming the types of caregivers on your unit (Anderson, Twibell, & Siela, 2006).

Use simple terms. For example, you could say, "Hello, Mr. Hanson. My name is _____and I'm a registered nurse. I'll be overseeing your care until _____a.m./p.m. My nursing assistant, Ray, will be checking your vital signs and checking your urine. If you have any discomfort or any questions, please ask Ray to let me know. We work as a team, but I have primary responsibility for your care."

Summary

In summary, use the following steps to delegate tasks to assistive personnel:

- Check your state nurse practice act for delegation information.
- Check state law and facility policy to find out which tasks lie within the scope of your practice and which tasks are delegable.
- Assess the client, and evaluate current needs.
- Assess the UAP's abilities, and answer his or her questions. (Anderson, Twibell, & Siela, 2006)

Then ask yourself these questions:

- Can I supervise the UAP?
- Would another nurse delegate this task?
- Have I communicated clearly to the UAP? (Anderson, Twibell, & Siela, 2006)

If you answered no to any of those last items, you are not ready to delegate. Go back to the first list, and complete those steps until you can answer yes to the final three questions.

Key Term Review

- **Delegation** is "transferring responsibility for the performance of an activity . . . while retaining accountability for the outcome" (ANA, 1995).
- **UAPs** are unlicensed assistive personnel, such as nursing assistants.

Leadership Development Exercises

- **Leadership Development Exercise 9-1**

Look up your nurse practice act, and find out what tasks you can delegate to UAPs.

- **Leadership Development Exercise 9-2**

Look up hospital policies where you are a student. Find job descriptions for UAPs.

- **Leadership Development Exercise 9-3**

Consult your state board of nursing rulings about what can be delegated. Also see whether it provides job descriptions for UAPs.

- **Leadership Development Exercise 9-4**

For each of the following client conditions, formulate a statement to delegate an associated task to a UAP:

   a. Dehydration
   b. Depression
   c. Uncontrolled diabetes
   d. Parkinson's
   e. Abdominal surgery
   f. Bacterial pneumonia
   g. Congestive heart failure
   h. Labor and delivery
   i. Chronic pain
   j. Bipolar disorder
   k. Urinary tract infection
   l. Asthma

- **Leadership Development Exercise 9-5**

   a. Role-play with at least three other students the delegation statements you developed in Leadership Development Exercise 9-4.
   b. Ask for feedback, using Box 9-1 as your guide.

■ **Leadership Development Exercise 9-6**

You are going to introduce yourself and a UAP to a client.

   a. What exactly would you say?
   b. Role-play with at least two other students.
   c. Obtain feedback from the other students.

■ **Leadership Development Exercise 9-7**

The UAP you're working with does not follow through on the special skin care regime for clients with spinal cord injuries.

   a. What do you do and say?
   b. Role-play with at least three other students.
   c. Obtain feedback on what you said, and repeat role-playing, if necessary.

Advanced Leadership Development Exercises

■ **Leadership Development Exercise 9-8**

Teach delegation skills to student nurses in an undergraduate leadership course.

■ **Leadership Development Exercise 9-9**

Formulate a problem statement for a nursing project related to delegation.

■ **Leadership Development Exercise 9-10**

Design a research project related to delegation.

References

American Nurses Association. (1995). Position statement on registered nurse utilization of assistive personnel. *American Nurse, 25*(2), 7–8.

American Nurses Association. (2005). *Principles for delegation.* Silver Spring, MD: Author.

Anderson, P. S., Twibell, R. S., & Siela, D. (2006). Delegating without doubts. *American Nurse Today, 1*(3), 54–57.

Boucher, M. A. (1998). Delegation alert! *American Journal of Nursing, 98*(2), 26–33.

Center for American Nurses. (2006). *Registered nurse utilization of nursing assistive personnel: Statement for adoption.* Retrieved May 2, 2007, from http://www.centerfor americannurses.org/positions/finalassistivepersonnel.pdf

Clark, C. C. (2003). *Holistic assertiveness skills for nurses: Empower yourself and others!* New York: Springer.

Lugo, N. R. (2007, May 7). For high-quality care, team up with techs. *Nursing Spectrum,* 36–37.

National Council of State Boards of Nursing & American Nurses Association. (2006). *Joint statement on nursing delegation.* Retrieved May 2, 2007, from https://www.ncsbn .org/1056.htm

Parkman, C. A. (1996). Delegation, are you doing it right? *American Journal of Nursing, 96*(9), 43–48.

Acting Legally, Ethically, and Politically

CHAPTER OBJECTIVES

After reading this chapter, answering the leadership challenges, and participating in the leadership development exercises, you will be able to:

- Discuss legal issues that impact nurse leaders
- Describe the relationship between legal, ethical, and political issues
- Discuss legal issues that impact the nursing profession
- Debate ethical issues affecting nursing practice

Advanced nurses will be able to:

- Teach legal, ethical, and political skills to student nurses in an undergraduate leadership course
- Formulate a problem statement for a nursing project related to a legal, ethical, or political issue
- Design a research project related to a legal, ethical, or political issue

Introduction

Law is a result of the minimum level of shared values or ethics of a community of people—in this case, nurses. Nursing law is specific to every state and is published in nurse practice acts (Trott, 1998).

> **KEY TERM**
>
> **Law** is a result of the minimum level of shared values or ethics of a community of people.

> **KEY TERM**
>
> When working as a **client advocate**, a nurse leader supports professional nursing goals that benefit consumers even when those goals conflict with institutional or medical priorities or the leader's personal ethics.

Law and ethics are related. Nurses may act in ways that are legal but not ethical. Both law and ethics are related to politics. Nurses may believe that politics conflicts with ethical principles.

A significant part of a nurse leader's responsibilities is to act as a **client advocate.** In that capacity, a nurse leader may have a duty to support professional nursing goals that benefit consumers even when those goals are not in agreement with institutional or medical priorities or the leader's personal ethics (Des Jardin, 2001).

Political-ethical conflicts can mean choosing between client care, your job, and your personal ideals. You may never have considered it your place to challenge the existing structure of health care or the rules guiding that system, but supporting political action sometimes entails demanding a change in the present system. Often, the individual client takes precedence over society as a whole, but could there be times when you support social interventions over one person's needs?

This chapter examines dilemmas that nurse leaders and managers may face and provides guidelines for thought and action related to legal, ethical, and political approaches in leadership situations.

LEADERSHIP IN ACTION

Laurel R., a director of nursing, learns that Sarah R., a young nurse had falsified narcotics records. Sarah R, a new graduate, was terrified: she thought that she had made a mistake in the dosage of a narcotic and that she didn't fully inform the client about the drug's risks. Sarah refused to take a drug screen, even though she hadn't taken the narcotics. She stated that she would rather leave nursing than be caught up in a scandal. (She'd named the client in an e-mail after promising not to disclose the client's prior status as a drug addict and feared that information might come out.)

This incident occurred in a state where rules of administrative procedure for the board of nursing held that a nurse could be disciplined for refusing to take a "for cause" drug screen. Usually, a nurse would not be disciplined in this situation unless random screening was part of facility policy.

Laurel tried to weigh the various facets of the situation. Even though she didn't know all the particulars of the case, she believed the nurse might actually leave nursing. The administrative code requires licensees to report illegal, substandard, unethical, unsafe, or incompetent nursing practice to the board of nursing. Laurel knew this, but she reasoned that the client suffered no harm as a result of the Sarah's action and finally decided against reporting the situation to the board of nursing.

LEADERSHIP CHALLENGE Should Laurel or Sarah receive disciplinary action? Provide a justification for your answer.

Falsification of records is a serious infraction, and the failure to report by a director of nursing (DON) like Laurel would warrant disciplinary action (Eddins, 2004). Sarah should have probably consulted with Laurel or at least talked with someone with more nursing experience and knowledge before falsifying the records. That could have prevented the problem. Sending an e-mail to a novice colleague about the client only added to the problem.

Nurse leaders like this DON can be placed in difficult positions. They must find a comfortable place between overlooking infractions of the law and losing their own license (Eddins, 2004).

Legal Issues for Nurse Leaders

Legal issues of interest to nurse leaders include standard of care, scope of practice, liability and negligence, informed consent, confidentiality, and malpractice.

Standard of Care

A different **standard of care** or conduct applies to nurses than to the public. Once you take care of a client, any future inter-action between the two of you now falls in the category of a professional relationship. This means you must speak, write, and act legally, ethically, and responsibly. This applies wherever care is provided, including classrooms where nursing approaches are taught (Hutchinson, 1997).

> **KEY TERM**
>
> **Standard of care** means a professional nurse must speak, write, and act legally, ethically, and responsibly.

Scope of Practice

Your state nurse practice act defines **scope of practice,** or what you can and cannot do in your state. Nurse practice acts define three categories of nurses—LVNs, RNs, and APNs—and their functions. You must read your nurse practice act to find out what actions are allowed. It is especially important that you know what is acceptable practice in terms of diagnosis and treatment. There is another reason to keep up to date on your state nurse practice act: as a nurse leader or manager responsible for supervising other employees, you need to know the distinctions in practice for various levels of nurses to monitor against potential liability.

> **KEY TERM**
>
> **Scope of practice** is spelled out in state nurse practice acts and must be carefully monitored to reduce potential liability.

> **KEY TERM**
>
> **Liability** means that your actions or words caused harm to a client.

> **KEY TERM**
>
> **Negligence** means that you did not act as another reasonable professional with your training, skills, and experience would.

Liability and Negligence

As a nurse leader, you are responsible for your actions and words. If either your actions or your words cause harm to a client, you can be held **liable** in a court of law. In addition, you can be held **negligent** if you do not act as another reasonable professional with equivalent training, skills, and experience would (Hutchinson, 1997).

LEADERSHIP CHALLENGE Is the DON liable or negligent in the Leadership in Action vignette at the beginning of the chapter? What about the nurse who gave the medication? Give a rationale for your answer.

> **KEY TERM**
>
> **Informed consent** means that clients fully understand a treatment and its benefits and risks before agreeing that it be done.

Informed Consent

Informed consent means clients fully understand any treatment and its benefits, including any risks or side effects, before agreeing that it be done. Options related to the treatment must be fully explained as well. Hospitals usually require that clients sign a general consent for standard nursing procedures and then sign for any specific treatments, allowing them to withdraw consent at any time (Hutchinson, 1997).

Confidentiality

Confidentiality means that you, as nurse a leader, do not disclose information about clients. If you read a chart, look up results on a computer, talk to a client, or discuss the client with another provider, you should not share information; you should maintain confidentiality. Confidentiality issues between nurses or between a nurse and other healthcare professional may also apply. Potential liability can be reduced by providing access to client data on a need-to-know basis. At all times, clients have a right to copies of their healthcare records, although they may be charged a copying fee.

As of 1996, when the Health Insurance Portability and Accountability Act was passed, healthcare facilities must provide clients with a documented notice of privacy rights, explaining how their healthcare records will be used or shared with other entities. (Find more information on the act at http://www.cms.hhs.gov/HIPAAGenInfo.)

Confidentiality also applies to incident reports. They should contain pertinent care information only—no finger-pointing and no interpretation. This will also reduce liability.

LEADERSHIP CHALLENGE What, if any, confidential issues may have been involved in the DON's decision in the Leadership in Action vignette at the beginning of this chapter? Give a rationale for your answer.

Malpractice

Nurses have a duty to act in a specific way toward clients. Malpractice occurs when that standard of care is breached, causing an injury to a client that would not have occurred had the nurse acted in a reasonable and prudent fashion (Trott, 1998).

Legal Trends

According to Trott (1998), major trends that affect healthcare settings include:

- *Documentation of change in a client's condition.* The process—what you do and say in a nursing situation—is of the utmost importance and must be clearly represented in written client records. Two parts of the client assessment process to focus on are documentation and communication. Remember that no part of client assessment can be delegated. It is your responsibility to always personally check out any change in a client's condition, and then clearly chart what you found.
- *Client falls.* Client falls are a leading source of litigation. Important sources of information involve the client's previous assessment, the time frame before the fall, client mentation, and procedures or medication that may have changed the client's mental status. When assessing the client's risk for a fall, a key factor in legal cases is the RN's assessment and what was done to prevent the fall. Some questions to ask include: Did you ensure the client received assistance while getting out of bed and walking? Did you ensure the client wore non-slip footwear? Did you assess strength, lack of dizziness, and ability to stand and move prior to allowing a client to walk without a walker or wheelchair?
- *Physician communication.* Communication between nurses and physicians can be problematic in many instances. Talking over the phone creates a high level of liability exposure. Once your communication with a physician ends, you must document the event and the conversation (Trott, 1998). If you haven't heard a particular complaint from a client before, notify the physician, keep the physician informed of the client's status, make sure you fully understand instructions, and document everything. Never ignore a reported symptom (Eskreis, 1998).

Eskreis (1998) cites the following common legal pitfalls in nursing:

- *Medication errors.* Medication errors kill at least one person a day and thousands each year. As a nurse, you're not protected simply because you followed a physician's order. You remain accountable for your own actions. If you're unfamiliar with a medication, consult *Physician's Desk Reference* or a pharmacist, your supervisor, or the physician who ordered the drug. Pay special attention to the dosage, the potential adverse effects, and the route of administration. (Many medication errors occur when giving oral drugs by IV; in those situations, the drugs are administered at 100 or more times the suggested amount.)
- *Improper use of equipment.* Always read brochures and directions that accompany equipment before using it, and obtain necessary orientation or training. If the equipment appears to be defective or you have a sense that it is not operating correctly, demand that it be inspected before use. Monitor clients using equipment to ensure that it is operating as expected. Take special care when the client is especially young, sedated, anesthetized, or lacking body sensation/interpretation. Burns are common, as are lacerations.
- *Failure to remove foreign objects.* Operating room nurses are most apt to be accused of failing to remove a foreign object. Abide by hospital policy and procedure to protect yourself against liability.
- *Failure to provide sufficient monitoring.* In addition to carefully and regularly monitoring clients' physical status, nurses are also responsible for monitoring their psychological status. If you fail to document such monitoring and the client sustains an injury, you can be charged with neglect. For example, if a client is at risk for aspiration, lung and respiratory status must be assessed and documented, including the client's ability to swallow and response to medication, as well as how often assessments were made.
- *Failure to communicate.* Communication is essential to safeguarding client well-being and must be thoroughly documented. If you are not familiar with a particular somatic complaint, notify a physician and document the information. Nurses can fail to communicate not only with physicians but also with clients and other healthcare professionals. In each case, failure to communicate could result in legal repercussions. Use your communication skills to communicate clearly and often with clients and other healthcare staff.

LEADERSHIP CHALLENGE Which of those pitfalls are exemplified by the following situation? A nurse was assigned to care for a client with a history of stroke and unstable angina. When the client experienced respiratory failure, the nurse called for assistance and then called a code. The client record made no indication that prescribed drugs were given that evening or that the client's physician was notified.

Eskreis (1998) suggested the following preventive procedures:

- Develop a caring, respectful, and attentive relationship with each client, including careful assessment, intervention, and documentation.
- Familiarize yourself with any equipment that is used.
- Follow physician's orders and hospital procedures unless you deem them to be detrimental, and then discuss the situation immediately with your supervisor or a member of the risk management department and document your conversation.
- Notify the physician immediately of any change in client status and document the call or conversation.

Nurse Leader Responsibility for Legal Issues

Although nurses in administration, education, and research have relationships with clients that are less direct, in assuming the responsibilities of any of these roles, you share responsibility for the care provided by those whom you supervise or instruct.

When functioning in management or administrative roles you have a particular responsibility to provide an environment that supports and facilitates appropriate assignment and delegation. This includes providing appropriate orientation to staff members, assisting less experienced nurses to develop the skills and competencies they need, and establishing policies and procedures that protect client and nurse from inappropriate assignment or delegation of nursing activities (American Nurses Association, 2001).

Some areas of legal responsibility you may encounter as a nurse leader include clear communication and documentation, corporate liability, all forms of harassment, and following the Family and Medical Leave Act and the Americans with Disabilities Act.

Communication and Documentation

Nurse leaders have a clear responsibility to educate and support their staff about communicating over the phone with physicians and clients and about appropriately documenting those conversations. Complete and thorough documentation is important because state statutes, insurance standards, and regulatory agencies (such as the Joint Commission on Accreditation of Healthcare Organizations) demand it for accreditation and reimbursement, and the client record is the physical demonstration of continuity of care (Trott, 1998).

Depending on your job description, as a nurse leader, it may be your responsibility to teach and monitor staff so that they:

- Write legibly and clearly
- Avoid defaming the client or other healthcare personnel, which only reinforces a case and makes nurses and the organization look bad from a legal/ethical viewpoint

- Include a listing of what was done to protect the client and the client's response to the intervention
- Document the client assessment and what the client told the RN
- Document all other issues, such as nurse-physician conflict, through the appropriate channels (if there are no appropriate and helpful channels, the nurse leader should develop a procedure and put it in operation, making sure that all staff know how to use it; if nurse-physician conflict is high, expect poor client outcomes [Forte, 1997])

Other Legal Responsibilities of the Nurse Leader

Other legal responsibilities nurse leaders must take on include:

1. Knowing about current legal trends, such as corporate liability for not suspending nurses or physicians who have many complaints lodged against them.
2. Encouraging nurses to speak up when they make clinical errors. More and more nurses are facing criminal charges when mistakes occur. By establishing an atmosphere of trust and learning, nurses will be more likely to take responsibility for their errors and learn from each event.
3. Having a zero-tolerance policy for all forms of harassment can also protect agencies against litigation problems.
4. Following the Americans with Disabilities Act (for more information, see **Box 10-1**) and the Family and Medical Leave Act (for more information, see **Box 10-2**) can provide nurses with support and protect the institution from law suits.
5. Practicing ethical leadership and establishing ongoing relationships with human resources and risk management can help ensure ethics and laws are followed (Trott, 1998).

KEY TERM
Nursing ethics are based on a set of values derived by the nursing profession.

Ethics and Values

Successful application of ethical decision making and action is integral to nurse satisfaction and nurse retention. As a nurse leader, you are key to helping nurses develop these skills and use them in the professional setting (Andrews, 2004).

Ethics in nursing includes making moment-to-moment decisions that are morally responsible and positive. Ethics focuses on doing more good than harm to clients (Clements & Averill, 2006). **Nursing ethics** are based on a set of values derived by the profession.

According to Trott (1998), nursing values include:

- **Beneficence:** doing good by caring for the client
- **Nonmaleficence:** doing no harm to the client

BOX 10-1   FACTS ABOUT THE AMERICANS WITH DISABILITIES ACT

The Americans with Disabilities Act (ADA) took effect July 26, 1992. It prohibits private employers, state and local governments, employment agencies, and labor unions from discriminating against qualified individuals with disabilities in job application procedures, hiring, firing, advancement, compensation, job training, and other terms, conditions, and privileges of employment. An individual with a disability is a person who fits at least one of the following conditions:

- Has a physical or mental impairment that substantially limits one or more major life activities
- Has a record of such an impairment
- Is regarded as having such an impairment

A qualified employee or applicant with a disability is an individual who, with or without reasonable accommodation, can perform the essential functions of the job in question. Reasonable accommodation may include but is not limited to:

- Making existing facilities used by employees readily accessible to and usable by persons with disabilities
- Restructuring jobs, modifying work schedules, or reassigning the person to a vacant position
- Acquiring or modifying equipment or devices; adjusting examinations, training materials, or policies; and providing qualified readers or interpreters

An employer is required to accommodate a qualified applicant's or employee's known disability if it would not impose an "undue hardship" on the business's operation. Undue hardship is defined as an action requiring significant difficulty or expense when considered in light of factors such as a company's size, financial resources, and the nature and structure of its operation. An employer is not required to lower quality or production standards to make an accommodation, nor is an employer obligated to provide personal-use items, such as glasses or hearing aids.

Medical Examinations and Inquiries

Employers may not ask job applicants about the existence, nature, or severity of a disability. Employers may, however, ask applicants about their ability to perform specific job functions. A job offer may be conditioned on the results of a medical examination—but only if the examination is required for all entering employees in similar jobs. Employee medical examinations must be job related and consistent with the employer's business needs.

Drug and Alcohol Abuse

Employees and applicants currently engaged in the use of illegal drugs are not covered by the ADA when an employer acts on the basis of such use. Tests for illegal drugs are not subject to the ADA's restrictions on medical examinations. Employers may hold illegal drug users and alcoholics to the same performance standards as other employees.

Enforcement of the ADA

The US Equal Employment Opportunity Commission (EEOC) issued regulations to enforce the provisions of Title I of the ADA on July 26, 1991. The provisions originally took effect on July 26, 1992, and covered employers with 25 or more employees. On July 26, 1994, the threshold dropped to include employers with 15 or more employees.

Source: EEOC (1997).

BOX 10-2 THE FAMILY AND MEDICAL LEAVE ACT

What Is the Family and Medical Leave Act, and to Whom Does It Apply?

(a) The Family and Medical Leave Act of 1993 (FMLA or Act) allows "eligible" employees of a covered employer to take job-protected, unpaid leave, or to substitute appropriate paid leave if the employee has earned or accrued it, for up to a total of 12 workweeks in any 12 months because of the birth of a child and to care for the newborn child, because of the placement of a child with the employee for adoption or foster care, because the employee is needed to care for a family member (child, spouse, or parent) with a serious health condition, or because the employee's own serious health condition makes the employee unable to perform the functions of his or her job. In certain cases, this leave may be taken on an intermittent basis rather than all at once, or the employee may work a part-time schedule.

(b) An employee on FMLA leave is also entitled to have health benefits maintained while on leave as if the employee had continued to work instead of taking the leave. If an employee was paying all or part of the premium payments prior to leave, the employee would continue to pay his or her share during the leave period. The employer may recover its share only if the employee does not return to work for a reason other than the serious health condition of the employee or the employee's immediate family member, or another reason beyond the employee's control.

(c) An employee generally has a right to return to the same position or an equivalent position with equivalent pay, benefits and working conditions at the conclusion of the leave. The taking of FMLA leave cannot result in the loss of any benefit that accrued prior to the start of the leave.

(d) The employer has a right to 30 days advance notice from the employee where practical. In addition, the employer may require an employee to submit certification from a health care provider to substantiate that the leave is due to the serious health condition of the employee or the employee's immediate family member. Failure to comply with these requirements may result in a delay in the start of FMLA leave. The employer may also require that an employee present a certification of fitness to return to work when the absence was caused by the employee's serious health condition. The employer may delay restoring the employee to employment without a certificate relating to the health condition that caused the employee's absence.

Source: [60 FR 2237, Jan. 6, 1995; 60 FR 16383, Mar. 30, 1995] From *What is the Family and Medical Leave Act?* U.S. Department of Labor. Retrieved May 10, 2007, from http://www.dol.gov/dol/allcfr/ESA/Title_29/Part_825/29CFR825.100.htm

- *Justice:* being fair to the client
- *Autonomy:* preserving the freedom of the client and the nurse
- *Loyalty:* keeping promises made to the client
- *Veracity:* telling the client the truth
- *Confidentiality:* not sharing what was told in private
- *Life:* treasuring the client's existence

Guidelines based on these values come from established standards of care, the nurses code of ethics, and state laws that regulate nursing practice. Legal difficulties can arise when nurses make decisions based on emotion or intuition or when their personal values clash with those professional values (Trott, 1998). For example, if you as a nurse leader hold specific religious or cultural values that differ from any of the professional values listed, you may face an ethical dilemma. There can even be conflict between the values listed. Take the leadership challenge to see how accepted values can conflict.

LEADERSHIP CHALLENGE Which value should a nurse support—autonomy or life—when a client wants to obtain an abortion or refuses care that could sustain life?

Conceptual Frameworks for Ethical Practice

Moral development is an important issue in nursing because nurses increasingly face ethical dilemmas. As a nurse leader, it is your job to help nurses attain higher levels of moral development so they can deal effectively with such dilemmas.

Many developmental psychologists use stage theories to explain moral development. Kohlberg (1981), probably the best-known theorist, developed six stages of moral development.

Stage 1 and 2 of Kohlberg's moral development are **preconventional stages**. Stage 1 is characterized by avoiding punishment and deferring to power without question; nurses who attain a moral level no higher than stage 1 are apt to do whatever anyone in power tells them to do, regardless of its effect on patient care. At stage 2, right action consists of what is satisfying to oneself or what is based on reciprocal sharing.

KEY TERM

The **preconventional stage of moral development** is exemplified by nurses who do whatever anyone in power tells them to do (stage 1) and by nurses who do what is satisfying or what is based on reciprocal sharing (stage 2).

Reciprocal sharing is the idea that "you scratch my back, and I'll scratch yours"; it is not based on loyalty, gratitude, or justice. Nurses at this development level may help clients or doctors only if they are helped in return.

The **conventional level of moral reasoning** includes stages 3 and 4. At stage 3, people choose to behave well so that others will approve of them; nurses at this level will most likely seek out approval and try to be nice to others. At stage 4, the keeping of rules, the completion of one's duty, and the maintenance of the status quo are important. Nurses at this stage are apt to give medications on the dot, not to question rules, and to live up to their job descriptions.

KEY TERM

The **conventional stage of moral reasoning** is exemplified by the nurse who seeks out approval and tries to be nice to everyone (stage 3) and the nurse who maintains the status quo (stage 4).

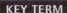

KEY TERM

The **postconventional or autonomous level of moral reasoning** is exemplified by the nurse who contracts with clients about healthcare issues (stage 5) and the nurse who acts based on logical, consistent, comprehensive, and universal ethical principles (stage 6).

Stages 5 and 6 are **postconventional or autonomous levels of moral reasoning.** Since nursing seems to be moving toward independent practice, it would seem reasonable to expect nurses to function at the postconventional level, yet many do not. At stage 5, right action is chosen after a critical examination of all the ethical factors in the situation and coming to an agreed upon action with the client....

The nurse may use a written or verbal agreement. Contracts and free agreements bind obligation. Nurses at this developmental level tend to contract with clients about healthcare issues.

At stage 6, right action is defined by individual conscience in accordance with self-chosen ethical principles based on logical comprehensiveness, universality, and consistency. Universal principles of justice, equal rights, and respect for the dignity of individuals are used as measures.

LEADERSHIP CHALLENGE According to Kohlberg's theory, what stage of moral development is the DON in the Leadership in Action vignette at the beginning of this chapter? Give a rationale for your answer.

Gilligan (1982) proposed a theory of moral development for women. Gilligan took umbrage at basing the theory on justice and guilt. From her careful interviews with women making momentous decisions in their lives, Gilligan concluded that these women thought more about the caring thing to do rather than the just thing to do.

Gilligan's five stages, which she called the "ethic of care," included:

1. *Preconventional stage.* The woman's goal is survival.
2. *Transitional stage* is from selfishness to responsibility to others.
3. *Conventional stage.* The woman recognizes that self-sacrifice is good.
4. *Transitional stage* is from goodness to truth that she is a person too.
5. *Postconventional stage.* This stage may never be attained. It's marked by the principle of nonviolence: do not hurt others or oneself.

LEADERSHIP CHALLENGE According to Gilligan's theory, what stage of moral development is the DON in the Leadership in Action vignette at the beginning of this chapter? Give a rationale for your answer.

Ethical Issues for Nurse Leaders

A survey of nurse executives (Cooper, Frank, Gouty, & Hansen, 2002) found the following ethical issues presented significantly greater problems for nurse leaders than they did for vice presidents of health organizations:

- Perceived failure of healthcare organizations to provide service of the highest quality (because nurses did not follow nursing standards, failed to provide honest information, experienced economic constraints in their departments, showed partiality toward clients or providers who were perceived to be influential, lacked knowledge or skills to competently perform their duties [reflecting the hiring of less qualified nurses because of nursing shortages and limited resources for continuing education])
- Failure of healthcare executives to effectively manage conflict between organizational and professional philosophy and standards
- Offering or soliciting payments or contributions to influence legislation, regulations, or accreditations
- Discrimination
- Drug and alcohol abuse in the workplace
- Employee theft

Being certified as a CAN or CNAA did not improve ethical responses. Those who were certified viewed failure to provide services to insurance companies as being a greater ethical problem than those who were not certified by the American Nurses Credentialing Center (ANCC). Those not credentialed by ANCC viewed employee theft as a greater ethical problem than those certified. This led Cooper, Frank, Gouty, and Hansen (2002) to question whether the current effort to put scarce resources into credentialing really mattered, at least in terms of ethics training. They concluded that putting resources into programs that focus on preparing employees to identify and deal effectively with ethical problems is a key responsibility of nurse leaders.

Principles for Ethical Leadership

Curtin (2000) proposed 10 ethical principles based on universal values and adapted to fit nurse leaders' responsibilities. Those principles appear in **Box 10-3.**

Ethical and predictable decision making and action helps nurse leaders walk the talk and establish trust and cooperation with their staff. Trust and sense of cooperation are the anchors that forestall anger and alienation, which can disrupt continuous and safe client care (Curtin, 2000).

BOX 10-3   TEN ETHICAL PRINCIPLES FOR NURSE LEADERS

1. **Frugality and therapeutic elegance:** includes promoting economy while using the right amount of resources to ensure competent care
2. **Clinical credibility through organizational competence:** requires balancing practice guidelines, peer evaluation, teaching and counseling, and policies that advance the welfare of employees and are designed to provide safe client care
3. **Providing presence:** involves promoting trusting and beneficent relations with peers, colleagues, clients, families, and the general public by communicating decisions in person and altering them as necessary
4. **Representing ethical concerns:** requires that nurse leaders make sure that nurses' concerns are heard at the highest levels of organizational decision making

5. **Loyalty:** forbids advancing one's own career by exploiting the organization
6. **Delegating ethically:** requires an act of faith and demands that nurse leaders delegate sufficient authority when delegating duties
7. **Responsible innovation:** requires that change be examined for its affect on client care and employee morale before implementation
8. **Fiduciary accountability:** ensures that clients receive safe, quality, and relevant services for their money
9. **Self-discipline:** forbids making decisions out of anger, fear, retribution, or vengeance
10. **Continuous learning:** invests time and resources to ensure continued competence of care (Curtin, 2000)

LEADERSHIP CHALLENGE Which, if any, of Curtin's ethical principles did the DON in the Leadership in Action vignette at the beginning of this chapter exemplify? Give a rationale for your answer.

Ethical Helps and Challenges

Research can provide some suggestions for dealing with ethical dilemmas. Cooper, Frank, Gouty, and Hansen (2003) found that resources reported for solving ethical dilemmas differed by position and/or work setting.

Vice presidents viewed a management philosophy that emphasized ethics and clear communication of appropriate ethical behavior by management as significantly more helpful than did directors. Participants employed by for-profit healthcare organizations (HCOs) viewed family and friends as significantly more helpful in dealing with ethical dilemmas at work than those working for non-profit HCOs. Participants who weren't credentialed viewed help from coworkers as significantly more helpful in dealing with ethical dilemmas than did participants who were credentialed.

Important challenges Cooper et al. (2003) identified included that management training programs to help nurse leaders develop skills in identifying and handling ethical challenges were needed. Another important challenge involved conflict between duty to one's employer and duty to one's employees and clients.

According to study findings, one of the best things HCOs can do is to refrain from pressuring managers and employees to compromise their own personal values. HCOs also should ensure that managers are equipped with ways to deal with their own ethical dilemmas and those of their supervisees. Ethics programs in HCOs are most successful in organizations that have three components: codes of conduct, ethics training, and ethics offices. As a result of their study, Cooper et al. (2003) suggested that preparing leaders to identify and manage ethical challenges is the responsibility of the healthcare setting.

Developing an Ethical Work Culture

Silverman (2000) suggested that to achieve organizational integrity, it's important to engage in several processes, including:

- Reexamining vision and guiding values to help employees own the final values statement and ethics program, thus ensuring commitment, rather than just compliance
- Developing an ethics infrastructure, including a code of ethics; forums that address ethics issues at each level of the organization; administrative case rounds in which corporate decisions can be displayed and argued from an ethical viewpoint; an appeals process (to encourage principled organizational dissent to some practice or policy and alignment of performance appraisals and other appraisal and reward systems with ethical matters); provision of ethics training at all levels of the organization; appointment of a high-ranking ethics officer who would ensure that ethics is a corporate priority; an organizational ethics committee that would provide a forum for ethical reflection; a strong ethical climate to support leadership; and monitoring and evaluating ethical performance

Encouraging Nurses to Participate in Ethical Decision Making

A review of the literature on nurses' participation in ethical decision making concluded that nurses play various roles, from being recognized as powerful members of a team that makes decisions to being physician surrogates with little autonomy. Dodd, Jansson, Brown-Saltzman, Shirk, and Wunch (2004) found that nurses were more likely to engage in ethical assertiveness (i.e., coach clients about questions to ask physicians about ethical choices, advocate for clients' requests about ethical issues with physicians, call ethical issues to the attention of physicians, participate in ethical deliberations, and withdraw from ethical situations unless specifically requested to participate) than ethical activism (i.e., seek written protocol to promote nurse participation in ethics deliberations, seek multidisciplinary training sessions in ethics, and educate physicians about nursing roles in ethics).

Nurses were more apt to engage in ethical assertiveness and activism if they received ethics education during nursing courses, and they more likely to do so in settings that were already receptive to their involvement. The researchers suggested that nurse leaders take action to further enhance nurse assertiveness and activism by:

- Generating administrative support for nurse involvement in ethical behaviors with clients and physicians
- Encouraging daily discussions around ethical issues
- Enhancing participation in the writing of protocols for ethics deliberations
- Ensuring that work settings are receptive to nurse participation in ethics deliberations (Dodd et al., 2004)

Political Issues

To effect change, you must often take a political stance. This section examines the importance of political action, a theory of political development, areas of political influence in which nurses can effect change, and guidelines for political action.

The Importance of Political Development

Although many nurses may believe that political action conflicts with professional practice, nurses as a group are now being encouraged to engage in political action (Albarran, 1995; Winter, 1991).

The push for nurses to take political action is understandable. After all, a significant part of every nurse's responsibility is to act as a client advocate. This goal may not always be in agreement with institutional goals, which is where political action comes in. Sources of political-ethical tension include clashes between cost-effectiveness and quality of care and between personal values and professional ethics and goals (Des Jardin, 2001).

> **KEY TERM**
>
> **Political–ethical conflict** is the pressure you feel as a result of a difference between your ethical belief system and what you are told to do by someone in a position of power.

A negative view of politics and politicians can interfere with political action and create ethical tension. **Political-ethical conflict** can result when you believe one thing is right but someone in a position of power pressures you to do something else.

Before engaging in political action, you may have to pass through one or more preparatory stages. One theorist (Wilson, 2002), tested four stages of political development developed by Cohen (1996). These stages were:

1. Understanding that political action is important
2. Using political expertise for self-interest

3. Effectively using political activism

4. Providing leadership in the political arena

The researcher found that nurses can be anywhere in the process, but they are more apt to engage in political action to advocate for the public than nonnurses (Wilson, 2002).

LEADERSHIP CHALLENGE Identify what stage of political development you are in. Give a rationale for your answer.

Guidelines for Examining Political-Ethical Dilemmas

A political-ethical dilemma may be more perceived than real. Believing that politics and nursing do not mix may be related to outdated images of fear of power and lack of knowledge about how to proceed. Even if that is the case, guidelines can help you understand when and how to get involved in political processes and determine which public policy issue takes priority (Des Jardin, 2001).

You can use the following process to examine political-ethical dilemmas and decide what to do:

- Identify the problem, including its background and associated issues.
- Choose a potential ethical conflict.
- Identify individuals who might be affected by political action.
- Explore all options and consequences of taking action.
- Proceed with confidence, knowing that you are taking unbiased, informed action.

Developing Coalitions

Coalitions are temporary groups of individuals or organizations that join together to effect change. Everyone involved must have the same need or goal, or the coalition will not be successful.

LEADERSHIP IN ACTION

Dr. Saran, a nurse leader with a PhD in nursing, was tired of the physicians referring to themselves as "doctor" but calling nurses by their first name. Every time it happened, Dr. Saran cringed and fell into an angry, depressed mood. She wasn't sure what to do about it until she brought the issue up at a local nursing meeting. One member told her to just ignore it; another said she should start introducing herself as "Dr. Saran" in meetings and appointments. Another nurse suggested that she form an empowerment committee and ask physicians and nurses to join to discuss the issue of how they could empower each other to help clients.

LEADERSHIP CHALLENGE Which approach would you choose? Give a rationale based on information in this chapter.

Negotiating

Negotiating or bargaining is the process of making trade-offs to attain an objective. To get something in a political process, it is necessary to give up something. At the start of a negotiation, the individuals involved may have radically different positions. As the negotiation proceeds, they may move closer together and find a way to compromise. Negotiators are more likely to be successful if they are well informed about the pros and cons of the opposing side.

KEY TERM

Collective bargaining is a form of negotiation regulated by state and federal labor laws and requires representation from a union or the state nurses association.

Collective bargaining is a special type of negotiation. It is regulated by state and federal labor laws (National Labor Relations Act or NLRA and the Labor Management Relations Act). Section 7 of the NLRA states that employees have the right to self-organize; to form, join, or assist labor organizations; and to bargain collectively through representatives of their own choosing (Michigan Nurses Association, 2007).

LEADERSHIP IN ACTION

Betty T., a nurse practitioner, had been working at the healthcare agency for 10 years. She had heard complaints from other nursing staff about being treated poorly by management regarding work time, salary and related pay, fringe benefits, discipline, grievance procedure, health and safety, discrimination, inservice education, continuing education, leaves of absence, holidays, management rights, layoffs, retraining and termination, staffing, professional practice committees, tuition reimbursement, mandatory overtime, and even benefits after retirement. Betty decided to initiate a collective bargaining procedure to help nurses like her obtain better treatment. The first thing she did was ask voting nurses to sign a petition to obtain formal recognition from their employer. They elected a negotiating committee and reached a tentative agreement for the membership to ratify, because of the need for mediation and the option of establishing boards of inquiry prior to a work stoppage.

Usually a representative of a union or the state nurses association must attend when collective bargaining is involved.

While collective bargaining requires progression through successively high levels of administration and ending in binding arbitration, negotiation may not.

LEADERSHIP IN ACTION

Jennifer S., a nurse leader, organized a meeting with the department director during the budget-planning process to negotiate additional training hours on legal, ethical, and political processes for her nursing staff.

LEADERSHIP CHALLENGE What obstacles might Jennifer face, and how could she overcome them? Give a specific answer and provide a rationale for your response.

Guidelines for Political Action

Many guidelines exist for public policy and political action. A major one is the Code for Nurses with Interpretive Statements (American Nurses Association, 1995). It says, "The nurse collaborates with members of the health professions and other citizens in promoting community and national efforts to meet the healthcare needs of the public." This means that as a nurse, you must make collaborative efforts outside the clinical arena to improve health care. The code goes on to state that nurses should actively participate in political arenas.

The World Health Organization (WHO) speaks of the safeguarding of health and human rights as a top responsibility. Included in its 2007 agenda is the ethical principle of equity: access to lifesaving or health-promoting interventions should not be denied for unfair reasons, including those with economic or social roots. Commitment to this principle ensures that WHO activities aimed at health development give priority to serving poor, disadvantaged, or vulnerable groups; preventing and treating chronic diseases; and using collective action to reduce health security threats because of environmental mismanagement, the way food is produced and traded, and the way antibiotics are used (or misused).

The United Nations Office of the High Commissioner for Human Rights also provides guidelines for nurses. Although you may think of war-torn countries in terms of human rights, abuses, such as elder abuse, occur in the United States in long-term settings and in the general community at large (Des Jardin, 2001). The declaration appears at http://www.unhchr.ch/udhr/lang/eng.htm and should be integrated into your nursing practice.

Political Action Strategies

From Florence Nightingale to Margaret Sanger and Lillian Wald, nurses have always been champions of activism. Although you may believe you need to focus on client care and let someone else make political decisions, ask yourself, "Who should be making decisions about needle-stick prevention, mandatory overtime, whistle-blowing, environmental hazards, part-time nurses and unlicensed assistants, faulty equipment, the nursing shortage, nursing practice, educating the public about their health and preventing illness, and incompetent healthcare workers?"

Because the American health system is in a crisis of soaring costs and epidemics of preventable disease, new strategies may be necessary. Poor health literacy contributes to many of the healthcare system's problems. One strategy is to establish an office of the national nurse. Like the surgeon general, the **national nurse** would practice at the highest political level, leading the way to public health education. Nurses calling for innovation, leadership, and inspiration are uniting behind this proposal to provide accessible health information to all Americans and reduce the incidence of preventable diseases (Mills & Schneider, 2007). For more information, go to http://www.national-nurse.blogspot.com.

KEY TERM

The **national nurse** will provide health information to all Americans to reduce the incidence of preventable disease.

As a nurse leader, you must participate in political action strategies if you hope to control your practice and practice environment. How and to what extent you do that is your choice. Choose from among the list of political strategies that appear in **Box 10-4**, and make a contract with yourself to begin pursuing your top priority today.

Summary

This chapter has explored legal, ethical, and political issues—from autonomy to beneficence to coalitions—that affect nurse leaders. Moral reasoning, informed consent, ethics, veracity, confidentiality, the national nurse, scope of practice, and collective bargaining were explored. Be sure to complete the leadership development exercises to help integrate your learning, and then move on to Part III, which focuses on advanced skills needed to creatively lead and manage.

BOX 10-4   POLITICAL STRATEGIES

Prioritize these strategies, and start working on your number one priority today.

____Serve on a nursing organization committee

____Write to elected officials about a healthcare issue

____Write a letter to the editor of a local newspaper about your healthcare views

____Assist local or national politicians or nurses who support nursing views by answering telephones, assisting with mailings, providing written support, or other ways

____Run for a local or national office

____Attend the American Nurses Association's Annual Legislative Day

____Start a Web site or e-zine to keep clients apprised of an important health issue

____Circulate a petition for some healthcare or working condition issue that's close to your heart

____Offer your services to a local hospital decision-making committee

____Join and become an active member of the League of Women Voters or the national nurse effort

____Serve on the legislative committee of a professional or environmental organization

____Join a committee of a local political organization

____Join a quality improvement, ethics, or policy committee at your workplace

____Become an informed voter; avoid listening to paid political announcements; Google the candidates, and find out what they've done in the past, not what they say they will do in the future

Key Term Review

- **Autonomy** includes preserving the freedom of the client and the nurse.
- **Beneficence** means doing good by caring for the client.
- When working as a **client advocate,** a nurse leader supports professional nursing goals that benefit consumers even when those goals conflict with institutional or medical priorities or the leader's personal ethics.
- **Coalitions** are temporary groups of individuals or organizations that join together to effect change.
- **Collective bargaining** is a form of negotiation regulated by state and federal labor laws and requires representation from a union or the state nurses association.
- **Confidentiality** means not sharing what was told in private.
- The **conventional stage of moral reasoning** is exemplified by the nurse who seeks out approval and tries to be nice to everyone (stage 3) and the nurse who maintains the status quo (stage 4).
- **Informed consent** means that clients fully understand a treatment and its benefits and risks before agreeing that it be done.
- **Justice** means being fair to the client.
- **Law** is a result of the minimum level of shared values or ethics of a community of people.
- **Liability** means that your actions or words caused harm to a client. You can be held negligent if you do not act as another reasonable professional with equivalent training, skills, and experience would (Hutchinson, 1997).
- **Life** is the value that includes treasuring the client's existence.
- **Loyalty** means keeping promises made to the client.
- The **national nurse** will provide health information to all Americans to reduce the incidence of preventable diseases.
- **Negligence** means that you did not act as another reasonable professional with your training, skills, and experience would.
- **Nonmaleficence** includes doing no harm to the client.
- **Nursing ethics** are the result of a set of values derived by the nursing profession.
- **Political-ethical conflict** can result when you believe one thing is right but someone in a position of power pressures you to do something else.
- The **postconventional or autonomous level of moral reasoning** is exemplified by the nurse who contracts with clients about healthcare issues (stage 5) and the nurse who acts based on logical, consistent, comprehensive, and universal ethical principles (stage 6).
- The **preconventional stage of moral development** is exemplified by nurses who do whatever anyone in power tells them to do (stage 1) and by nurses who do what is satisfying or what is based on reciprocal sharing (stage 2).

- **Scope of practice** is spelled out in state nurse practice acts and must be carefully monitored to reduce potential liability.
- **Standard of care** means a professional nurse must speak, write, and act legally, ethically, and responsibly.
- **Veracity** includes telling the client the truth.

Leadership Development Exercises

Leadership Development Exercise 10-1

Discuss the most ethical response to the following situations with at least three other learners, and give a rationale for your answer based on information in this chapter.

    a. A new RN who believes in information taught in class but observes a teacher breaking technique

    b. An RN who observes a physician acting in such a way that could result in a misdiagnosis

    c. A nurse leader who observes another nurse or physician displaying inappropriate behavior with a client or family member of a client

    d. A nurse leader who observes a nurse who is a friend of a physician performing procedures outside her scope of practice

Leadership Development Exercise 10-2

Go back and see if your answers were different based on whether they included an RN observer or a nurse leader observer. If they were different, give a rationale for your answers based on information in this chapter. If they were not different, explain why you believe RNs and nurse leaders should be held to the same code of ethics.

Leadership Development Exercise 10-3

    a. Choose a belief or value you hold.

    b. Write down as many ways as you can to demonstrate that value or belief.

    c. Seek opportunities for modeling your beliefs and values even when they differ from those of others.

    d. Journal about your experiences.

    e. Share what happened with at least two other nursing students or nurses.

    f. Have you considered it your place to challenge either the structure of your healthcare system or the official or unofficial rules guiding that system? Discuss with at least two other nursing students or nurses why such action may be part of a nurse's role and how the idea may create tension among nurses.

■ **Leadership Development Exercise 10-4**

a. Perform a negotiation process with a client, supervisor, supervisee, friend, or family member.
b. During the negotiation, look for the other person's point of view, and try to understand it. Ask questions until you thoroughly understand.
c. Help the other person understand your point of view by discussing it directly and honestly and giving any information to back up your viewpoint.
d. Indicate to the other person that you have heard the other point of view by maintaining good eye contact and summarizing the key points that you agree on.
e. Write down what happened, and share your experience with at least two other students; ask for feedback and suggestions.

■ **Leadership Development Exercise 10-5**

If you haven't already, investigate the proposal for a national nurse at http://www
.nationalnurse.blogspot.com. Then:

a. Choose an activity to become involved in.
b. Share your experience with at least three other colleagues.
c. Obtain feedback.

Advanced Leadership Development Exercises

■ **Leadership Development Exercise 10-6**

Teach legal, ethical, and/or political skills to student nurses in an undergraduate leadership course or LPN students. Share your results with at least two other students in your leadership class, and ask for feedback.

■ **Leadership Development Exercise 10-7**

Formulate a problem statement for a nursing project related to legal, ethical, or political issues. Share your results with at least two other learners in your class, and ask for feedback.

■ **Leadership Development Exercise 10-8**

Design a research project related to a legal, ethical, or political issue. Share your design with at least two other learners in your class, and ask for feedback.

References

Albarran, J. W. (1995). Should nurses be politically aware? *British Journal of Nursing, 4,* 461–465.

American Nurses Association. (1995). *Nursing's social policy statement.* Washington, DC: Author.

American Nurses Association. (2001). *ANA Code of Ethics for nurses with interpretive statement.* Silver Spring, MD: Author.

Andrews, D. R. (2004). Fostering ethical competency: An ongoing staff development process that encourages professional growth and staff satisfaction. *Journal of Continuing Education in Nursing, 35*(1), 27–33.

Clements, P. T., & Averill, J. B. (2006). Finding patterns of knowing in the work of Florence Nightingale. *Nursing Outlook, 54*(5), 269–274.

Cooper, R. W., Frank, G. L., Gouty, C. A., & Hansen, M. C. (2002). Key ethical issues encountered in healthcare organizations: Perceptions of nurse executives. *Journal of Nursing Administration, 32*(6), 331–337.

Cooper, R. W., Frank, G. L., Gouty, C. A., & Hansen, M. C. (2003). Ethical helps and challenges faced by nurse leaders in the healthcare industry. *Journal of Nursing Administration, 33*(1), 17–23.

Curtin, L. L. (2000). The first ten principles for the ethical administration of nursing services. *Nurse Administration Quarterly, 25*(1), 7–13.

Des Jardin, K. (2001, November 1). Political involvement in nursing: Politics, ethics, and strategic action. *AORN Journal,* 1–4.

Dodd, S.-J., Jansson, B. S., Brown-Saltzman, K., Shirk, M., & Wunch, K. (2004). Expanding nurses' participation in ethics: An empirical examination of ethical activism and ethical assertiveness. *Nursing Ethics, 11*(1), 16–28.

Eddins, D. (2004, March–May). Legal corner. *Alabama Nurse,* 1–2.

Equal Employment Opportunity Commission. (1997). *Facts about the Americans with Disabilities Act.* Retrieved May 9, 2007, from http://www.eeoc.gov/facts/fs-ada.html

Eskreis, T. R. (1998). Seven common legal pitfalls in nursing. *American Journal of Nursing, 98*(4), 34–41.

Forte, P. S. (1997). The high cost of conflict. *Nursing Economics, 15*(3), 19.

Gilligan, C. (1982). *In a different voice: Psychological theory and women's development.* Cambridge, MA: Harvard University Press.

Hutchinson, D. (1997). *The Internet workbook for health professionals.* Sacramento, CA: New Wind.

Kohlberg, L. (1981). *Essays on moral development: Vol. 1. The philosophy of moral development.* New York: Harper & Row.

Michigan Nurses Association. (2007). *Nurses and collective bargaining: Basic facts and considerations.* Retrieved November 15, 2007, from http://www.minurses.org/Labor/nursescollectbgn.shtml

Mills, T., & Schneider, A. (2007). The office of the national nurse: Leadership for a new era of prevention. *Policy, Politics, & Nursing Practice, 8*(1), 64–70.

Silverman, H. (2000). Organizational ethics in health care organizations. *Hospital Ethics Committee Forum, 12*(3), 202–215.

Trott, M. C. (1998). Legal issues for nurse managers. *Nursing Management, 29*(6), 39–42.

Wilson, D. M. (2002). Testing a theory of political development by comparing the political action of nurses and nonnurses. *Nursing Outlook, 50*(1), 30–34.

Winter, K. (1991). Educating nurses in political process: A growing need. *Journal of Continuing Education in Nursing, 22,* 143–146.

World Health Organization. (2007). *The WHO agenda.* Retrieved May 13, 2007, from http://www.int/aboutwho/en/good.html

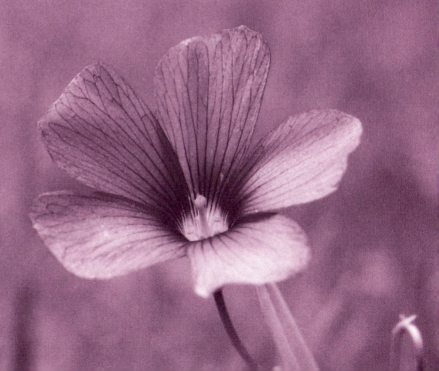

Part III

Advanced Skills to Creatively Lead and Manage

Motivating and Team Building

Introduction

Motivating employees is a key nurse leader responsibility, and it would seem to be a simple thing: just offer higher pay and generous benefits. But motivation is not based solely on monetary rewards. Less tangible motivators are often more effective. This chapter provides theories of motivation that you can use to help build a cohesive team, research that examines what motivates nurses, stages of team development that can assist you in moving your team along, and suggestions for interdisciplinary teams.

LEADERSHIP IN ACTION

After hospital management changed, Elise, a nurse leader, noticed that her team wasn't working together well. Team members berated and teased each other, gossiped, and weren't motivated to do their best work. She knew the behavior was self-destructive and considered talking to her boss about giving them each a raise in exchange for doing better work. She knew that there might be better solutions, but she was at a loss about what else to do.

LEADERSHIP CHALLENGE What would you do if you were Elise?

Motivational Theories

Motivate means to energize others to action, to help them move forward when they are blocked or confused, to get them excited about their work. But you, as a creative leader, must also be motivated.

> **KEY TERM**
>
> **Motivating** includes inspiring or energizing yourself or others to action.

When you are motivated, you are willing to pause and consider all the alternatives. These alternatives can help you create new ways of handling situations that you can teach your staff. If your horizons are limited to a thought pattern of fixing things, you may not be able to develop a highly motivated team.

Motivational theories provide a starting point for creative leadership. Theories we will examine include attribution theory, choice theory, ERG theory, expectancy theory, extrinsic and intrinsic motivation, goal-setting theory, Herzberg's motivation-hygiene theory, reactance theory, and self-efficacy theory.

Attribution Theory

Heider (1958) first proposed a theory of attribution, but Jones et al. (1972) and Weiner (1974, 1986) developed the framework for this major paradigm of social psychology. This theory examines how individuals explain events and how that relates to thinking and behavior. An assumption of this theory is that individuals seek to understand others' behavior. For some reason, human beings need to understand and explain what happens to them. Attribution theory helps explain why that is so.

Core Assumptions and Statements of Attribution Theory

Heider (1958) found two kinds of attributions:

1. **Internal attribution.** This is the idea that an individual behaves a certain way because of his or her attitude, character, or personality. When people develop an internal attribution for their actions, they change their attitudes and beliefs to match.

> **KEY TERM**
>
> In attribution theory, **internal attributions** relate to attitudes, character, or personality, and **external attributions** relate to how behavior is caused by a situation.

2. **External attribution.** This is the idea that a person behaves in a specific manner because of something about the situation. If you use external attributions, it may be more difficult to get staff to change their behavior because they will only act as desired when there is an external reward for doing so. This illustrates the problem with rewarding staff or punishing them. Both behaviors prevent individuals from developing an internal attribution that will invoke the desired behavior. Instead, staff may expect some external agent, such as you, to cause their action (Booth-Butterfield, 1996).

Emotional and motivational drives—such as blaming others (including the victim), avoiding personal recrimination, defending against attacks, and seeing ourselves as more multifaceted and less predictable than others—can also influence attributions.

Research and Attribution Theory

Attribution theory has been used to measure attributions. Open-ended questions have been used, as have ratings on a 5-point scale related to attribution dimensions. Using the direct rating method, participants are asked to state their reasons for a specific event and map those reasons to attribution dimensions.

LEADERSHIP IN ACTION

Elise decided to use attribution theory to motivate her staff. First, she collected some data to find out what was affecting the staff's motivation. She met with the staff in small groups and asked for anonymous information about what was interfering with work. When she tallied the responses, she found out that many of the day staff were mad at the night staff, and vice versa, because the other shift was leaving used supplies around and not ordering replacements. Elise concluded that her staff's attributions were faulty and needed to be changed. Elise attended the next shift reports and complimented the staff when the unit was tidy, hoping that they would start to think about why Elise was saying that they were tidy. The obvious answer was because they cleaned up their messes. By the end of the week, when she observed the nursing staff members on both shifts, they were more motivated to work with the other shift and even wrote notes to each other thanking each other for being so tidy.

Elated with the results, Elise decided to go a step further. This time she told each staff member, "You are really motivated to work hard, and you're very good at it. I'm proud of your work." By the end of the next week, Elise evaluated the staff's progress. She noted that the staff was beginning to change their attributions, bringing those attributions in line with the comments she had made.

LEADERSHIP CHALLENGE   Was Elise working on internal or external attributions? Give a rationale for your answer.

Application of Attribution Theory

Attribution theory can explain the difference in motivation between high and low achievers. According to this theory, high achievers will approach tasks related to succeeding because they think success is a result of their ability and effort, which they're confident about. Failure does not affect high achievers' self-esteem because they think failure is not their fault. Low achievers tend to avoid success-related chores because they tend to doubt their ability or assume that success is related to whom you know or to factors beyond their control. Even when successful, low achievers do not feel rewarded because they do not feel responsible, so their sense of pride and confidence do not increase (Lewis & Daltroy, 1990).

LEADERSHIP CHALLENGE   How could Elise apply the high/low achievers application of attribution theory with her staff? Give a rationale for your answer.

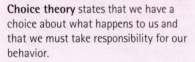

KEY TERM

Choice theory states that we have a choice about what happens to us and that we must take responsibility for our behavior.

Choice Theory

Choice theory implies that we take an active role in our behavior. According to Glasser (1999), all behavior is an attempt to satisfy powerful forces within us. The needs that drive most people are:

- The need to survive and reproduce
- The need to belong (love, share, and cooperate)
- The need for power
- The need for freedom
- The need for fun

This theory of motivation proposes that behavior is never caused by a response to an outside stimulus but inspired by one of those needs.

Sometimes, that behavior is ineffective and leads to bad decisions and subsequent misery. Examples of bad choices include psychosomatic illness, alcoholism, drug addiction, and other radical behaviors that are futile attempts to gain control over one's life. For Glasser, there are four reasons why we choose misery. They include:

1. To keep anger under control
2. To get others to help us out
3. To excuse our unwillingness to do something more effectively
4. To gain powerful control

What people do not realize is that if they made better choices, they would not have to feel miserable and could have more control of their lives.

When we feel that we've lost control of our lives, we feel hopeless about a situation. According to Glasser, even in these situations we can choose to feel miserable, or we can learn to make better choices—that is, choose to view situations as challenges and not as overwhelming events. By using choice theory, we can learn to put our energy into attacking the problem, rather than blaming it.

Glasser explained that our behavior is an attempt to reduce the difference between what we want (the pictures we carry around in our heads of what will satisfy us) and what we have (the way we see situations in the world). Although we may have little or no ability to separate how we feel from what we do or think, we have almost complete ability to change what we do. We are not controlled by external events; we must take responsibility for our action. By viewing situations as challenges, we can choose not to be overwhelmed.

LEADERSHIP CHALLENGE How could Elise use choice theory with her staff? Give specific examples and a rationale for your answers.

ERG Theory

Clayton Alderfer (1972) extended and simplified Maslow's hierarchy of needs (see Chapter 2) into a shorter list: existence, relatedness, and growth (ERG). Unlike Maslow, Alderfer did not view these as a hierarchy but more of a continuum.

Existence needs include staying alive and safe. When existence needs are satisfied, we feel safe and physically comfortable. This need encompassed Maslow's physiological and safety needs.

Relatedness needs are concerned with relationships with people and what they think of us. When these needs are met, we feel a sense of identity and position within our immediate group. Relatedness encompasses Maslow's love/belonging and esteem needs.

> **KEY TERM**
>
> **Existence needs** include staying alive and feeling safe.

> **KEY TERM**
>
> **Relatedness needs** include feeling a sense of identity and position within a group.

Growth needs include being creative for ourselves and for our environment. Successful growth means that we have a sense of wholeness, achievement, and fulfillment. Growth encompasses Maslow's self-actualization needs.

ERG theory can help a nurse leader assess the relative state of another person's needs for existence, relatedness, and growth and find ways to satisfy those needs. Nurse leaders must also be aware of their own needs in each category and make sure that their own needs are met. It is also important for nurse leaders to protect against a threat to any of these three needs.

LEADERSHIP CHALLENGE How can Elise use ERG theory for herself and her staff? Provide some specific ideas, and give a rationale for each one.

Expectancy Theory

Expectancy theory focuses on likely futures. As humans, we are constantly predicting how the future will likely turn out. We create expectations about future events, and certain specific futures are more apt to motivate us to act. They are:

- The future seems reasonably likely to happen.
- We know how to get there.
- We believe that we can make a difference. (Vroom, 1964)

In this theory, motivation becomes a combination of:

- *Valence:* The value of the perceived outcome or "What's in it for me?"
- *Instrumentality:* The belief that if I complete certain actions, I will achieve the outcome.
- *Expectancy:* The belief that I am able to complete the actions.

GUIDED LEADERSHIP TIP

USING EXPECTANCY THEORY

As a nurse leader, you can use expectancy theory to motivate staff or clients by:
- Showing them something desirable
- Indicating how straightforward it is to obtain
- Supporting their belief that they can attain it (Vroom, 1964)

LEADERSHIP CHALLENGE How can Elise use expectancy theory with her staff? Provide specific things that she can do or say to motivate them.

Extrinsic Motivation

Extrinsic motivation occurs when you motivate others using external factors, such as rewards or pressure, as opposed to internal factors, such as fun or satisfaction with accomplishment. Extrinsic motivation drives us to do things for tangible rewards or pressures (Petri, 1991).

Extrinsic motivation for nurses occurs when they are offered signing bonuses to work at specific hospitals or medical centers, when they receive extra pay for working extra hours, or when they are given awards for nursing excellence.

As a nurse leader, you can use extrinsic motivation by offering rewards (positive motivators) to staff or by using threats or guilt (negative motivators) to encourage them to accomplish their goals. Extrinsic motivation is easy to use and can often be effective. The downside is that it focuses people on a reward, not on the action. When you stop giving the reward, the behavior usually ends. Sometimes, this effect can be useful, especially when you want a behavior to stop. To use extrinsic rewards this way, first give a staff member a reward for doing the unwanted behavior and then remove the reward.

LEADERSHIP CHALLENGE How can Elise use extrinsic motivation with her staff? Give specific examples.

Intrinsic Motivation

Intrinsic motivation drives us to actions because they are fun or because we believe they are a good thing or the right thing to do (Deci & Ryan, 1991). Intrinsic motivation is far superior to extrinsic motivation because it is stronger. For example, many people are highly motivated to do work outside their jobs; they may volunteer to help others with a zeal that they do not carry into the workplace.

To use intrinsic motivation:

- Find a way to get staff to align their values with what you want.
- Find a way to make the staff feel good about what you want.
- Minimize extrinsic motivation by making sure workers are paid fairly. (Deci & Ryan, 1991)

Goal-Setting Theory

A goal is something you want to accomplish or you want someone else to accomplish. Goal-setting theory focuses on the clarity, challenge, achievability, directionality, accuracy, and feedback of goals. To direct ourselves most effectively, we need goals that are:

- Clear, not vague
- Understandable, so we know what to do and what to avoid doing
- Challenging, so we will not be bored
- Achievable, so we are unlikely to fail
- Self-developed, so we will be motivated to work hard

We all need feedback to tell us whether we are succeeding or whether it is time to change direction. Feedback must be sympathetic and encouraging. This includes feedback from ourselves: negative self-talk can be just as demoralizing as negative statements from other people.

KEY TERM

A **directional goal** motivates us toward a particular conclusion by narrowing our beliefs and enhancing optimism.

KEY TERM

An **accuracy goal** motivates us toward the most accurate conclusion. **Performance goals** focus on avoiding mistakes and being judged, and **mastery goals** focus on developing new skills.

There are several kinds of goals that influence our choice of beliefs and decision-making rules: directional goals, accuracy goals, performance goals, and mastery goals (Locke & Latham, 1990). A **directional goal** motivates us to arrive at a particular conclusion. A directional goal forces us to narrow our thinking and select beliefs that support a specific conclusion. Because we do not waste time deliberating, we are most optimistic when using a directional goal.

An **accuracy goal** motivates us to arrive at the most accurate possible conclusion; such goals are especially important when the cost of being inaccurate is high. **Performance goals** focus on avoiding mistakes; they usually include a concern about being judged. **Mastery goals** focus on developing new skills.

Some tips for using goal-setting theory include:

- Focus on the meaningful aspects of learning.
- Design learning tasks for novelty, variety, diversity, and interest.
- Help staff and clients develop their own short-term goals; they will be more motivated to succeed and will have a higher rate of success.
- Actively engage staff or clients in achieving their goals.
- Provide constructive feedback regularly.
- Strive to provide an atmosphere of belonging. (Wang, 2001)

LEADERSHIP CHALLENGE How can Elise use goal-setting theory with her staff? Provide a rationale for your answer.

KEY TERM

Herzberg's motivation-hygiene theory examined satisfying and dissatisfying factors of a job.

Herzberg's Motivation-Hygiene Theory

Herzberg developed his **motivation-hygiene theory** to help understand employee attitudes and motivation. He conducted studies to determine which factors in the work environment lead to worker satisfaction or dissatisfaction (Herzberg & Mausner, 1993).

His studies included interviews and asking employees what pleased and displeased them. He called the satisfying factors "motivators" (including achievement, recognition, the work itself, responsibility, and advancement/growth) and the dissatisfying factors "hygiene factors" or "maintenance factors" (including policies, supervision, relationships with boss and peers, work conditions, and salary). According to Herzberg, maintenance factors are kick-in-the-butt items that provide incentives or a threat of punishment, and he insisted that they reap only short-run success. He said that satisfaction is intrinsic to the job itself, not from carrot-and-stick incentives (Herzberg & Mausner, 1993).

Herzberg argued that job enrichment is required for motivation to occur and is a continuous management process. The job has to provide a sufficient challenge so that workers use their full abilities.

Herzberg also believed that once employees demonstrate an ability, they should be given a higher level of responsibility. If a job does not fully use an employee's abilities, that employee will always have a motivation problem.

Although Herzberg's theory has been criticized, it endures because of the recognition that true motivation comes from within, not from external force.

To achieve satisfaction with workers, a nurse leader must:

- Be concerned with hygiene factors to avoid employee dissatisfaction and provide motivators intrinsic to the work itself
- Provide sufficient challenge to workers
- Provide increasing levels of responsibility once ability has been demonstrated or replace the employee with one who has a lower level of skill to ward off motivation problems

LEADERSHIP CHALLENGE How could Elise use Herzberg's motivation-hygiene theory with her staff?

Reactance Theory

Reactance theory deals with pushing too hard to get what you want from the staff or clients. If you do, you will get the opposite of what you want. Pennebaker and Sanders (1976) put one of two signs on college bathroom walls. One read, "Do not write on these walls under any circumstances." The other sign read, "Please don't write on these walls." A couple of weeks later, the signs bearing the first message had far more graffiti on them. Using a message that is too strong only invites opposition.

> **KEY TERM**
>
> **Reactance theory** proposes that if you push too hard for a reaction, you may get the opposite result.

To avoid receiving a negative reaction to your ideas or orders, avoid pushing too hard or persuading too overtly or too much. If staff or clients get the idea that they are being railroaded, they will do the opposite of what you want.

KEY TERM

Self-efficacy is the belief in one's ability to perform adequately.

Self-Efficacy Theory

Bandura (1977, 1986, 1997, 2001) developed a social cognitive theory that has been widely used and accepted (Graham & Weiner, 1996). In Chapter 4, Bandura's theory was applied to stress reduction. In this chapter, Bandura's theory is discussed as a tool for nurse leaders.

According to Bandura (1986) staff possess beliefs about themselves that enable them to exercise control over their thoughts, feelings, and actions.

Self-efficacy, or the belief in one's ability to perform adequately, has proved to be a more consistent predictor of behavioral outcomes than other motivational constructs (Graham & Weiner, 1996). Employees with high self-efficacy expect higher performance from themselves and put forth the effort to achieve it as do their leaders. They approach difficult tasks as challenges, rather than as situations to be avoided.

In order to help your staff perform in concert with their beliefs and abilities, you must:

- Provide an incentive
- Provide the necessary resources
- Help remove social constraints

Bandura (1977; 1986) emphasized the importance of modeling behaviors, attitudes, and emotional reactions. By role modeling appropriate behaviors, attitudes, and emotional reactions, you can help staff learn new ways to act.

LEADERSHIP CHALLENGE Based on what you know about Bandura's theory, what specific actions are important for nurse leaders to model for staff?

Using Bandura's Social Cognitive Theory

Some principles of Bandura's (1997) theory that hold relevance for nurse leaders include the following:

- Rehearse the modeled behavior in your head and then enact it.
- For better retention, code modeled behavior for staff by providing key words, labels or images.
- Provide information that has functional value for staff and they're more apt to adopt the behavior.

- Tell staff that you have confidence they can perform adequately; their beliefs are more important than what is objectively true.

LEADERSHIP IN ACTION

Jason, a seasoned nurse leader, had been using Bandura's social learning theory for many years. Just recently, he'd been experimenting with several of the principles from Bandura's theory. Jason set up a role-playing situation he wanted to use at a staff meeting. He planned to ask participants to wear signs around their necks indicating the main concept they were portraying.

LEADERSHIP CHALLENGE Which of Bandura's principles was Jason demonstrating?

Implications of Social Cognitive Theory

The implications of Bandura's social cognitive theory are that nurse leaders should:

- Take care to model positive behaviors, attitudes, and emotional reactions when teaching learners
- Provide a learning environment that allows learners to extract meaning from it
- Use social persuasion based on attainable success to help learners create and develop high self-efficacy beliefs
- Remove real or imagined social or resource constraints to increase incentive to produce competent performances
- Help learners use self-reflection and self-evaluation to alter their thinking and behavior toward high self-efficacy
- Provide learning incentives and adequate resources

LEADERSHIP IN ACTION

Devon, a seasoned nurse leader, planned to model the most effective way to obtain an intake interview, allow nurses to practice small segments of the interview process, and ask them to evaluate their learning experience in a journal.

LEADERSHIP CHALLENGE Which of Bandura's principles did Devon overlook, and how would you change Devon's approach so that it included them?

Nursing Research on Motivation

A number of studies examined motivational factors affecting nurses.

Shindul-Rothschild, Berry, and Long-Middleton (1996) surveyed 7,560 nurses about their perceptions of the quality of client care, the amount of involvement they had with their clients, their involvement in decisions about care, and their opportunities to improve practice. Fifty percent of the nurses reported that part-time or temporary nurses had been substituted for full-time RNs, and 40% reported the use of unlicensed assistive personnel. Twenty-five percent of the nurses planned to leave nursing because they could not provide clients with adequate care. Most respondents (85%) reported they saw a decrease in the quality of care, and an overwhelming number said they had less time to teach, comfort, and talk to clients and their families; provide basic nursing care and document it; and consult and participate in care with other healthcare team members. More than 50% of the RNs stated that less continuity of care and an increase in readmissions and complications occurred secondary to the admitting diagnosis.

Lyons (2003) examined the job satisfaction of nursing and allied health graduates from a mid-Atlantic university. Participants who returned mailed surveys reported that there have been many more negative than positive changes in the healthcare system—including less job security, efficiency, and time to spend with individual clients—and increases in workload, paperwork, and control of health care by insurance companies. Even with these changes, respondents reported a high level of satisfaction with their jobs. What made them feel most satisfied included:

- Having a feeling of worthwhile accomplishment from their job
- Being offered opportunities for personal and professional growth
- Receiving recognition for, and having satisfaction with, their workload

Lewis (2007) provided a report of acute care hospital-based staff nurses from a survey conducted by Brewer and Kovner. This survey investigated factors related to RN job satisfaction in a nationally representative sample of 553 RNs. The researchers found that the *perception* of rewards being tied to performance was significantly related to job satisfaction.

In a study of extrinsic and intrinsic work values and their impact on Australian nurses' job satisfaction, Hegney, Plank, and Parker (2006) found:

- Over 53% of nurses who worked in geriatrics believed that their pay rate was extremely poor or quite poor.
- In addition to a lack of parity between nurses working in the public and private sectors, respondents noted that other similarly educated and accountable professions, such as teaching, were paid more than nurses.
- Nurses believed their skills and experience were extremely unrewarded or quite unrewarded (36% in geriatrics, 42% in public care, and 42% in private care).

- Nurses employed in management positions were more likely to believe their skills and experience were rewarded adequately.
- Perception of poor collegial support and teamwork were more evident with nurses in geriatrics than with those in the public or private sectors.

A dissertation by Beech (1995) on patient satisfaction and nursing staff satisfaction in an urban public teaching hospital in Texas reported a low level of satisfaction with the dimensions of work (autonomy, pay, professional status, interaction, task requirements, and organizational policies). Only one dimension of work—professional status—received a positive score. Staff members were also unanimously dissatisfied with their salaries and frequently mentioned the following work-related problems: staffing shortages, heavy patient loads, and excessive paperwork.

LEADERSHIP CHALLENGE **For each of the studies described, what were the intrinsic and extrinsic motivators for nurses?**

Ways to Increase Staff Motivation

To increase motivation in staff members, consider:

- Rewarding staff nurses who give good nursing care
- Giving staff nurses more power by helping them achieve leadership positions
- Helping meet staff needs for achievement by challenging them to succeed and by providing training and orientation
- Helping meet the need for affiliation by providing opportunities to enjoy social relationships, empathize with others in trouble, and work side by side with a nurse leader to decide on client care
- Improving physical working conditions to satisfy basic needs for safety
- Increasing the level of training and skills to raise self-esteem
- Placing staff in positions that help fulfill their self-actualization needs
- Providing assignments that satisfy and give value to employees, encouraging them to perform well
- Enhancing positive motivation by using a democratic leadership model, rewarding good work, and encouraging positive peer group interaction
- Providing annual awards for best client care and other nursing actions
- Avoiding scolding in front of others or humiliating staff
- Stating what was not completed adequately and demonstrating a better performance
- Observing (not hovering over) staff carefully to make sure that they are taking responsibility
- Providing warmth and support and respecting individual capabilities (Bashir, 2005)

Team Building

A **team** is a small number of people with complementary skills who share a common purpose and are committed to a set of performance goals and an approach to which they hold themselves accountable (Katzenbach & Smith, 1993).

As the saying goes, there is no "I" in teamwork. Everyone works together for the common good. When team members finish their work early, they offer to help others. When team members have information that pertains to the team, they share it.

One type of team is the self-managed team, which has unprecedented responsibility (Gross, 1995). Self-managed teams:

- Set priorities and goals
- Prepare and manage budgets and schedules
- Develop and choose work methods
- Assign tasks to members (e.g., vacation scheduling, performance appraisals, training, and hiring and firing)

That list is impressive and may be more wishful thinking than reality in most settings (Gross, 1995).

LEADERSHIP CHALLENGE Which, if any, of these tasks could Elise help her team fulfill?

Methods of Maximizing a Team

There are numerous ways to maximize teams, including building a vision, establishing shared goals and expectations, keeping employees well informed, promoting a caring environment that's conducive to teamwork, encouraging and modeling positive interactions, teaching supportive behavior, assessing and building self-esteem, encouraging stability, listening, setting an example, accepting responsibility, and sharing the spotlight.

Building a Vision

A **vision** gives a team an overall picture of what the final product will be, whether it means providing quality cost-effective health care for your setting or community or making your department the best in the field. A vision is a unique and ideal image of the future and should be consistent with the organization's vision (Allman, 1998).

Establishing Shared Goals and Expectations

Teams establish goals that encompass more than just providing care for clients. Some valid team purposes are:

- To provide optimal care to decrease incidents of future hospitalization
- To prevent infections
- To assist clients in becoming more independent (Allman, 1998)

Once a goal is established, team members can sign a document indicating their support (Carver, 1996).

LEADERSHIP CHALLENGE How could Elise use this information about goals and expectations with her staff?

Keeping Employees Well Informed

As a nurse leader, it is your responsibility to share information about how organizational plans affect your staff and their work area. Knowledgeable staff can provide ideas about meeting organizational goals and help promote positive outcomes (Carver, 1996).

LEADERSHIP CHALLENGE How could Elise keep her staff better informed?

Promoting a Caring Environment That's Conducive to Teamwork

It is important to get to know your staff as individuals and respond to their needs when possible. When that is not possible, it is important to discuss the reasons why. Staff will appreciate your honesty and learn to trust you. This adds a sense of humanity to the workplace; but it must be sincere, or the staff will know (Carver, 1996).

LEADERSHIP CHALLENGE How can Elise promote a more caring environment with her staff?

Encouraging and Modeling Positive Interactions

By insisting on and demonstrating positive interactions, you can prevent wasting time on addressing hurt feelings and rude behavior. Even a negative message or criticism can be given in a positive way, especially if it is preceded by several positive points.

LEADERSHIP CHALLENGE How could Elise encourage and model positive interactions with her team?

Teaching Supportive Behavior

Being supportive is more than telling team members that they are doing a good job and that it is OK to fail occasionally. Being supportive means:

- Not blaming a coworker or supervisee without knowing all the facts
- Pointing out how destructive behavior can lead to work problems instead of overlooking it
- Discouraging derogatory discussions and gossip
- Always expecting the best (Allman, 1998)

One other thing to keep in mind when providing support for staff is that not all workers benefit from support (Shirey, 2004). When type A workers are involved with a heavy workload and under stress, even social support can be stressful because it may be viewed as a distraction from concentrating on the job at hand.

LEADERSHIP CHALLENGE **Which of these behaviors can Elise practice to support the team?**

Assessing and Building Self-Esteem

Positive self-esteem gives team members a feeling of their own worth. A quick way to diagnose self-esteem is to recall how often a team member responds to mistakes and kids others. Team members who berate themselves for mistakes or tease others about their weaknesses have low self-esteem (Rinke, 1988).

LEADERSHIP CHALLENGE **How could Elise use this information with herself and her staff?**

Encouraging Stability

According to research, there are several actions nurse leaders can take to encourage unit stability and mitigate the teamwork obstacles in a typical hospital setting. They include:

- Creating smaller teams
- Establishing consistent schedules
- Creating all 8-hour or all 12-hour shifts
- Decreasing turnover and absences
- Offering rewards and incentives
- Physically clustering teams so they can coordinate action (Kalisch & Begeny, 2005)

LEADERSHIP CHALLENGE Which of these measures should Elise consider with her team? Give a rationale for your answer.

Listening

Listen effectively means that you allow the other person to talk 80% of the time and that you have only 20% of the time to talk and/or prepare to speak. In many conversations, both participants are thinking ahead to what they want to say next and are not listening. To reverse that common process, train yourself to listen and not think ahead. The benefits of listening are numerous, including:

- Improved relationships
- Enhanced productivity and work performance
- Increased team spirit and morale
- Better understanding from the staff of their mission as healthcare providers (Eade, 1996)

See **Box 11-1** for more tips on communicating effectively.

Setting an Example

People, including your staff, learn by example. Not only can you operationalize goals and supportive behaviors by setting a good example, but you can teach your staff how to lead by example. Begin by following the rules that you have negotiated with team members, and do it in a respectful and kind way. Learn to keep cool during a crisis, spreading calm as you go. If you get upset, your negative feelings will be contagious. Always keep your word. Nothing undermines trust more quickly than breaking a promise (Eade, 1996).

Accepting Responsibility

Accepting responsibility for someone else's behavior can be scary. Human beings, including you, make mistakes. Never pass blame to your supervisees. You are in charge; the buck should stop with you. The staff will respect you for that (Eade, 1996).

Sharing the Spotlight

Always give staff members credit for everything that goes right, and never take credit for their work. Mention the names of staff to your boss and others, drawing attention to their excellent performances (Eade, 1996).

BOX 11-1 TIPS FOR EFFECTIVELY COMMUNICATING WITH STAFF

- Ask short, simple questions that draw staff out that cannot be answered with yes or no (e.g., "What are you thinking?" "What do you suggest?").
- Ask questions in a concerned, nonthreatening style and tone.
- Allow staff to vent when upset, and then acknowledge their feelings (e.g., "You look upset. Want to talk about it?" "I can see why you'd be upset about that.").
- No matter what is said, stay open and nondefensive, realizing that the other person is your teammate and wants to improve things but may not know how.

Stages of Team Development

Once goals, roles, and processes have been established, teams usually pass through four stages of development:

1. *Forming.* During this initial stage, confusion, boundary testing, and orientation reign. Team members are unsure about how to proceed and what role they will play. Goals and processes are unclear, and members tend to think in terms of "me," not "we."

2. *Storming.* Conflict and turmoil are prominent during this stage. Team members' work styles become more evident, and differences may not be as readily tolerated as before. Members may still lack a "we" perspective and may advance their own agendas.

3. *Norming.* Team members begin to think in terms of "we," not "me," and have accepted and internalized the goals and roles, share information openly, and work together.

4. *Performing.* Individuals fully commit to the team and cooperate to improve team functioning. Team members are accountable to each other and believe they have the power to meet agreed-upon goals and objectives. (Gross, 1995)

LEADERSHIP CHALLENGE What stage of development is Elise's team in?

Not all teams pass through all these steps. When a team does not progress, it is less effective. According to Gross (1995), teams fail because their goals are not clear; their objectives keep changing; they have inadequate management support, ineffective team leadership, inadequate team member priority, and lack of mutual accountability; or because they are inadequately compensated.

Interdisciplinary Teams

Teamwork is recommended by the Institute of Medicine as a way to minimize the nursing shortage's effect on client outcomes, efficiency, and quality improvement. Not all healthcare workers agree with this suggestion. RNs, MDs, CEOs, and chief nursing officers (CNOs) have different perceptions of nurses, the nursing shortage, and the effect of staffing on client care and safety. The majority of RNs and CNOs express concern about the impact of the shortage on early detection of client complications and nurses' ability to maintain safety. On the other hand, according to a survey, the majority of physicians and CEOs do not agree that the nursing shortage has frequently or often impaired safety for clients (Steefel, 2007).

This gap in perception could be addressed by forming interdisciplinary teams in colleges and universities and on units to jointly offer information on improving client care quality and safety. Such coordination could foster a sense of understanding, value for each other's contributions, and teamwork (Steefel, 2007).

Summary

This chapter examined theory and interventions important to motivating staff, including motivational theories, nursing research about motivating nurses, and ways to increase staff motivation. This chapter also provided information on how to build effective teams, including methods of maximizing a team, the stages of team development, and information for interdisciplinary teams. The next chapter focuses on budgeting and managing resources.

Key Term Review

- An **accuracy goal** motivates us toward the most accurate conclusion.
- **Choice theory** states that we have a choice about what happens to us and that we must take responsibility for our behavior.
- A **directional goal** motivates us toward a particular conclusion by narrowing our beliefs and enhancing optimism.
- **Existence needs** include staying alive and feeling safe.
- **Expectancy theory** examines future events and what situations are most apt to motivate us to act.
- **External attributions** relate to how behavior is caused by a situation.
- **Extrinsic motivation** occurs when you motivate others using tangible rewards or pressure.
- **Growth needs** include being creative and experiencing a sense of wholeness, achievement, and fulfillment.
- **Herzberg's motivation-hygiene theory** examined satisfying and dissatisfying factors of a job.
- **Internal attributions** relate to attitudes, character, or personality.
- **Intrinsic motivation** comes from within and drives people to act on things that they think are right, good, or fun.
- **Mastery goals** focus on developing new skills.
- **Motivating** includes inspiring or energizing yourself or others to action.
- **Performance goals** focus on avoiding mistakes and being judged.
- **Reactance theory** proposes that if you push too hard for a reaction, you may get the opposite result.
- **Relatedness needs** include feeling a sense of identity and position within a group.
- **Self-efficacy** is the belief in one's ability to perform adequately.
- A **team** is a small number of people with complementary skills who share a common purpose and are committed to a set of performance goals and an approach to which they hold themselves accountable.
- A **vision** gives a team an overall picture of what the final product will be and is a unique and ideal image of the future that should be consistent with the organization's vision.

Leadership Development Exercises

- **Leadership Development Exercise 11-1**

Work with at least two other colleagues on the following tasks:

a. Each person provides information about one motivation theory to the rest of the group.

   b. Together, the team discusses the pros and cons of using each of those theories with staff or teams and develops a plan for using each one.

   c. All team members take 15–20 minutes to write down what they learned about motivation theories and plans for their use with their classmates or write a paper.

■ Leadership Development Exercise 11-2

Discuss nursing research on motivation found in this chapter with at least two other colleagues. After a study is presented, discuss among you how (or if) the findings can be applied in nursing situations.

■ Leadership Development Exercise 11-3

Role-play the following situations:

   a. Giving negative criticism in a positive way
   b. Pointing out how destructive behavior can lead to work problems
   c. Discouraging derogatory discussions and gossip
   d. Expecting the best
   e. A team in the forming stage
   f. A team in the storming stage
   g. A team in the norming stage
   h. A team in the performing stage

■ Leadership Development Exercise 11-4

Diagnose your own level of self-esteem based on the measures presented in the chapter.

Advanced Leadership Development Exercises

■ Leadership Development Exercise 11-5

Teach motivational and team-building skills to student nurses in an undergraduate leadership course. Share your findings and observations with your class, or write up your results in a paper.

■ Leadership Development Exercise 11-6

Formulate a problem statement for a nursing project related to motivation or team building. Share your statement with at least two other colleagues. Ask for feedback on whether your statement is testable. Revise your problem statement based on the feedback you receive.

■ Leadership Development Exercise 11-7

Design a research project related to motivation or team building. Obtain feedback from at least two other colleagues about the adequacy of your design. Revise your project based on their feedback.

References

Alderfer, C. (1972). *Existence, relatedness & growth*. New York: Free Press.

Allman, C. (1998). Teamwork: The keys to success. *Continuing education for nurses*. Sarasota, FL: Burt Rodgers Schools.

Bandura, A. (1977). *Social learning theory*. New York: General Learning Press.

Bandura, A. (1986). *Social foundation of thought and action: A social cognitive theory*. Englewood Cliffs, NJ: Prentice Hall.

Bandura, A. (1997). *Self-efficacy: The exercise of control*. New York: W. H. Freeman.

Bandura, A. (2001). Social cognitive theory: An agentic perspective. *Annual Review of Psychology, 52*, 1–26.

Bashir, M. (2005). Motivation for better nursing management. *Nursing Journal of India, 96*(9), 209–210.

Beech, B. M. (1995). *Patient satisfaction and nursing staff work satisfaction in an urban public teaching hospital*. Unpublished doctoral dissertation, University of Texas HSC at Houston School of Public Health, Houston, TX.

Booth-Butterfield, S. (1996). *Attribution theory*. Retrieved May 21, 2007, from http://www.as.wvu.edu/~sbb/comm221/chapters/attrib.htm

Carver, I. G. (1996, January). The six elements of team building. *Nursing Spectrum, 29*, 5.

Deci, E.L., & Ryan, R.M. (1991). Intrinsic motivation and self-determination in human behavior. In R.M. Steers & L.W. Porter (Eds.), *Motivation and work behavior* (pp. 44–58; 5th ed.). New York: McGraw-Hill.

Eade, D. M. (1996, November/December). Motivational management: Developing leadership skills. *Clinician Reviews*, 115–125.

Glasser, W. (1999). *Choice theory: A new psychology of personal freedom*. New York: HarperCollins.

Graham, S., & Weiner, B. (1996). Theories and principles of motivation. In D. C. Berliner & R. C. Calfee (Eds.), *Handbook of Educational Psychology*. New York: Simon & Schuster/Macmillan.

Gross, S. E. (1995). *Compensation for teams*. New York: American Management Association.

Hegney, D., Plank, A., & Parker, V. (2006). Extrinsic and intrinsic work values: Their impact on job satisfaction in nursing. *Journal of Nursing Management, 14*(4), 271–281.

Heider, F. (1958). *The psychology of interpersonal relations*. New York: Wiley.

Herzberg, F., & Mausner, B. (1993). *The motivation to work*. Edison, NJ: Transaction.

Jones, E. E., Dannouse, D. E., Kelley, H. H., Nisbett, R. E., Valins, S., & Weiner, B. (Eds.). (1972). *Attribution: Perceiving the causes of behavior*. Morristown, NJ: General Learning Press.

Kalisch, B., & Begeny, S. (2005). Improving nursing unit teamwork. *Journal of Nursing Administration, 35*(12), 550–556.

Katzenbach, J., & Smith, D. K. (1993, March/April). The discipline of teams. *Harvard Business Review*, 111.

Lewis, D. (2007, February). Multiple factors affect job satisfaction of hospital RNs. *Robert Wood Johnson Research Highlight, 22*, 1–2.

Lewis, F. M., & Daltroy, L. H. (1990). How causal explanations influence health behavior: Attribution theory. In K. Glanz, F. M. Lewis, & B. K. Rimer (Eds.), *Health education and health behavior: Theory, research, and practice.* San Francisco: Jossey-Bass.

Locke, E. A., & Latham, G. P. (1990). *A theory of goal setting and task performance.* Englewood Cliffs, NJ: Prentice Hall.

Lyons, K. J. (2003). A study of job satisfaction of nursing and allied health graduates from a mid-Atlantic university. *Journal of Allied Health, 32,* 10–17.

Pennebaker, J. W., & Sanders, D.Y. (1976). American graffiti: Effects of authority and reactance arousal. *Personality and Social Psychology Bulletin, 2,* 264–267.

Petri, H. (1991). *Motivation: Theory, research and application* (3rd ed.). Belmont, CA: Wadsworth.

Rinke, W. J. (1988, March). Maximizing management potential by building self-esteem. *Managements Solutions,* 11–16.

Shindul-Rothschild, J., Berry, D., & Long-Middleton, E. (1996). Where have all the nurses gone? *American Journal of Nursing, 96,* 25–39.

Shirey, M. R. (2004). Social support in the workplace: Nurse leader implications. *Nursing Economics, 22*(6), 313–319.

Steefel, L. (2007, May 21). Surveys reveal differing views. *Nursing Spectrum,* 20–21.

Vroom, V. H. (1964). *Work and motivation.* New York: John Wiley.

Wang, S. (2001). Motivation: General overview of theories. In M. Orey (Ed.), *Emerging perspectives on learning, teaching, and technology.* Retrieved May 24, 2007, from http://www.coe.uga.edu/epltt/Motivation.htm

Weiner, B. (1974). *Achievement motivation and attribution theory.* Morristown, NJ: General Learning Press.

Weiner, B. (1986). *An attribution theory of motivation and emotion.* New York: Springer-Verlag.

Budgeting and Managing Resources

CHAPTER OBJECTIVES

After reading this chapter, answering the leadership challenges, and participating in the leadership development exercises, you will be able to:

- List the financial/budget competencies required of nurse leaders
- Read a financial statement
- Develop a business plan
- Describe the budgeting process
- Apply budgeting principles to Leadership in Action vignettes
- Discuss the principles of three different types of budgets

Advanced nurses will be able to:

- Teach budgeting and resource management skills to student nurses in an undergraduate leadership course
- Formulate a problem statement for a nursing project related to budgeting or resource management
- Design a research project related to budgeting or resource management

Introduction

As a nurse leader, you should be able to read a financial statement, develop a business plan, and track nursing costs. You may have to develop and justify a budget each year. Depending on the setting you work in, you may use an incremental model, a redistribution model, formula budgeting, responsibility-centered management, or activity-based cost management.

This chapter explores each of these methods in turn and suggests ways budget methods can be used by nurse leaders. Senior nurse leader competencies related to resource and finance management are also presented.

LEADERSHIP IN ACTION

Sheila M., a nurse leader, was asked to develop a business plan for her unit and to track nursing costs. She was also given a financial statement for the previous year and asked to incorporate some of the information into her plans. She had no idea how to do any of these tasks, so she looked up some articles on the Internet and started to learn about business plans and nursing costs. For the first time, she received a copy of the medical center's annual report and was able to understand it.

Budget/Financial Competencies for Senior Nurse Leaders

According to the American Health Care Association (2001), senior nurse leaders should:

- Continually collect and assess staffing, equipment, and supply data to note budget implications
- Make budget projections
- Consider clinical profit-and-loss information
- Develop a realistic budget for the nursing department that meets objectives and falls within financial parameters
- Monitor revenues and expenses throughout the year
- Use regular reports (daily, weekly, monthly, and quarterly) to track expenditures
- Modify budget priorities based on budget variances

LEADERSHIP CHALLENGE Based on the Leadership in Action vignette about Sheila, which of these competencies did she demonstrate? Which does she still need to cover?

Hospital Nursing Costs, Billing, and Reimbursement

Although nursing has 24-hour accountability for care of hospitalized clients, current hospital billing practices list nursing services as room-and-board fees that are billed as flat daily rates for private, semiprivate, intermediate, and intensive care rooms. Yet nursing care accounts for 25% of a hospital's total operating budget and 44% of direct care costs (McCue, Mark, & Harless, 2003; Welton, Fischer, DeGrace, & Zone-Smith, 2006). One of the problems with billing for nursing services is that reimbursement for hospital care is based on medical diagnosis, especially diagnostic-related groups (DRGs) and principal procedures.

LEADERSHIP CHALLENGE What could nursing do to obtain more reliable billing for its services?

Hospitals are not reimbursed for different levels of nursing care even though nursing intensity and estimated direct nursing costs vary greatly within and across similar nursing units. A nurse-centric billing model could be a better solution (Welton et al., 2006).

The New York State Nurses Association successfully incorporated a nursing intensity weight (NIW) for each DRG category (Ballard, Gray, Knauf, & Uppal, 1993). The NIW does not address the variability of nursing care for a particular diagnosis nor acknowledge the independence of nursing care from medical care (Welton et al., 2006).

Some other billing systems that could provide more accurate billing include using:

- Actual nursing time (intensity), which would move some clients to the intermediate room rate and others to the private room rate and provide an evidence-based strategy (Welton et al., 2006)
- An existing nursing classification system to bill directly for nursing services (Titler et al., 2005)

LEADERSHIP CHALLENGE Is there evidence that nursing care costs differ significantly from medical costs? Cite your source.

One study showed that nursing diagnosis, when collected daily and summarized on the hospital bill, predicted length of stay, hospital charges, and mortality. Nursing diagnoses also enhanced the explanatory power of diagnosis-related groups by twofold (Welton & Halloran, 2005).

Reading Financial Statements

Reading a financial statement is like reading a nutrition label. The US Securities and Exchange Commission (2007) provided tips to reading three basic kinds of financial statements: balance sheets, income statements, and cash flow statements.

Balance Sheets

Balance sheets provide detailed information about an organization's assets, its liabilities, and shareholders' equity.

$$\text{Assets} = \text{Liabilities} + \text{Shareholder's equity}$$

Assets are anything the organization owns that has value, such as trucks, equipment, inventory, cash, and investments. Current assets are things, like inventory, that can be converted to cash within one year. Noncurrent assets take more than a year to sell. Fixed assets—including furniture, property, and equipment—are used to operate the service but are not available for sale.

Liabilities are money that an organization owes to others, including rent, money owed to suppliers, payroll owed to employees, environmental cleanup costs, taxes, and obligations to provide goods or services to clients in the future.

Shareholder's equity includes the amount owners invest in the organization's stock plus or minus earnings or losses since inception. Sometimes, organizations distribute earnings as dividends.

Income Statements

Income statements show the money that was earned for a specific period of time and the costs and expenses associated with earning that revenue. Think of an income statement as a set of chairs. At the top is the total amount of sales/services made during the accounting period. It is called "gross revenues" or "gross sales" because expenses have not yet been deducted from it. At each step down, deductions are made for certain costs or operating expenses, such as salaries, research costs, and marketing. Depreciation—including the wear and tear on machinery or equipment, tools, and furniture—is also deducted from gross profit. At the bottom of the stairs, after deducting all the expenses, you learn how much the company earned or lost. This is called the "bottom line."

Cash Flow Statements

Cash flow statements report an organization's inflows and outflows of cash. You need to know this because it is important to have enough cash on hand to pay expenses and purchase assets.

A cash flow statement shows changes over time and is divided into three main parts:

- *Operating activities.* The first part of a cash flow statement discriminates cash flow from net income or losses. This section of the statement reconciles the net income (as shown on the income statement) to the actual cash that the organization received from or used during operation.
- *Investing activities.* The second part of a cash flow statement shows purchases or sales of long-term assets—such as property, plants, and equipment—as well as investment securities.
- *Financing activities.* The third part of a cash flow statement shows cash raised by selling stocks and bonds and the status of any bank loans.

Remember: whenever reading a financial statement, always read the footnotes carefully. They are packed with information about accounting policies, income taxes, pension and/or retirement programs, and stock options.

Developing a Business Plan

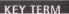

A **business plan** provides a clear understanding of an organization's customers, strengths, and competition as well as provides a strategy for future expansion. A business plan has several components, including an executive summary and information on the product or service, the market, the competition, operations, and the management team.

A business plan contains:

- A brief description of the organization's history
- The organization's objectives
- A description of and marketing plan for the organization's services or products
- A persuasive statement about why the organization will succeed, including its competitive advantage
- Projected growth for the organization and the market
- A brief description of the key management team and its experience
- An organizational chart with chain of command and listing of duties
- Information on salaries and benefits
- Employees' required skill sets and their job descriptions
- A bookkeeping system
- Supporting documents and a summary

Sheila M., a nurse leader, was asked to sit on the budget committee for her organization. She was very nervous about the first meeting and had no understanding of finance and budgets. As the meetings progressed and Sheila learned more about the method in place, she realized that receiving a standard 3% increase per year would not meet the needs for documented growth in enrollment.

LEADERSHIP CHALLENGE What should Sheila do to learn more?

KEY TERM

Budgeting is a process of making plans and quantifying the expected results. A budget is a concrete expression of how well a unit or project is managed and how resources are used.

Budgets and Budgeting

Budgeting refers to the process of making fiscal plans and quantifying the expected results (Finkler, 2001). A **budget** is a concrete expression of how well a unit or project is managed. The budget documents how resources are used to fund growth, day-to-day operations, and strategic initiatives (Donnelly, 2005).

Once a budget is place, it can be a powerful tool for controlling what happens in an institution and for measuring success (Finkler, 2001). Budgets are always based on assumptions. They require participants to predict spending changes or usage rates (Finkler, 2001).

Managing a Unit-Level Budget

As a nurse leader at the unit level, you will probably receive monthly reports of operations that show profits and losses and may be asked to explain the underlying causes of variances (the budgeted amount versus the actual money spent) if it is more than 5%. Many factors can lead to such variances, including salaries, staffing levels, cost of supplies or equipment, staff meetings or workshops, client census or acuity, vacation and benefit time, illness, and orientation needs.

LEADERSHIP CHALLENGE Which of the many factors that can lead to variances would you, as a nurse leader, have any control over?

Table 12-1 shows a statement of operation for one unit, including the budgeted, actual, and variance amounts for various revenues and expenses.

TABLE 12-1 PROFIT-AND-LOSS STATEMENT

REVENUES

	Current Month			Year-to-Date		
	Budget	Actual	Variance		Budget	Actual	Variance

Client Revenues

Budget	Actual	Variance		Budget	Actual	Variance
22,000	20,000	2,000	Insurance payment	40,000	45,000	(5,000)

Nonclient Revenues

Budget	Actual	Variance		Budget	Actual	Variance
2,500	2,500	0	Rent	5,000	5,000	0
25,000	24,500	500	Family donations	47,000	43,000	4,000
49,500	47,000	2,500	Net revenues	92,000	93,000	(1,000)

EXPENSES

Personnel

Budget	Actual	Variance		Budget	Actual	Variance
20,000	21,500	(1,500)	Managerial/ professional	40,000	41,000	(1,000)
5,000	4,800	200	Clerical/technical	10,000	9,800	200
25,000	23,300	1,700	Net salaries/wages	50,000	50,800	(800)
3,750	3,495	255	Benefits	7,500	7,620	(120)
53,750	53,095	655	Net personnel	57,500	58,420	(920)

Nonpersonnel

Budget	Actual	Variance		Budget	Actual	Variance
2,600	2,600	0	Office expenses	5,200	5,200	0
3,450	3,300	150	Supplies	7,500	7,400	100
6,050	5,900	150	Net nonpersonnel	12,700	12,600	100
12,100	11,800	300	Net expenses	25,400	25,200	200
14,700	14,805	(105)	Net income	29,400	28,600	800

Budgeting in Academic Settings

Tradition and status often supersede documented need in academic settings. Leaders of nursing programs may not always be able to obtain the monies needed to maintain quality programs and grow. A budget can be a crucial tool that documents and quantifies program needs and how the program contributes to the overall college or university. Budget models can track expenses and income (revenue) and analyze the relationship between the two. If you are a nurse leader in an academic setting or plan to be one, remember to pay as much attention to financial outcomes as to educational outcomes (Donnelly, 2005).

There is a myth that nursing programs are excessively expensive as compared to other academic majors. Analyzing the relationship between revenue and expenses can dispel this myth (Donnelly, 2005). No matter the method of budgeting and resource allocation used by the parent institution, this type of analysis can prove useful.

As you will see next, a budget can be built in a number of ways.

The Incremental Budget

KEY TERM

The **incremental budget model** provides a standard yearly increase per year.

The **incremental budget model** is based on the assumption that financial needs of different departments vary only slightly from year to year and that previous budgets are good indicators of future budgetary needs. If you are a nurse leader using this budget model, your department might receive a standard 3% increase even if you were underfunded in the preceding year and/or documented growth shows that this amount of increase will not be enough (Donnelly, 2005).

The Redistribution Model

KEY TERM

The **redistribution model** of budgeting allows the nurse leader to redistribute funds across different line items.

The **redistribution model** combines the incremental model (i.e., a standard increase each year) with an understanding that the nurse leader can redistribute funds across line items, such as faculty salaries, research growth, or program development. Although this model provides some flexibility, if you use it, it may not allow you the ability to adapt to rapidly changing times (Donnelly, 2005).

LEADERSHIP CHALLENGE Should Sheila take information to the committee about the redistribution model? Give a rationale for your answer.

KEY TERM

Formula budgeting distributes money based on the number of full-time students and may be subject to state policies and past performance.

Formula budgeting distributes money based on the number of full-time students. Although this may seem like a big step forward, this type of budgeting is often subject to the influences of state policies and may reward past performance rather than projected growth or future initiatives (Donnelly, 2005).

Responsibility-centered management (RCM) shifts responsibility for generating revenue from central administration to the unit or department. If you are the leader of a unit and that unit uses RCM, you would be accountable for fiscal performance. If you go over your budget, that amount of money would be deducted from your next year's budget. This method can be damaging if your unit or department experiences negative enrollment cycles (Donnelly, 2005).

No matter what type of nursing program you are affiliated with, it is important to understand the type of budget model used and the financial underpinnings of your program. When you are clear about these matters, you can make logical decisions about resources.

Developing a Nursing Program Budget

LEADERSHIP IN ACTION

Sheila decided to develop a nursing program budget. She read an article that informed her that for most nursing programs, the greatest source of revenue was tuition and student fees.

LEADERSHIP CHALLENGE What would you tell Sheila to do with this new bit of information?

The first step in building an academic budget is to gather information about the program's total tuition revenue, either from the finance office or by estimating revenue earned from information available on tuition rates and enrollment. Add the revenue generated by nursing students who take support courses in other departments (Donnelly, 2005).

The next step is to calculate tuition discounts. Find out what kind of agreements the nursing department has with hospital systems or corporations to discount tuition for groups of employees.

Next divide expenses into full-time and part-time faculty and support staff salaries plus fringe benefits for each program. (Human resources can help calculate fringe benefits.)

The next step is to calculate each program's operating expenses, which includes instructional equipment and supplies, travel, accreditation fees, membership fees, and other expenses. (Grant monies are not included because they represent a money-in/money-out situation.)

Total expenses per program = Instructional expenses + Operating expenses

Net revenue (income) – Total expenses from net revenue =
The surplus generated by each program and for the college or school as a whole
(Donnelly, 2005)

Analyzing a Program's Contribution to Revenue

The ratio of net revenue to expenses (NRE) can show you which programs are generating enough revenue to cover expenses. To compute the NRE ratio, divide the total expenses into the net revenue. A ratio above 1.0 indicates that the program is profitable and not only covers expenses but also contributes to the college or school. Many undergraduate nursing programs generate a high NRE ratio because they are a blend of full-time and part-time faculty. The NRE ratio, especially if it is healthy, can show that nursing programs are of fiscal worth to their academic institutions (Donnelly, 2005).

Activity-Based Cost Management

Traditional accounting methods provide little information about factors that incur costs in healthcare management. Organizations have become more complex, and information systems have expanded the potential for analyzing data. Both of these factors have opened the door for more useful accounting methods (Stortjell & Jessup, 1996).

> **KEY TERM**
>
> **Activity-based cost management** means that you know the inputs, purpose, and performance for an activity.

Traditional budgets are organized according to payroll, fringe benefits, equipment, supplies, or rent. If you want to reduce costs or add value, your organization must start to manage activities, not categories (Stortjell & Jessup, 1996), which is called **activity-based cost management.**

How would that work? If you consider the admissions process (an activity), it is possible to determine that specific factors—such as availability of accurate information, prior admission, payment source, or client diagnosis—influence costs. For example, how much time is spent by nurses when financial or demographic data is not accurate (Stortjell & Jessup, 1996)?

Managing an activity means that you know the answers to the following questions:

- What inputs (people, equipment, space) does the activity consume?
- What is the activity's purpose or output?
- How well is the activity being performed?

Developing a Facility Maintenance Budget

Leaders in nursing homes have to develop and justify a budget. Twenty-five percent of costs can be attributed to building and system operations. Costly system failures can result if you are a nursing home administrator and make a plan for scheduled maintenance costs but do not know the facility's current condition (Jones, 1998).

Although no facility maintenance budget plan is 100% accurate, it can be an essential tool for keeping a facility in peak condition. The first step in developing a budget is to develop targeted goals like the following:

- Financial growth
- Ongoing maintenance
- Renovation
- Expansion
- Facility utilization

Once goals are delineated, develop a written outline of the program that links to your facility's strategic or long-range plan. This is the time to meet with your accountant or chief financial officer to work out the details (Jones, 1998).

To develop a comprehensive facility study, you will need structural and civil engineers, planners, and interior designers who have had experience in settings similar to yours.

If you have multiple facilities, it is wise to assemble a team of design professionals to help conduct an audit and space analysis, detailing what needs to be repaired, replaced, or maintained regularly. Drawings, specifications, and a standard worksheet may all need to be developed. When using today's dollars, be sure to build in depreciation, taxes, inflation, and future replacement costs (Jones, 1998).

Keep your facility information dynamic by updating it quarterly. You can track and monitor maintenance work orders in terms of time, cost, and occurrence daily to establish a reference point for present and future planning. Choose computer software that is easy to use and can be linked to computer-assisted design programs (Jones, 1998).

Summary

This chapter examined budgeting and resource use, including budget/financial competencies for senior nurse leaders; hospital nursing costs, billing, and reimbursement; reading financial statements; developing a business plan; managing a unit-level budget; budgeting in academic settings; activity-based cost management, and developing a facility maintenance budget. The next chapter focuses on the effectiveness of health care.

Key Term Review

- **Activity-based cost management** means that you know the inputs, purpose, and performance for an activity.
- **Assets** are anything the organization owns that has value, such as trucks, equipment, inventory, cash, and investments. Fixed assets—including office furniture, property, and equipment—are used to operate the service but are not available for sale.
- **Balance sheets** provide detailed information about an organization's assets, its liabilities, and shareholders' equity.
- A **budget** is a concrete expression of how well a unit or project is managed and how resources are used.
- **Budgeting** is a process of making plans and quantifying the expected results.
- A **business plan** provides a clear understanding of an organization's customers, strengths, and competition as well as provides a strategy for future expansion.
- **Cash flow statements** report an organization's inflows and outflows of cash.
- **Formula budgeting** distributes money based on the number of full-time students.
- **Income statements** show the money that was earned for a specific period of time and the costs and expenses associated with earning that revenue.
- The **incremental budget model** provides a standard yearly increase per year.
- **Liabilities** are money that an organization owes to others, including rent, money owed to suppliers, payroll owed to employees, environmental cleanup costs, taxes, and obligations to provide goods or services to clients in the future.
- The **redistribution model** of budgeting allows the nurse leader to redistribute funds across different line items.
- **Responsibility-centered management** shifts responsibility for generating revenue from central administration to the unit or department.
- **Shareholder's equity** includes the amount owners invest in the organization's stock plus or minus earnings or losses since inception; earnings can be distributed as dividends.

Leadership Development Exercises

Leadership Development Exercise 12-1
What existing nursing classification system could be used to bill directly for nursing services? Give a rationale for your answer.

Leadership Development Exercise 12-2
Develop a balance sheet for your personal finances.

■ **Leadership Development Exercise 12-3**
Develop a cash flow statement for your personal finances.

■ **Leadership Development Exercise 12-4**
Develop a business plan for a nursing service.

■ **Leadership Development Exercise 12-5**
Discuss why leaders of a nursing program may not be able to obtain the money needed to maintain quality programs.

■ **Leadership Development Exercise 12-6**
Interview a nursing leader for tips on budgeting. Share what you find with at least three other colleagues.

■ **Leadership Development Exercise 12-7**
Look at Table 12-1. For each revenue and expense, examine the variance, and determine which items vary more than 5%. For each of those items, describe at least two steps that could be taken to reduce the variance.

Advanced Leadership Exercises

■ **Leadership Development Exercise 12-8**
Teach budgeting and resource management skills to student nurses in an undergraduate leadership course or to nurses on your team.

■ **Leadership Development Exercise 12-9**
Formulate a problem statement for a nursing project related to budgeting or resource management.

■ **Leadership Development Exercise 12-10**
Design a research project related to budgeting or resource management.

References

American Health Care Association. (2001). *Competencies for senior nurse leaders in LTC vision statement.* Retrieved June 1, 2007, from http://www.ahca.org/qualities/competencies_report.pdf

Ballard, K. A., Gray, R. F., Knauf, R. A., & Uppal, P. (1993). Measuring variations in nursing care per DRG. *Nursing Management, 24,* 33–36.

Donnelly, G. (2005). A budget model to determine the financial health of nursing education programs in academic institutions. *Nursing Leadership Forum, 9*(4), 143–151.

Finkler, S. A. (2001). *Budgeting concepts for nurse managers* (3rd ed.). Philadelphia: W. B. Saunders.

Jones, G. A. (1998, August). Developing a facility maintenance budget. *Nursing Homes,* 1–3.

McCue, M., Mark, B. A., & Harless, D. W. (2003). Nursing staffing, quality, and financial performance. *Journal of Health Care Finance, 29,* 54–76.

Stortjell, J. L., & Jessup, S. (1996). Bridging the gap between finance and clinical operations with activity-based cost management. *Journal of Nursing Administration, 26*(1), 12–17.

Titler, M., Dochterman, J., Picone, D. M., Everett, L., Xie, X. J., & Kanak, M. (2005). Cost of hospital care for elderly at risk of falling. *Nursing Economics, 23,* 290–306.

US Securities and Exchange Commission. (2007). *Beginners' guide to financial statements.* Retrieved June 1, 2007, from http://www.sec.gov/investor/pubs/begfinstmtguide.htm

Welton, J. M., Fischer, M. H., DeGrace, S., & Zone-Smith, L. (2006). Hospital nursing costs, billing and reimbursement. *Nursing Economics, 24*(5), 239–246.

Welton, J. M., & Halloran, E. J. (2005). Nursing diagnoses, diagnosis-related group, and hospital outcomes. *Journal of Nursing Administration, 35,* 541–549.

Resources

Mark, B. A., Harless, D. W., McCue, M., & Xu, Y. (2004). A longitudinal examination of hospital registered nurse staffing and quality of care. *Health Services Research, 39,* 279–300.

Virtual Advisor. (2003). *Developing a business plan.* Retrieved June 1, 2007, from http://va-interactive.com/inbusiness/editorial/bixdev/ibt/business_plan.html

Demonstrating Effectiveness and Quality Care

CHAPTER OBJECTIVES

After reading this chapter, answering the leadership challenges, and participating in the leadership development exercises, you will be able to:

- Discuss the National Healthcare Quality Report
- Describe uses for the National Database of Nursing Quality Indicators
- Give examples of healthcare outcomes research
- Describe uses of the Health Care Report Card Compendium
- Discuss how to use patient registries to determine healthcare effectiveness
- Describe disparities in healthcare provision
- Discuss the benchmarking process
- Describe client evaluations of the health care they received
- Apply healthcare effectiveness principles to Leadership in Action vignettes
- Discuss the pros and cons of Magnet hospital accreditation and its relationship to healthcare effectiveness

Advanced nurses will be able to:

- Teach effectiveness measurement skills to student nurses in an undergraduate leadership course or to nurses on a unit
- Analyze a real or hypothetical benchmarking process
- Formulate a problem statement for a nursing project related to demonstrating healthcare effectiveness
- Design a research project related to demonstrating effectiveness management

Introduction

As a nurse leader, you will need to be familiar with healthcare effectiveness research and to participate in procedures to increase effectiveness. This chapter focuses on the 2006 National Healthcare Quality Report, the National Database of Nursing Quality Indicators, outcomes research and how it relates to healthcare effectiveness, a Web tool called the Health Care Report Card Compendium, disparities in health care, patient evaluations of health care, the use of patient registries to improve health care and public health, the pros and cons of Magnet recognition as a way to improve care, how the presence of nursing students affects quality of care, and how to use benchmarking to analyze care and set improvement goals.

LEADERSHIP IN ACTION

Clarisse, a nurse leader, had implemented many leadership initiatives. Her next goal was to assess and increase effective healthcare provision, but she wasn't sure where to begin.

LEADERSHIP CHALLENGE What advice do you have for Clarisse? Be specific, listing the exact steps she needs to take.

KEY TERM

The **National Healthcare Quality Report** examines and tracks the quality of health care in the United States, including effectiveness, client safety, timeliness, and client-centeredness.

The 2006 National Healthcare Quality Report

The Agency for Healthcare Research and Quality (AHRQ) released the fourth annual **National Healthcare Quality Report** (NHQR) on behalf of the US Department of Health and Human Services (HHS) and in collaboration with an HHS-wide interagency work group. Like previous reports, the 2006 NHQR (AHRQ, 2007a) received significant guidance from AHRQ's leadership and national advisory committee. The NHQR examines and tracks the quality of health care in the United States, using the most scientifically credible measures and data sources available.

Twenty-two core measures of healthcare quality address the extent to which providers and hospitals deliver evidence-based care for specific services as well as the outcomes of the care provided. The measures are organized around four dimensions of quality (effectiveness, client safety, timeliness, and client-centeredness) and cover four stages of care (staying healthy, getting better, living with illness or disability, and coping with the end of life).

Most measures of quality are improving, but the pace of change remains modest. Quality improvement varies by setting and phase of care. Hospitals demonstrate the highest rates of improvement (7.8%) as compared to ambulatory care (3.2%) and nursing home and home health care (1.0%).

Improvements in hospital care may have resulted from public reporting of healthcare quality measures, focused quality improvement programs, and policies that support improvement initiatives. For example, the Centers for Medicare and Medicaid Services' Quality Improvement Organization (QIO) measures for good heart attack care showed the greatest improvement of all core measures, at 15.0% per year. This rate of improvement is markedly better than the 9.2% rate reported in 2005, and it's more than five times the 2.6% overall rate of improvement for all nonhospital core measures. QIO measures of the quality of hospital care for pneumonia care and for heart failure also showed high rates of improvement compared with all other measures—11.7% and 8.4%, respectively.

New core client safety measures for postoperative complications from certain procedures and adverse events from central venous catheters improved 7.3% and 4.5%, respectively.

The median rate of improvement for acute care measures of quality is 4.3%, about twice as high as that for preventive care and chronic care, which are 2.4% and 1.8%, respectively. Improvements in the quality of acute care were more than twice as high for hospital care (7.8%) as they were for ambulatory care (3.1%). Except for vaccinations for children, adolescents, and the elderly, which have demonstrated high rates of improvement overall (5.8%), the improvement rate for other preventive measures—including screenings, advice, and prenatal care— is relatively low (1.7%).

Chronic care for ambulatory conditions—such as diabetes, end-stage renal disease, and pediatric asthma—improved over three times more than chronic care for clients in nursing homes and home health care (3.6% versus 1.0%).

These core measures went from a flat trend in the 2005 report to a significantly improved trend in 2006:

- ■ *Client-centeredness.* This composite measure shows when providers sometimes or never listened carefully, explained things clearly, respected what clients had to say, or spent enough time with them. The percentage of clients' reporting sometimes or never having good communication experiences with providers declined at an average annual rate of 9.3%.

> **KEY TERM**
>
> **Client-centeredness** is a composite measure of when providers sometimes or never listened carefully, explained things clearly, respected what clients had to say, or spent enough time with them.

- ■ *Respiratory diseases.* Two measures went from showing no change in 2005 to showing an improvement in 2006. The percentage of tuberculosis clients who did not complete a curative course of treatment within 12 months of the initiation of treatment decreased at an average annual rate of 2.2%. The percentage of visits at which an antibiotic was prescribed for the diagnosis of a common cold for children decreased at an average annual rate of 7.0%.

- *Diabetes.* The percentage of adults with diabetes who did not receive three important screening tests for the management of that disease decreased by an average annual rate of 3.9%. Hospital admissions for lower-extremity amputation—which can result from suboptimal management of diabetes—decreased by an average annual rate of 7.5%.
- *Heart disease.* The percentage of smokers who had a routine checkup and did not receive advice to quit smoking decreased at an average annual rate of 3.8%.

These measures continued to show significant deterioration:

KEY TERM

Timeliness is a measure of the percentage of emergency room visits during which the client left without being seen.

- *Timeliness.* The percentage of emergency room visits during which the client left without being seen increased by 48% between 1997 and 1998 (1.2% of visits) and between 2003 and 2004 (1.8% of visits).
- *Suicides.* The suicide death rate increased by an average of 1.3% per year between 2000 and 2003.

Other core measure information included:

- The core measure with the highest degree of variation between states, as computed by the ratio of the best-performing state to the worst-performing state, is the percentage of chronic nursing home clients who were physically restrained. It varies by a multiple of 8.4 across the states, ranging from 1.7% to 14.6%.
- Other core measures with at least a threefold variation across the states are hemodialysis clients with adequate dialysis, pediatric asthma hospital admissions, prenatal care in the first trimester, appropriate heart attack hospital care, and the suicide death rate.
- Overall, quality continues to improve, as the NHQR documented in 2003, 2004, and 2005. An acceleration in improvement is evident across a wide range of diseases, including heart disease, diabetes, respiratory diseases, and colorectal cancer.
- Communication between providers and clients show marked improvements. Hospital care has shown demonstrable improvements relative to other settings, especially on the QIO measures.

The pace of change is slow overall, and there is a long way to go to achieve the best quality possible across most measures. What is also clear from this report, and others, is that sustained focus, public reporting, and active and persistent interventions seem to make a significant difference in the quality of health care, especially in the areas of patient safety and hospital measures. Examples of programs that appear to be making an impact in these areas include:

- The Institute for Healthcare Improvement's successful campaign to reduce over 100,000 preventable hospitalizations
- The public and private endorsement of hospital measures for heart attacks, heart failure, and pneumonia by the Centers for Medicare & Medicaid Services, the Joint Commission on Accreditation of Healthcare Organizations, and the National Quality Forum
- Implementation programs, such as the voluntary public reporting of performance demonstration programs associated with the Medicare Modernization Act
- Innovations in the private sector that reward delivery of high-quality care, such as the Premier Hospital Quality Incentive Demonstration (a pay-for-performance program)

Other AHRQ Resources

To support quality improvement efforts, AHRQ has developed a variety of information products that are derived from data gathered for the annual production of the NHQR and the National Health Disparities Report (NHDR). These products seek to translate information into practical applications for use by state and local health policymakers.

State Snapshots

State Snapshots is an interactive Web-based tool, produced annually by AHRQ using data from the NHQR and NHDR, and is designed to help state officials and their public- and private-sector partners understand healthcare quality and disparities in their state, including strengths, weaknesses, and opportunities for improvements. These snapshots provide information on healthcare quality measures for each state using user-friendly graphs and customized tables.

> **KEY TERM**
>
> **State Snapshots** is an interactive Web-based tool, produced annually by AHRQ using data from the NHQR and NHDR, and is designed to help state officials and their public- and private-sector partners understand healthcare quality and disparities in their state.

Diabetes and Asthma Resource Guides

Designed in partnership with the Council of State Governments and for elected state leaders, state executive branch officials, and other nongovernmental state and local healthcare leaders, *Diabetes Care Quality Improvement: A Resource Guide for State Action* provides background information on why states should consider diabetes as a priority for action, presents analysis of state and national data and measures of diabetes quality and disparities, and gives guidance for developing a state quality improvement plan. A companion interactive workbook provides review exercises for state leaders on the resource guide's key skills and lessons to use in making the case for diabetes care quality improvement, in learning from improvement efforts that are already under way, in measuring diabetes quality and disparities, and in implementing diabetes care quality improvement plans using a state-led quality improvement framework.

Like the diabetes resources, *Asthma Care Quality Improvement: A Resource Guide for State Action* and its companion workbook provide information about asthma quality and disparities and present exercises to hone skills that are useful for developing a state asthma care quality improvement plan.

State and Community Partnerships

AHRQ also supports dozens of state and community projects that engage public and private stakeholders to improve the quality of care for people with diabetes and asthma, to develop quality improvement action plans, and to evaluate innovative implementations of state and community efforts to improve quality and reduce disparities. These partnerships go beyond collecting and reporting on quality measures; they actively address problems with quality and disparities and include:

- *National Health Plan Learning Collaborative to Reduce Disparities and Improve Quality.* This partnership with nine of America's foremost health plans (Aetna, CIGNA, Harvard Pilgrim Health Care, HealthPartners, Highmark, Kaiser Permanente, Molina Healthcare, UnitedHealth Group, and WellPoint) is testing ways to improve the collection and analysis of data on race and ethnicity, matching these data to existing quality measures in the Health Plan Employer Data and Information Set and developing quality improvement interventions that close gaps in care. Lessons learned by plans in the collaborative will be shared with other health plans so that they too can improve the care that they provide.
- *Aim setting and state plans for quality improvement.* This partnership with five states (Maine, Rhode Island, Massachusetts, West Virginia, and Arkansas) reviews the State Snapshots in the context of these states' needs to develop new tools that will help them use data for quality improvement.
- *Improving diabetes care in communities.* This partnership with three of the nation's leading business coalitions (the Greater Detroit Area Health Council, Mid-Atlantic Business Group on Health, and Memphis Business Group on Health) supports local communities in their efforts to reduce the rate of obesity and other risk factors that can lead to diabetes and its complications and to work together to ensure that people with diabetes receive appropriate healthcare services. These coalitions have convened stakeholders—including businesses, providers, health plans, insurers, consumers, and academics—to set priorities in their efforts to improve diabetes care, reduce disparities, and develop solutions that fit within the communities' needs and capabilities.

- *Improving implementation of diabetes improvement programs through ongoing evaluation.* This partnership with Vermont supports the state's Blueprint for Health to improve diabetes care by developing dashboards to continuously monitor activities and progress, by designing and conducting patient and provider satisfaction surveys, by providing learning and collaborative opportunities to advance pay-for-performance programs and by documenting knowledge learned so that it is available to other states.

- *Decreasing disparities in pediatric asthma.* This partnership with coalitions in six states (Arizona, Maryland, Michigan, New Jersey, Oregon, and Rhode Island) focuses on developing action plans to improve disparities in pediatric asthma by addressing racism and cultural competency; using data to target needs, coordinate resources, and make the case for policy action; and increasing access and improving the quality of care for underserved populations.

For more information, consult the AHRQ Web site (http://www.ahrq.gov) for announcements about the availability of the State Snapshots as well as the agency's tools at http://ahrq.gov/qual/diabqualoc.htm and http://www.ahrq.gov/qual/asthmaqual.htm.

LEADERSHIP CHALLENGE **What advice would you give Clarisse about information that's available from AHRQ and how to use it?**

National Database of Nursing Quality Indicators

Nurses have been collecting independent data about nursing practice for years. The National Center for Nursing Quality at the University of Kansas School of Nursing is an example. Nurse researchers at the center conduct research on clinical and healthcare effectiveness. One of the tools used at the center is the **National Database of Nursing Quality Indicators** (NDNQI). This database was developed by the American Nurses Association, and today is one of the most powerful tools available to nurse leaders (Nevada Nurses Association, 2006).

> **KEY TERM**
>
> The **National Database of Nursing Quality Indicators** allows nursing leaders to compare information with other healthcare facilities and use quality improvement activities to improve effectiveness.

NDNQI participants have seen positive results and achieved better client outcomes. The database can also help nurse leaders target nursing resources where they are most needed, which is often when they are most cost-effective.

Currently, data include client outcomes related to the following units:

- Critical care
- Step down

- Medical
- Surgical
- Medical/surgical
- Pediatrics
- Psychiatry and rehabilitation (Nevada Nurses Association, 2006)

LEADERSHIP TIP

As a nursing leader, you can use the NDNQI to mark progress, understand and improve care (as well as nurses' work environments), avoid costly complications, and assist in marketing the quality of your efforts.

A major advantage of the NDNQI is the ability to trend data. Instead of isolated and possibly misleading snapshots of performance, the NDNQI provides quarter-by-quarter and unit-by-unit comparisons of nursing care. This kind of data provides information about the complex kind of care nurses offer.

The NDNQI allows you to compare your unit to others nationally for events like falls and pressure ulcers. Such information can help you:

- Quantify elements of the quality of nursing care in your facility
- Estimate the value of nursing in achieving high-quality client outcomes in a cost-effective manner
- Demonstrate the link between quality nursing care and client safety (Nevada Nurses Association, 2006)

LEADERSHIP CHALLENGE How can Clarisse use the NDNQI with her staff and unit to improve morale and team efforts?

Outcomes Research and Healthcare Effectiveness

At the request of providers and consumers, AHRQ developed a Web tool that demonstrates a variety of approaches to health quality report cards.

KEY TERM

The **Health Care Report Card Compendium** is a searchable directory of over 200 samples of report cards that are produced by a variety of organizations and that show formats for and approaches to providing comparative information on the quality of health plans, hospitals, medical groups, individual physicians, nursing homes, and other care providers.

The **Health Care Report Card Compendium** is a searchable directory of over 200 samples of report cards produced by a variety of organizations. The samples show formats for and approaches to providing comparative information on the quality of health plans, hospitals, medical groups, individual physicians, nursing homes, and other care providers. The Health Care Report Card Compendium can be found at http://www.talkingquality.gov/compendium.

The purpose of the AHRQ Health Care Report Card Compendium is to inform and support the various organizations that develop healthcare quality reports, to provide easy access to examples of different approaches to content and presentation, and to meet the needs of health services researchers. It also provides related Web sites and sample pages when possible.

AHRQ makes no judgment concerning the effectiveness or value of reports in the compendium; it offers the reports to users for their consideration. The inclusion of a report in the compendium does not constitute an endorsement of the report, or of any elements in the report, by AHRQ.

The compendium was developed to supplement guidance provided on AHRQ's TalkingQuality Web site (http://www.talkingquality.gov). TalkingQuality informs and supports current and potential sponsors of healthcare performance reports by sharing the lessons learned by researchers and experienced report developers.

Public reporting regarding the performance of healthcare providers and plans is expanding as standards for measuring quality grow and reports of the quality of healthcare providers and services become more available to consumers. Public reporting about the quality of care is also a central feature of a value-driven health care initiative. Other private and public employers are likewise committing to quality reporting for enrollees in their health plans, as well as to public reporting on the costs of care (AHRQ, 2007).

More information about the initiative on value-driven health care is available at http://www.hhs.gov/transparency. For more information, contact AHRQ at 301-427-1244 or 301-427-1862.

Improving Healthcare Disparities

Not all Americans receive the same level of care. The 2006 NHDR highlighted four key themes for policymakers, researchers, clinicians, administrators, and community leaders who seek information to improve healthcare services for all Americans:

1. Disparities remain prevalent.
2. Some disparities are diminishing while others are increasing.
3. Opportunities for reducing disparities remain.
4. Information about disparities is improving, but gaps still exist.

Disparities Remain Prevalent

The 2006 report shows that disparities related to race, ethnicity, and socioeconomic status still pervade the American healthcare system. Although they vary in magnitude by condition and population, these disparities are observed in almost all aspects of health care, including:

- Effectiveness, patient safety, timeliness, and patient-centeredness
- Facilitators and barriers to care and healthcare utilization

- Preventive care
- Treatment of acute conditions
- Management of chronic diseases
- Many clinical conditions, including cancer, diabetes, end-stage renal disease, heart disease, HIV, mental health and substance abuse, and respiratory diseases
- Many care settings, including primary care, home health care, hospice care, emergency departments, hospitals, and nursing homes
- Many subpopulations, including women, children, the elderly, residents of rural areas, and individuals with disabilities and other special healthcare needs

For a sizable number of measures, racial and ethnic minorities and the poor receive lower-quality care. African Americans received poorer-quality care than Caucasians for 73% (16/22) of core measures. Asians received poorer-quality care than Caucasians for 32% (7/22) of core measures. American Indians and Alaska Natives received poorer quality care than Caucasians for about 41% (9/22) of core measures and better quality care for 14% (3/22) of core measures. Hispanics received poorer quality care than non-Hispanic whites for 77% of core measures (17/22). Poor people received lower quality care than high-income people for 71% (12/22) of core measures (AHRQ, 2007b).

For most of the six core measures of access to care, racial and ethnic minorities and the poor fared the worst:

- African Americans and Asians had worse access to care than Caucasians.
- American Indians and Alaska Natives had worse access to care than whites for 17% (1/6) of core measures.
- Hispanics had worse access than non-Hispanic whites for 83% (5/6) of core measures.
- Poor people had worse access to care than high-income people for all six core measures.

Some Disparities Are Diminishing While Others Are Increasing

For the poor, most disparities are worsening. Of disparities in quality experienced by blacks, Asians, American Indians and Alaska Natives, and Hispanics, about a quarter were improving and about a third were worsening. Two-thirds of quality disparities experienced by poor people (8/12) were worsening. Examples of these changing disparities in the quality of health care include the following:

- From 2000 to 2003, the percentage of adults who received care for illness or injury as soon as they wanted decreased for Caucasians (from 16.2% to 13.4%) but increased for African Americans (from 17.5% to 18.4%), corresponding to an increase of 9.8% per year in this disparity.

- From 2000 to 2004, the rate of new AIDS cases remained about the same for Caucasians (from 7.2 to 7.1 per 100,000 population age 13 and over) but decreased for African Americans (from 75.4 to 72.1 per 100,000 population), corresponding to a decrease of 7.9% per year in this disparity.
- From 1999 to 2004, the percentage of adults age 65 and over who did not receive a pneumonia vaccine decreased for Caucasians (from 48% to 41%) but increased for Asians (from 59% to 65%).
- From 1998 to 2004, the percentage of children ages 19–35 months who did not receive all recommended vaccines decreased for Caucasians (from 26% to 17%) but decreased even more for Asians (from 31% to 17%).
- From 2000 to 2003, the percentage of adults who had not received a recommended screening for colorectal cancer decreased for Caucasians (from 49% to 47%) but increased for American Indians and Alaska Natives (from 51% to 58%).
- From 2002 to 2003, the percentage of adults that reported communication problems with providers decreased somewhat for Caucasians (from 10.4% to 9.4%) but decreased even more for American Indians and Alaska Natives (from 18.4% to 8.3%).
- From 2001 to 2003, the rate of pediatric asthma hospitalizations remained the same for non-Hispanic whites (139 hospitalizations per 100,000 population) but increased for Hispanics (from 188 to 226 per 100,000 population).
- From 2001 to 2003, the percentage of children who did not have a vision check decreased somewhat for non-Hispanic whites (from 40% to 38%) but decreased even more for Hispanics (from 48% to 42%).
- From 2000 to 2003, the percentage of adults age 40 and over who did not receive three recommended services for diabetes decreased substantially for high-income persons (from 54% to 41%) but decreased less so for poor persons (from 68% to 63%).
- From 2001 to 2003, the percentage of children whose parents or guardians reported communication problems with providers remained about the same for high-income persons (from 3.6% to 3.3%) but decreased for poor persons (from 12.5% to 9.5%).
- For racial minorities, most trackable disparities in access to care are improving; for Hispanics and the poor, most disparities are worsening. Of trackable core measures of access, most disparities experienced by Hispanics (4/5) and by poor people (3/5) were worsening. (AHRQ, 2006)

Opportunities for Reducing Disparities Remain

Some disparities are diminishing, but there still are many opportunities for improvement. For all groups, measures could be identified for which the group not only received lower-quality care than the reference group but for which this difference was getting worse rather than better. For example:

- For African Americans, Asians, and Hispanics, these disparities involved all trackable domains of quality: preventive services, treatment of acute illnesses, management of chronic diseases and disabilities, timeliness, and patient-centeredness.
- For American Indians and Alaska Natives, disparities were concentrated in the treatment of acute illnesses and the management of chronic diseases and disabilities. (AHRQ, 2006)

Some disparities in quality of care were prominent for multiple groups; these disparities included:

- Colorectal cancer screening
- Vaccinations
- Hospital treatment of heart attacks
- Hospital treatment of pneumonia
- Services for diabetes
- Children hospitalized for asthma
- Treatment of tuberculosis
- Nursing home care
- Problems with timeliness
- Problems with patient-provider communication

The 2006 NHDR also found that Hispanics and the poor faced many disparities in access to care that were getting worse:

- For Hispanics, not having health insurance and not having a usual source of care were getting worse.
- For the poor, not having a usual source of care and experiencing delays in care were getting worse.

Information about Disparities Is Improving, but Gaps Still Exist

The 2006 NHDR provides more information about disparities than previous reports. Improvements include the addition of new data sources and measures that have allowed for the analyses of new disparities, including those related to obesity, asthma management, hospice care, patient safety, client-centeredness in hospital care, Hispanic subpopulations, language assistance, and uninsurance.

Obesity

New measures of counseling of overweight and obese persons from the National Health and Nutrition Examination Survey and the Medical Expenditure Panel

Survey were added to the 2006 NHDR report. One of these measures is whether obese adults were given advice about exercise.

Only 68% of obese adults age 20 and over reported being told by their provider that they were overweight. Obese African Americans and Mexican Americans were less likely to be informed than obese non-Hispanic whites; obese persons with less than a high school education were less likely to be informed than obese persons with any college education.

Only 37% of overweight children and teens ages 2–19 reported being told by their provider that they were overweight. (Disparities were not observed.)

Only 58% of obese adults reported being counseled about exercise. Among obese adults, counseling was reported less often by Hispanics compared with non-Hispanic whites; by poor, near-poor, and middle-income persons compared with high-income persons; and by persons with a high school education or less compared with persons with any college education.

Asthma Management

Supplemental measures from the 2003 National Asthma Survey—coordinated by the National Heart, Lung, and Blood Institute at the National Institutes of Health—were included in the 2006 NHDR.

The **National Asthma Education and Prevention Program** develops and disseminates science-based guidelines for the diagnosis and management of asthma. It recognizes assessment and monitoring, controlling factors that contribute to symptom exacerbation, pharmacotherapy, and education for partnership in care as four essential components of asthma management.

> **KEY TERM**
>
> The **National Asthma Education and Prevention Program** develops and disseminates science-based guidelines for the diagnosis and management of asthma.

Considerable variation was observed. Among persons with asthma, only 70% were taught to recognize early signs of an attack, 49% were told how to change their environment, 40% were given a controller medication, and 27% were given an asthma management plan. Compared to persons with any college education, persons with less education were less likely to report receiving information about assessing their asthma and controlling environmental triggers. African Americans were less likely than Caucasians to receive controller medications.

Hospice Care

Hospice care was examined in terms of providing medication for pain and giving care consistent with stated end-of-life wishes. Only 6% of families with a relative in hospice care reported that hospice providers did not provide the right amount of medication for pain. Rates were higher among African Americans and Asian and Pacific Islanders compared with Caucasians and among Hispanics compared with non-Hispanic whites. Only 5% of families reported that hospice providers gave care inconsistent with stated end-of-life wishes. Rates were higher among

African Americans, Asian and Pacific Islanders, and American Indians and Alaska Natives compared with Caucasians; among Hispanics compared with non-Hispanic whites; and among persons with a high school education or less compared with persons with any college education.

Client Safety

Postoperative complications occur at a rate of 6 per 100 Medicare clients who have surgery. According to the 2006 NHDR, rates are higher among African Americans compared with Caucasians.

Timing of prophylactic antibiotics for surgery is appropriate 58% of the time. African Americans, American Indians and Alaska Natives, and Hispanics were less likely than non-Hispanic whites to receive prophylactic antibiotics at the correct times.

Although rates of in-hospital death following complications of care are falling, they remained higher among Asian and Pacific Islanders compared with non-Hispanic whites.

About 10% of hospital clients receiving anticoagulant or hypoglycemic medications experienced complications. African Americans were more likely than Caucasians to experience complications from hypoglycemic medications.

Client-Centeredness in Hospital Care

Only 6% of hospitalized clients reported communication problems with doctors, and 7% reported communication problems with nurses. Twenty-six percent of hospitalized clients reported problems with communications about medications, and 21% reported problems with discharge information.

Hispanic Subpopulations

Mexicans reported the lowest rates of being advised to quit smoking (42.4%) and the highest rates of delayed care for illness or injury (24.1%) and uninsurance (31.1%) of all Hispanic subpopulations.

Central or South Americans reported the highest rates of client-provider communication problems (18%).

Language Assistance

Nearly half (47%) of individuals with limited English proficiency reported that they do not have a usual source of care. An additional 47% of individuals reported having a usual source of care that offers language assistance.

Only 6% of individuals with limited English proficiency reported having a usual source of care that does not offer language assistance.

Uninsurance

For the total population and for every income group, the percentages of adults who reported receiving recommended colorectal cancer screening or a dental visit were lower for uninsured persons (21.8% and 18.7%, respectively) compared with privately insured persons (49.2% and 51.8%, respectively).

Being uninsured has a large negative impact on almost all aspects of healthcare quality and access. In fact, among adults, the negative effects of being uninsured are typically greater than the effects of race, ethnicity, income, and education. Multivariate analyses suggest that uninsurance is an important mediator of racial, ethnic, and socioeconomic disparities, although race, ethnicity, and socioeconomic position often have independent effects as well.

Unresolved Information Needs

The expanded capability of federal data sources has allowed researchers to make more reliable estimates for more populations, but considerable gaps still remain. Information gaps can relate to insufficient data to produce reliable estimates or, when estimates are possible, to inadequate statistical power to detect large differences.

For example, of the 22 core measures of quality, statistically reliable estimates were not possible for:

- Most measures for Native Hawaiians or other Pacific Islanders and persons of more than one race
- About half of the quality measures for American Indians or Alaska Natives
- About a third of the quality measures for Asians
- About two-thirds of the quality measures for the poor

Power issues were also a problem, particularly for American Indians and Alaska Natives, in core measures of access. Data collection that focuses on specific groups may be needed to yield reliable information about these populations.

Of the six core measures of access, statistically reliable estimates were not possible for:

- Most measures for Native Hawaiians and other Pacific Islanders
- A quarter of measures for American Indians and Alaska Natives

Additionally, statistical power was insufficient to detect a 20% difference relative to whites for:

- Over a third of access measures for Native Hawaiians and other Pacific Islanders and for Native American Indians and Alaska Natives
- A quarter of access measures for persons of more than one race

Nursing Data on Quality of Care

Nurse researchers have also been involved in eliminating healthcare disparities. Together, the National Institute of Nursing Research and the National Center on

Minority Health and Health Disparities created eight partnerships between nursing schools with established research programs in health disparities and minority-serving nursing schools. The following nursing schools are participating:

- The University of Washington and the University of Hawaii at Manoa focus on the health needs of Asian and Pacific Islanders.
- The University of Michigan and the University of Texas Health Science Center at San Antonio study health promotion and restoration in the Hispanic population.
- The John Hopkins University and North Carolina A&T State University address three areas of disparity: access to care, process of care, and health outcomes.
- The University of California, San Francisco, and the University of Puerto Rico explore the needs of minority groups living with HIV.
- The University of North Carolina at Chapel Hill, North Carolina Central University, and Winston-Salem State University focus on culturally competent nursing research.
- The University of Pennsylvania and Hampton University address the influence of culture, race, and ethnicity on health promotion and disease prevention.
- The University of Texas at Austin and New Mexico State University at Las Cruces explore the health needs of rural, low-income Mexican American and American Indian populations.
- Yale University and Howard University examine self-management and self-assessment strategies to promote positive health and lifestyle changes in minority populations. (Grady, 2003)

Table 13-1 provides information about outcomes research and how to measure the end results of health care.

LEADERSHIP CHALLENGE What advice would you give Clarisse about reducing disparities in health care?

Client Evaluations and Quality of Health Care

This section presents three major studies focused on client evaluations of health care: (1) the Shabrawy and Mahmoud

TABLE 13-1 EXAMPLES OF MEASURABLE HEALTH OUTCOMES

Measure	Example
Physiologic measures	Respiration rate
Clinical events	Stroke
Symptoms	Fatigue
Functional measures	SF-36, a 36-item health survey
Client experiences with care	Consumer Assessment of Health Plans survey; Caring Behavior Inventory

Source: Adapted from Clancy & Eisenberg (1998); Reichert (1998); Yang, Simms, & Yin (1998).

1993 study in Saudi Arabia; (2) the Beech study in the southwestern United States; and (3) the DAWN study in 13 countries in Asia, Australia, Europe, and North America.

The Shabrawy and Mahmoud Study in Saudi Arabia

The **Shabrawy and Mahmoud study** conducted in Saudi Arabia measured satisfaction with primary healthcare services. Fourteen primary healthcare centers were chosen randomly to represent various geographic areas of Riyadh, the capital of Saudi Arabia. Information was collected through a pretested questionnaire used by 30 well-trained final-year medical students. Systematic sampling of family files was conducted, and the household head was interviewed. Nine hundred respondents were interviewed concerning their satisfaction with the services delivered.

> **KEY TERM**
> The **Shabrawy and Mahmoud study** in Saudi Arabia measured satisfaction with primary healthcare services.

The findings were as follows: 40% were dissatisfied. One-third of the dissatisfied said that the health center was too far from their homes; 19.4% complained that the center's business hours were not suitable; 38.9% complained of the absence of specialty clinics; 19.4% encountered language barriers with the physicians; and 63.9% complained about delays at the center. Also, 16.7% of the satisfied and 38.9% of the dissatisfied complained that their physicians did not satisfactorily explain their health problems and treatments. In the dissatisfied category, 22.7% said that their physicians' explanations were neither clear nor understandable. Among the satisfied, 74.6% said that their primary healthcare center was their first choice if they felt sick; 61.1% of the nonsatisfied category gave the same response (Shabrawy & Mahmoud, 1993).

The Beech Study in the Southwestern United States

Another study, the **Beech study,** examined the level of client satisfaction and nursing staff work satisfaction at an urban public hospital in the southwestern United States. The study findings showed that clients experienced a moderate to low level of satisfaction with the dimensions of hospital care (e.g., the admissions process, daily care, information, nursing care, physician care, care from other hospital staff, living arrangements, and overall care).

> **KEY TERM**
> The **Beech study** examined the level of client satisfaction and nursing staff work satisfaction at an urban public hospital in the southwestern United States.

Of the eight dimensions of care, clients reported a 75% or better positive level of satisfaction with only one dimension: physician care. Ethnicity, perceived health status, and hospital image were significantly related to client satisfaction. Hispanic clients who were in good health and who thought that the hospital had a good image in their community were most satisfied with hospital care. Areas that were reported as needing the most improvement included the staff's attitudes, nursing care, and communication (Beech, 1995).

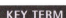

The **DAWN study** was a cross-sectional survey of 13 countries that sampled individuals diagnosed with diabetes and examined client reports of treatment.

The DAWN Study of 13 Countries

The Diabetes Attitudes, Wishes and Needs study (or **DAWN study**) was a cross-sectional survey of national samples of diabetes clients. The data were reports obtained through structured telephone or face-to-face interviews.

Respondents' home country, their demographic and disease characteristics, and healthcare features were all associated with client-reported outcomes, such as perceived diabetes control. Better client-provider collaboration was associated with more favorable ratings on all outcomes and with better access to providers.

Some of the findings included:

- Compared with clients in the United States, those in Germany, Spain, and the Netherlands generally reported outcomes that were significantly more positive.
- Participants in India reported significantly worse general well-being and medical regimen adherence than clients in the United States.
- Medical regimen adherence was better for Scandinavian participants for diabetes-related distress and for diabetes control and hyperglycemic symptoms.
- US clients reported better outcomes for general well-being and lifestyle and for medical regimen adherence.
- The quality of collaboration with the provider was the strongest predictor of client-reported outcomes; clients reporting better collaboration had more positive ratings on all six outcome measures.
- Clients who had easier access to their providers reported positive outcomes on measures of well-being and diabetes control but not on measures of self-care.

According to this study, spending time with clients to more fully inform them of treatment options and involve them in making treatment decisions are essential behaviors for improving regimen adherence; simple access to providers appears to be insufficient to improve these outcomes (Rubin, Peyrot, & Siminerio, 2006).

LEADERSHIP CHALLENGE What would you tell Clarisse to do about client collaboration?

Client Registries and Their Effect on Healthcare Practices

The data contained in registries can come from many sources, including hospitals, pharmacy systems, physician practices, and insurance companies. Information can concern clients with the same diagnosis or clients who have undergone a common surgical procedure or received the same newly approved medication.

An analysis of registry data offers insights that can improve health care and public health. For example, nurse leaders may analyze treatments to identify opportunities for quality improvement.

Many client registries are already in use. One of the best-known is the Surveillance, Epidemiology, and End Results Program, which is managed by the National Cancer Institute. That registry collects and publishes data on cancer clients, including demographics and information about their tumors, treatment, and follow-up status. Other registries analyze treatment outcomes for depression, emphysema, Parkinson's disease, and heart disease.

AHRQ released a handbook to help researchers and others use client registries to evaluate the real-life impact of healthcare treatments. This handbook identifies the best scientific practices for operating registries, including how to design a registry, what types of data sources may be accessed, how to encourage participation from clients and healthcare providers, how to detect adverse events, how to interpret data, and how to handle ethical and publications issues. The summary chapter serves as a checklist for best practices. The guide is downloadable from http://effectivehealthcare.ahrq.gov. Hard copies can be ordered from the AHRQ Publications Clearinghouse by e-mailing ahrqpubs@ahrq.gov or by calling 1-800-358-9295.

Pros and Cons of Magnet Recognition as a Way to Improve Care

Some experts believe that **Magnet status** can recognize the quality of nursing care and demonstrate the importance of nurses to an entire organization's success (American Nurses Credentialing Center [ANCC], 2006). Others, including the Massachusetts Nurses Association, disagree, claiming that Magnet status increases reimbursement for services by the federal government and private insurers but does nothing to guarantee a safe nurse-to-client ratio or safe working conditions. Clearly, there are both pros and cons to becoming a Magnet hospital.

> **KEY TERM**
>
> **Magnet status** recognizes the quality of nursing care but does not guarantee a safe nurse-to-client ratio or safe working conditions.

According to the ANCC (2006), which designates Magnet status, advantages to becoming a Magnet hospital include:

- Magnet designation helps with recruitment and retention of nurses.
- Costs are reduced because of low turnover, which results in greater institutional stability.
- A national survey found the 93% of the public would have more confidence in the overall quality of a hospital if it had passed the nursing standards required to be a Magnet hospital.

- The Magnet culture is believed to create a dynamic and positive milieu for professional nurses that includes empowerment, pride, mentoring, nurturing, respect, integrity, and teamwork.

The opposite position on Magnet accreditation is provided by the Massachusetts Nurses Association (MNA), whose board of directors oppose the Magnet program on the grounds that it is an industry strategy to avoid both safe nurse-to-client ratios and improved working conditions for nurses. The MNA provided a list of negatives that result from inadequate RN staffing levels, poor RN-to-patient ratios, mandatory overtime, dangerous working conditions, and dangerous administrative practices, such as using unlicensed personnel to provide care that only RNs should provide and floating nurses to units where they are ill prepared to practice competently and safely (MNA, 2004).

According to the MNA (2004), the effects of inadequate RN staffing include:

- Poor client outcomes
- An alarming number of preventable client deaths that are directly attributable to inadequate RN staffing levels
- A dramatic rise in medical errors

The MNA's objections to Magnet status are that:

- It is a ploy to increase market share by trading on nurses' trust and credibility with the public.
- The process is structured around the formation of nursing councils that give the illusion of shared governance and nurse empowerment without granting nurses equal power with management; nurses have no legally protected veto power, and all decisions are ultimately left to senior administrators.
- Providing quality nursing care and establishing standards of quality care for nursing services should not be a particular institution's choice; it should be a legal requirement and condition of licensure for practice.
- All hospitals, not just Magnet-designated ones, should be accountable for providing safe staffing and a satisfactory work environment for nurses.
- Money spent on Magnet status (thousands of dollars in fees to ANCC consultants and thousands of dollars in staff time) would be better spent on improving staffing conditions or on nursing salaries.
- The US inspector general and another government accounting office commissioned research on a different voluntary credentialing program—the Joint Commission on Accreditation of Healthcare Organizations (JCAHO)—and found that accredited hospitals had significant client safety problems that went undetected by the surveyors. The inspector general's report criticized JCAHO for the collegial relationship between surveyors and those surveyed. MNA stated that the same problems are being duplicated by the Magnet Recognition Program.

- The Magnet Recognition Program provides no specific recommendations for the establishment of safe staffing standards, nor does it grant nurses the protected right to refuse an unsafe patient assignment.
- In the unionized setting, the Magnet process undermines collective bargaining and true workplace democracy by proposing changes in policy without directly dealing with the nurses' elected union representatives, engaging in good-faith negotiations over those changes, or codifying them through enforceable language as part of the union contract.

The MNA (2004) provided the following principles for nurses to use when participating in the Magnet process:

- Frontline nurses should have the power to select, among themselves, who will represent them in the Magnet, or any other, process.
- When elected by peers to participate in the process, frontline nurses must have the right to recommend and approve changes in the criteria for Magnet status based on their institution's needs.
- In a unionized setting, all proposals that impact nurses' working conditions are subject to review, negotiation, and ratification by the union. The same should be true in Magnet institutions.
- The Magnet process should result in a written, legally binding document that guarantees nurses a voice and a real choice in all decisions that impact their work and that obligates the institution to adhere to the standards arrived at for the life of the Magnet recognition designation (i.e., 4 years).
- Nurses participating in the process should have access to all information and materials (financial documents, consultant studies, vendor contracts, merger or restructuring plans, etc.) that will assist them in making informed decisions.
- The process must adhere to collective bargaining, which is authorized and protected by law.

The Presence of Nursing Students and Quality of Care

Having nursing students present on hospital units can affect quality of care given by staff nurses, as the research in **Research Box 13-1** illustrates.

Although more research may be needed, this study adds to the knowledge of quality nursing practice. The results support the much-debated aspects of nursing education and practice. Based on this study, students should be considered a valuable asset to nursing care, not only as future professionals, but also as a means of improving the quality of care.

One use of these findings is to consider sending students to units with a low standard of care. Students generate knowledge because they are learning, asking questions, and making sure that they themselves are on top of things (Akinsanya, 1994; Idvall, Rooke, & Hamrin, 1997).

RESEARCH BOX 13-1   THE PRESENCE OF NURSING STUDENTS AND ITS INFLUENCE ON THE QUALITY OF CARE PROVIDED BY STAFF NURSES

- **Background.** Although it has been suggested that the presence of students may influence the behavior of practitioners, it has not been empirically validated.
- **Hypothesis.** The purpose of this study was to test the hypothesis that the presence of students in hospital units improves the quality of care given by nurses.
- **Conceptual framework.** The theoretical model used in this study focused on two concepts: self-focus and social role.
- **Method.** A strict protocol based on the Israeli Standard Nursing Procedure was used to carry out systematic observations on 15 hospital units. Observers graded nursing activities on a specially designed quality-of-care scale

that allowed for the computing of quality-of-care indexes. Each subject was compared with his or her own performance with and without students.
- **Results.** In the presence of students, nurses provided higher-quality care than when they were alone.
- **Conclusions.** The presence of students had a beneficial effect on nurse performance and quality of care. Data analysis supported the hypothesis.
- **Suggestions for future research.** The general influence of students on the unit is still to be examined in terms of organizational climate and overall functioning of nursing staff.

Source: Adapted from Zisberg, Bar-Tal, & Krulik (2003).

Benchmarking to Make Effective Care Decisions

Benchmarking includes measuring operational and clinical practices that lead to the best outcomes. Your team members will get the most value out of benchmarking by understanding day-to-day operations (Czarnecki, 1995).

Benchmarking is important to:

- Improve current practices
- Understand current performance levels
- Reduce costs
- Provide information for managed care organizations
- Find ways to collaborate with other healthcare providers
- Find gaps in performance
- Bring in ideas from other organizations and identify opportunities
- Rally the organization to create a consensus to move forward
- Offer quality products and services (Czarnecki, 1995)

Steps in the benchmarking process include identifying problems, comparing hospital performance to the benchmark, developing action plans, implementing plans and monitoring progress, and comparing the hospital's revised performance to recalibrated benchmarks (Czarnecki, 1995).

LEADERSHIP IN ACTION

Clarisse was part of a benchmarking team of nurses, physicians, and other staff that convened to study diagnostic-related group (DRG) 127: congestive heart failure. The diagnostic category had been chosen because it was one of the highest-admitting DRGs and because of the need for treatment improvement. The benchmarking team found that its clients with congestive heart failure (CHF) experienced a length of stay that was 2 days longer than other comparable hospitals. Another statistic that raised a red flag was that 38% of those clients in the high-risk CHF group were discharged to go home from the hospital. Clarisse raised the question that maybe this discharge rate could be related to the high readmission rates for clients with a CHF diagnosis.

After interviewing various staff members and studying how similar hospitals worked with this DRG, the benchmarking team made the following recommendations: develop and implement standing nursing orders for a direct admission for stable CHF clients to eliminate delays in beginning treatment; improve discharge planning by advising physicians of possible discharge options; and coordinate available client information about CHF by computerizing all educational materials. These changes were implemented. A follow-up project review revealed positive results in eliminating delays, improving discharge planning, and coordinating client education.

LEADERSHIP CHALLENGE What information about this benchmarking process would you advise Clarisse to share with her team? Give a rationale for your answer.

Summary

This chapter discussed the 2006 National Healthcare Quality Report, the National Database of Nursing Quality Indicators, outcomes research and healthcare effectiveness, improving healthcare disparities, nursing data on quality of care, client evaluations of quality of health care, client registries and their effect on health care, the pros and cons of Magnet recognition as a way to improve care, the presence of nursing students and quality of care, and benchmarking to make effective care decisions.

Key Term Review

- The **Beech study** examined the level of client satisfaction and nursing staff work satisfaction at an urban public hospital in the southwestern United States.
- **Benchmarking** includes measuring operational and clinical practices that lead to the best outcomes.
- **Client-centeredness** is a composite measure of when providers sometimes or never listened carefully, explained things clearly, respected what clients had to say, and spent enough time with them.
- The **DAWN study** was a cross-sectional survey of 13 countries that sampled individuals diagnosed with diabetes and examined client reports of treatment.
- The **Health Care Report Card Compendium** is a searchable directory of over 200 samples of report cards that are produced by a variety of organizations and that show formats for and approaches to providing comparative information on the quality of health plans, hospitals, medical groups, individual physicians, nursing homes, and other care providers.
- **Magnet status** recognizes the quality of nursing care but does not guarantee a safe nurse-to-client ratio or safe working conditions.
- The **National Asthma Education and Prevention Program** develops and disseminates science-based guidelines for the diagnosis and management of asthma.
- The **National Database of Nursing Quality Indicators** allows nursing leaders to compare information with other healthcare facilities and use quality improvement activities to improve effectiveness.
- The **National Healthcare Quality Report** examines and tracks the quality of health care in the United States, including effectiveness, client safety, timeliness, and client-centeredness.
- The **Shabrawy and Mahmoud study** in Saudi Arabia measured satisfaction with primary healthcare services.
- **State Snapshots** is an interactive Web-based tool, produced by AHRQ annually using data from the NHQR and NHDR, and is designed to help state officials and their public- and private-sector partners understand healthcare quality and disparities in their state.
- **Timeliness** is a measure of the percentage of emergency room visits during which the client left without being seen.

Leadership Development Exercises

- **Leadership Development Exercise 13-1**

Discuss the NHQR and NDNQI with at least three colleagues.

a. Strategize about at least three ways to improve healthcare effectiveness.
b. Try out one of your strategies in a real-life or hypothetical situation.
c. Present an oral report to a class or write a paper about your real or hypothesized findings.

■ Leadership Development Exercise 13-2
Give examples of healthcare outcomes research.

■ Leadership Development Exercise 13-3
Describe uses a nurse leader might make of the Health Care Report Card Compendium.

■ Leadership Development Exercise 13-4
Discuss how to use client registries to determine healthcare effectiveness.

■ Leadership Development Exercise 13-5
Describe disparities in healthcare provision.

■ Leadership Development Exercise 13-6
Discuss the four steps in the benchmarking process.

■ Leadership Development Exercise 13-7

a. Obtain permission from a nurse leader to interview at least three clients about the care they received.
b. Present your findings to at least three colleagues, and obtain feedback.
c. Decide on a strategy for presenting your findings to the nurse leader on the unit you surveyed.

■ Leadership Development Exercise 13-8
Debate the pros and cons of Magnet hospital accreditation with at least two other colleagues.

Optional: Write up the results, and submit it for publication.

Advanced Leadership Development Exercises

■ Leadership Development Exercise 13-9
Teach effectiveness measurement skills to at least three student nurses in an undergraduate leadership course or nurses on a unit team.

■ Leadership Development Exercise 13-10
Analyze a real or hypothetical benchmarking process.

■ **Leadership Development Exercise 13-11**

a. Formulate a problem statement for a nursing project related to demonstrating healthcare effectiveness.

b. Share your problem statement with at least three other colleagues, and obtain feedback.

c. Revise your problem statement based on the feedback you received.

■ **Leadership Development Exercise 13-12**

a. Design a research project related to demonstrating effective management.

b. Share your design with at least three other colleagues.

c. Obtain feedback, and revise your project based on what you learn.

■ **Leadership Development Exercise 13-13**

Design a registry to improve client care.

a. Download the AHRQ's handbook (see section on client registries).

b. Decide on the types of data sources to use.

c. Devise a plan to encourage client and healthcare provider participation.

d. Strategize about how to detect and use information about adverse events.

e. Decide on which ways to interpret data.

f. Design a plan for handling ethical and publication issues.

g. Develop a checklist for best practices.

References

Agency for Healthcare Research and Quality. (2006). *Outcomes research: Fact sheet*. Rockville, MD: Author. Retrieved June 3, 2007, from http://www.ahrq.gov/clinic/outfact.htm

Agency for Healthcare Research and Quality. (2007). *Key themes and highlights from the National Healthcare Quality Report*. Rockville, MD: Author. Retrieved June 2, 2007, from http://www.ahrq.gov/qual/nhqr06/highlights/nhqr06high.htm

Akinsanya, J. A. (1994). Commitment to nursing: The quest for quality education and practice. *Journal of Advanced Nursing, 20*, 983–985.

American Nurses Credentialing Center. (2006). *The benefits of becoming a Magnet designated facility*. Retrieved June 2, 2007, from http://www.nursingworld.org/ancc.magnet.html

Beech, B. M. (1995). *Patient satisfaction and nursing staff work satisfaction in an urban public teaching hospital*. Unpublished dissertation, University of Texas HSC at Houston School of Public Health, Houston, TX.

Clancy, C. M., & Eisenberg, J. M. (1998). Outcomes research: Measure the end results of health care. *Science, 282*, 245–6.

Czarnecki, M. T. (1995). *Benchmarking strategies for health care management*. Gaithersburg, MD: Aspen.

Grady, P. A. (2003). A NINR initiative to address health disparities. *Nursing Outlook, 11*, 5.

Idvall, E., Rooke, L., & Hamrin, E. (1997). Quality indicators in clinical nursing: Review of the literature. *Journal of Advanced Nursing, 25,* 6–17.

Kamien, M. (1992). Can first-year medical students contribute to better care for patients with a chronic disease? *Medical Education, 24,* 23–26.

Lublin, J. R. (1992). Role modeling: A case study in general practice. *Medical Education, 26,* 116–122.

Massachusetts Nurses Association. (2004). *Position statement on the "Magnet Recognition Program for Nursing Services in Hospitals" and other consultant-driven quality improvement projects that claim to improve care.* Retrieved June 2, 2007, from http://www.mass nurses.org/pubs/positions/magnet.htm

Nevada Nurses Association. (2006). National database of nursing quality indicators transferring data into quality care. *Nevada RNformation.* Retrieved June 7, 2007, from http://findarticles.com/p/articles/mi_qa4102/is_200602/ai_n17170216

Reichert, A. L. (1998, June 7). Postoperative nursing care contributions to symptom distress and functional status after ambulatory surgery. *Medsurg Nursing,* 148–158.

Rubin, R. R., Peyrot, M., & Siminerio, L. M. (2006). Health care and patient-reported outcomes: Results of the cross-national Diabetes Attitudes, Wishes and Needs (DAWN) study. *Diabetes Care, 29,* 1249–1255.

Shabrawy Ali, M. E., & Mahmoud, M. E. A. (1993). A study of patient satisfaction with primary health care services in Saudi Arabia. *Journal of Community Health, 18*(1), 49–54.

Wilson, A., & Startup, R. (1991). Nurse socialization: Issues and problems. *Journal of Advanced Nursing, 16,* 1478–1486.

Yang, K. A., Simms, L. M., & Yin, J. T. (1998). Factors influencing nursing-sensitive outcomes in Taiwanese nursing homes. *Online Journal of Issues in Nursing, 3*(2). Retrieved November 16, 2007, from http://nursingworld.org/MainMenuCategories /ANAMarketplace/ANAPeriodicals/OJIN/TableofContents/Vol31998/Vol3No21998 /TaiwaneseNursingHomes.aspx

Zisberg, A., Bar-Tal., Y., & Krulik, T. (2003). The presence of nursing students and its influence on the quality of care provided by staff nurses. *Nursing Outlook, 11,* 102–106.

Managing Change and Innovation

After reading this chapter, answering the leadership challenges, and participating in the leadership development exercises, you will be able to:

- Explain the nature of change in nursing
- Discuss planned-change theories and their relevance to nursing
- Assess your change agent capabilities
- Try out different change theory measures
- Discuss methods for dealing with resistance to change
- List innovation strategies

Advanced nurses will be able to:

- Teach peers or less experienced nurse leaders how to produce change
- Design a problem statement to study change or innovation
- Develop a research project to study change or innovation

Introduction

Change is inevitable, unpredictable, and constant. There is no way to escape it, so it is often best to view it as a challenge or an opportunity for learning. In this era of staff who are weary of the managed care environment, introducing change seems simple, but it requires outstanding communication skills and a keen sense of timing (Rich, 1998). This chapter explores theories of change, the nurse as a change agent, and innovation in nursing.

LEADERSHIP IN ACTION

Robert, a nurse leader working in a medical center, wanted to bring change to his unit and make the results consistent with nursing philosophy. Along the way, he wanted to build trust and avoid threatening the staff. When he observed staff, he found that they had become lackadaisical about giving care and had very little to suggest when he asked them for input.

LEADERSHIP CHALLENGE What advice would you give Robert to help him meet his goals?

You might tell him a number of things. One of them might be that before taking action, it is wise to construct a strategy based on theory. Planned-change models may be useful.

KEY TERM

In an **open systems framework**, change is possible in any work setting, and what happens in one part of the system will affect the whole system, including the nurse leader.

Open Systems Theory

Before we explore the different models for planned change, remember that, no matter which model you choose, in a **open systems framework** change in one part of the system affects the whole system. This can be helpful because it is not always necessary to work directly with the target person to effect change. Another thing to remember is that leaders who start a change process will also be affected by it.

Although change is everywhere, it is common to hear employees complain, "Nothing ever changes here. This is the way things were when I came, and they will be this way when I leave."

From a systems framework, change is inevitable, but it may not be sweeping, large-scale change. Some changes are barely perceptible; others can seem to be earth shaking. All systems have the potential to change, even though employees may not agree with the decision to change. As a nurse leader, it is important to keep this principle of systems theory in the forefront of your mind when employees resist change.

Systems have a tendency to resist change and to maintain integrity and identity. Bureaucracies have built-in resistances, but even these systems change over time. Change is neither inherently good or bad. Some changes have positive effects; others have negative effects.

LEADERSHIP CHALLENGE How can Robert use this information on systems theory to bring change to his unit?

Sometimes, resistance to change is a healthy response. The following example demonstrates how resistance can be healthy.

LEADERSHIP IN ACTION

City Hospital developed plans for a new nuclear medicine laboratory. Staff in the hospital joined forces with community residents. They picketed, wrote letters to the hospital administrator, and contacted radio and TV news to describe the negative effects that the materials in the new lab might have on the health of clients and staff. Staff saw this change as a threat to their own and others' health and opposed it.

Factors Affecting a System Influence Change

An open system responds to change according to the many factors influencing it. Knowing the positive effects of a proposed change is only one of those factors. That can affect staff. Even if they know what to expect, they may still resist the change. (That is why it is important to have more than one planned-change model in your repertoire.)

Another factor that influences a system's response to change is that knowledge alone may not be sufficient to effect change. The following example illustrates this point.

LEADERSHIP IN ACTION

Dolores, age 48, had emphysema after years of heavy cigarette smoking and living in a highly polluted area of the city. Despite the evidence to the contrary, Dolores insists that she has to continue to smoke because it is the only pleasure she has left. Attempts to convince her of the dangers of smoking result in resistance, and she refuses to accept smoking cessation information.

Another factor affecting acceptance of change is the rate of change. Nurse leaders who expect staff members to make a change quickly, even when given sufficient preparation, are in for a rude awakening. Any change that occurs rapidly is apt to evoke system resistance.

Other factors that can affect a system's response to change include:

- The perceived importance of the change
- The needs, values, and coping skills of individuals involved in the change

- Whether those expected to change are involved in planning for the change (if they are, you will encounter less resistance)

LEADERSHIP CHALLENGE   How can Robert use the information on system response when he implements change on the unit?

Models for Planned Change

Many planned-change models are available. The following models are presented in this chapter: the rational model, normative model, change process model, change agent model, power-coercive model, and paradoxical model.

> **KEY TERM**
>
> Assumptions underlying the **rational model for planned change** are that people are logical and behave rationally; ignorance and superstition are the main roadblocks to change; and once people are informed, they will adopt a change willingly.

Rational Model for Planned Change

You are probably most familiar with the **rational model for planned change.** The assumptions underlying this model are:

- People are logical and behave rationally.
- Ignorance and superstition are the main roadblocks to change.
- Once people are informed, they will adopt a change willingly.

> **KEY TERM**
>
> **Rogers's diffusion of innovation model** includes three steps: invention of the change, diffusion or communication of information about the change, and adoption or rejection of the change.

One of the best-known examples of this model is **Rogers's diffusion of innovation** (Rogers & Shoemaker, 1971). This model is frequently used in health education. Rogers's model has three steps:

1. Invention of the change
2. Diffusion or communication of information about the change
3. Adoption or rejection of the change

LEADERSHIP CHALLENGE   Is the rational model of change something Robert should consider using with his staff? Give a rationale for your answer.

The rational model is the method of choice when there is almost universal readiness for the change within the system. The following example illustrates a system that is ready for change and for which the rational model is a good choice.

LEADERSHIP IN ACTION

Samantha, a nurse leader in an HMO, was asked for her assistance in selecting foods to eat to prevent heart conditions. Samantha consulted references for the latest nutritional information and developed an outline and handout (invention of change). Next, Samantha contacted all clients and healthcare personnel who had asked for information, surveyed records from other possible candidates, and announced in the HMO's regular newsletter and in a radio spot (use of mass media for diffusion) that there would be a workshop on the subject in 2 weeks. Samantha also hung a poster and distributed fliers in all outpatient clinics for the next 2 weeks. She did a 1-month and 6-month follow-up on all workshop attendees to find out whether they had made changes in their daily eating habits as a result of the workshop (adoption or rejection of the change).

Normative Model for Planned Change

The **normative model for planned change** provides a more holistic approach. It recognizes and deals with the influence of needs, feelings, attitudes, and values on efforts to change. The assumptions underlying this model are:

- All members of the system are active participants in the change process.
- Rationality is only one of the many factors that influence change.
- The system can resist or modify change.
- Education alone is not enough to implement change.

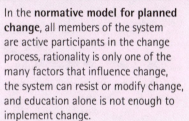

KEY TERM

In the **normative model for planned change**, all members of the system are active participants in the change process, rationality is only one of the many factors that influence change, the system can resist or modify change, and education alone is not enough to implement change.

LEADERSHIP TIP

Two types of normative models are the change process model and the change agent model.

LEADERSHIP CHALLENGE Is the normative model for planned change something Robert could use at this time? Give a rationale for your answer.

Change Process Model

The **change process model** was developed by Lewin (1951) and revised by Schein and Bennis (1975). It is divided into three phases:

1. Freezing
2. Changing
3. Refreezing

KEY TERM

The **change process model** is divided into three phases: freezing, changing, and refreezing.

Lewin (1951) recommended that a system be analyzed to identify forces for and against change before implementing the change process. For example, in attempting to help team members reduce stress, a nurse leader identified the following forces for change:

- Group members expressed a willingness to learn about stress management procedures.
- They gave lip service to the importance of role modeling.
- They had the ability to learn stress management procedures.

Forces against change included:

- Giving up their old methods of dealing with stress was a potential threat to group members.
- Team members had little or no previous knowledge of stress management methods.
- They refused to complete between-class stress management tasks because of a "lack of time."
- They did not participate in selecting the class materials or topics to cover.

Groups often need a push to begin the change process. Specific procedures can **unfreeze the system** so it will be ready to change. These include using disconfirmation, inducing guilt and anxiety, and providing psychological safety. In the previous example, participants had already come together as a group that planned to focus on stress management methods. The leader had yet to convince them to become appropriate role models in stress reduction methods, although they gave lip service to the idea.

The nurse leader brought research findings to the group that detailed how role modeling was a powerful teaching tool (using disconfirmation), indicated that team members may not be doing the best job possible if they do not model stress management (inducing guilt and anxiety), and assured team members that they would have ample time and opportunities to learn how to use the procedures in their own lives before using them at work (providing psychological safety).

During the **change phase** of the change process model, the nurse leader used planned-change theory when:

- Encouraging team members to practice and experiment with stress management procedures (so those procedures would become part of the system's regular patterns)
- Providing a supportive climate (to reduce resistance to change)
- Providing opportunities to vent about the guilt, anxiety, and/or anger aroused by the change process (to reduce resistance to change)

- Providing feedback on progress and clarifying goals (to reinforce change and keep the group on task)
- Preserving confidentiality (to reduce resistance to change)
- Energizing the group
- Returning to freezing tactics when resistance arose

The purpose of the **refreezing phase** is to make sure that the change becomes part of the system's everyday functioning. If you provide continuing education experiences for groups, you must pay particular attention to this phase to ensure that participants do not return to their work settings only to revert to previous behaviors. One way to do this is to provide follow-up workshops, interviews, letters, phone or e-mail discussions, or peer partnerships with specific reinforcement skills to assist with refreezing.

> **KEY TERM**
> The purpose of the **refreezing phase** is to make sure that the change becomes part of the system's everyday functioning.

When working with ongoing teams, complete the following functions during the refreezing phase:

- Show continued interest and support.
- Delegate responsibility to team members.
- Keep the change visible by stating observed changes or illustrating them through charts, letters, memos, newsletter items, and other concrete measures of change.
- Intervene when problems of implementing the new behavior occur.
- Designate specific team members as peer helpers for other members outside of team meetings.

LEADERSHIP CHALLENGE What would Robert have to do first before he tried to use the change process model on his unit? Give a rationale for your answer.

Change Agent Model

Havelock (1973) developed a **change agent model** that included the following steps:

- Building a relationship of trust
- Diagnosing the problem through a consensus of opinion
- Assessing resources for change
- Setting goals
- Selecting strategies
- Reinforcing change

> **KEY TERM**
> The **change agent model** includes building a relationship of trust, diagnosing the problem through consensus, assessing resources, setting goals, selecting strategies, and reinforcing change.

Take a moment, and answer the questions in **Table 14-1** to assess your change agent potential. Even if you do not know how to answer all the questions now, by the time you finish reading this chapter and complete the leadership development exercises, you will be able to provide answers.

Normative models like the change agent model work best when there is little resistance to change and participants are open to being persuaded and can problem-solve. Normative models do not work well when bosses or others are not open to persuasion, when conflicting values preclude consensus, or when those in power resist sharing it with others.

The example that follows shows how one nurse leader used the change agent model to implement planned change.

LEADERSHIP IN ACTION

Claudia took a position of authority in a community health agency. Initially, she spent a lot of time with the staff, meeting with them and finding out about their jobs, concerns, and dreams (building a relationship of trust). She listened, and the staff told her everything that was wrong with the agency. Almost everyone agreed that something had to be done about the referral system (diagnosing the problem). Claudia called a meeting to discuss the need to meet with physicians and other healthcare professionals involved in referrals. Claudia shared the referral process that she had used successfully when she was a nurse leader at a similar agency (assessing resources). Group members decided to invite healthcare professionals to a tea that they were holding to honor their 10th year in business and asked that everyone involved in referrals meet after the tea to decide on the best way to change the referral process (setting goals and selecting strategies).

Ninety percent of the healthcare professionals they invited showed up and were most eager to speak and ask questions about referrals. By the end of the meeting, they had all agreed to try Claudia's referral process and worked out a way and a time to begin testing it out (reinforcing the change). Claudia also agreed to be available to these healthcare professionals to provide direction and support as they moved forward.

Power-Coercive Model for Planned Change

The **power-coercive model** for change (Tappan, 1983) focuses on overcoming resistance to change. In this model, needs, feelings, attitudes, and values are recognized but not always respected. The assumptions underlying this model are:

- Consensus cannot be reached through persuasive methods.
- When change is needed and the target system is resistant, power must be seized.

TABLE 14-1 YOUR CHANGE AGENT CAPABILITIES

1. Change theory

    1. The change theory that I would choose in most instances is

    _____

2. Rationale for change theory

    2. The _____ change theory is best for

    where I work because _____

    _____

3. Change strategies

    3. To bring about change in another person, group, or

    organization, I would _____

    _____

    _____

    _____

    (List specific actions you would take.)

4. Reducing resistance to change

    4. The best ways to reduce resistance to change are to

    _____

    _____

    _____

    _____

5. Involving staff in change

    5. The best ways to involve staff in change efforts are to

    _____

    _____

    _____

    _____

Many different kinds of power exist, including physical force, public embarrassment, loss (or threat of loss) of prestige or popularity, money, practice acts (i.e., legal power), public recognition and support, establishing oneself as an expert in the eyes of the public, using an idea or symbol that has meaning (e.g., Gandhi used the power of passive resistance), strength in numbers (e.g., if all employees united, their voices would be heard), and control of access to resources (e.g., if a group of employees seized access to money, communication, or information in a healthcare agency, they would have a great deal of power). Threat of harm is also a source of power.

The basic steps in the power-coercive model are:

- Define the issue and identify the opponent.
- Begin an action phase.
- Keep the pressure on.
- Force a decision through struggle.

The power-coercive model uses sources of power that are most available to the have-nots. The example that follows illustrates the use of the power-coercive model.

LEADERSHIP IN ACTION

The chief of medicine was being pressured by two obstetricians and an oncologist not to allow nurses to teach their clients postpartum exercises or to talk with clients about parenting. This pressure began after one client had been found weeping after a talk with a nurse. The chief of medicine complained to the hospital administrator who asked the director of nursing to ask all nurses to cease teaching and counseling clients. The director of nursing refused and showed the hospital administrator a copy of their state's nurse practice act.

The administrator sent out his own memo to order the nurses to stop teaching clients. The head nurse on one unit was infuriated and decided that the issue was one of nurses' rights and that their opponent was the administrator (defining the issue and identifying the opponent). The head nurse met with two of her nurse colleagues. They decided to collect signatures and send a reasonable letter stating their position.

Signatures were collected, and key people who signed met with the head nurse to plan their next move. They identified their power by the many nurses who had signed the letter (i.e., strength in numbers). The nurse practice act (i.e., legal power) provides support of clients, most physicians, and staff for client teaching (i.e., public support). The fact that the nurses were good at their job (i.e., expert power) and had the potential to refuse work and paralyze the hospital system (i.e., threat of harm) was especially powerful.

Four nurses launched a campaign to publicize their fight and had buttons and fliers made up that read, "Nurses' Rights" (beginning an action phase). The nurses asked clients, physicians, and other nurses to call or stop by the administrator's office to tell him that they thought he was susceptible to physician influence (keeping the pressure on) and began to refer to the administrator as "chicken Chuck." By resorting to ridicule, the nurses hoped to keep the pressure on. By refusing to back down, the nurses forced a struggle.

The four nurses met with the director of nursing and asked for more direct support. Their next attack focused on making the administrator look foolish by obeying his rules while simultaneously bringing in pressure from outside the hospital. They stopped talking to clients, and the director of nursing canceled all prenatal classes and asked the local newspaper and radio stations to announce the cancellations. The president of the hospital called the administrator, demanding to know why they were going to be the only hospital in the city without "those popular prenatal classes" and ordered the administrator to stop the public announcements. The chief of medicine told the administrator to let the nurses get on with their work and stop being ridiculous so that physicians could get on with theirs.

Victorious, the nurses celebrated by agreeing to serve on the nurse advisory committee to make recommendations about anything that affected nurses or nursing. The director of nursing strengthened her position in relation to the administrator so that future policies affecting nursing would come only from her office.

Paradoxical Model for Planned Change

The paradoxical model is based on the brief therapy model of Haley (1973) and Watzlawick, Weakland, and Fisch (1974). Some assumptions underlying the model are:

- There are two kinds of change: first-order and second-order change.
- First-order change occurs within a given system. The individual or a variation of behavior may change, but the system remains the same. For example, a team may exhibit disturbance when several nurses are frequently absent. Over time, absenteeism may drop, but tardiness and resistance to change may increase. Using this model, these behaviors become symptoms of an underlying problem in the work system. The only change that has occurred is that the disturbance has moved from one worker to another. In this sense, first-order change does not alter system patterns and may even reinforce them.
- Second-order change is change of change. The system changes because it takes on a new perspective on the problem or situation. This new perspective is called "reframing," and it deals with the effects of the problem, not its cause. Insight is not essential in this approach.

Steps in the paradoxical model for change are:

- Forget about trying to understand the cause of the problem.
- Determine the symptom-solution cycle.

- Encourage resistance.
- Define goal behavior.
- Secure a commitment to change.
- Set a time limit for change.
- Prescribe the symptom.
- Include a variation.
- Reframe the situation in the client's language.
- Secure agreement to follow instructions.
- Predict a relapse.
- Demystify or disengage.

The example that follows illustrates one use of the paradoxical model in a healthcare setting.

LEADERSHIP IN ACTION

The members of a nursing team decided to discuss their fears of speaking up in interdisciplinary conferences. The nurse leader did not try to understand the underlying causes of their anxiety (forgetting about trying to understand the cause of the problem).

The nurse leader spent 15 minutes helping team members describe exactly what happened right before they attempted to speak up in an interdisciplinary conference. They described feeling a rush of anxiety, dry throats, butterflies in their stomachs, cracking voices, pounding hearts, and an inability to speak (determining the symptom-solution cycle).

One team member said that she would rather not talk about the problem and asked whether it was OK to just listen. The nurse leader smiled and said, "Sure. Just hold back until it seems like the right time to speak. Don't reveal anything until you're absolutely ready" (encouraging resistance while conveying the message that a time will come when it will feel all right to speak).

The nursing leader asked team members to define a behavioral goal to accomplish (defining goal behavior). The nurse leader asked them to think about their willingness to try a new solution. They all nodded and agreed that they were willing. The nurse leader told them, "I have a solution in mind, but I'll only tell you if you promise to carry out the instructions to the letter." The group agreed unanimously (securing a commitment to change). The nurse leader said, "Do you want the slow or fast method?" The team said in unison, "Fast!" (By asking an either-or question about time, the nurse leader is setting a time limit. The only choice is whether change will occur sooner or later.)

"The first thing you must do," the nurse leader told the group, "is to go ahead and be nervous when you walk into the next interdisciplinary conference. Notice how your heart pounds, how dry your throat is, how many butterflies you have in your stomach" (prescribing the symptom). The nurse leader next told the team, "Instead of whatever you plan to say at the meeting, announce, 'I'm so nervous that I'll probably blow this, but here it goes,' and then go on to say what you'd planned to say" (including a variation). "When you try to hide your nervousness, it's like a lie," the nurse leader told the team. "Tell them up front that you are nervous. It will help decrease your anxiety." (Several team members had indicated the importance of honesty and truthfulness, so by saying this, the nurse leader reframed the situation in their language.) The nurse leader reminded team members that they had agreed to try out the solution (securing agreement to follow instructions).

The next week, several team members reported speaking up in interdisciplinary conferences without difficulty. The group leader warned the team to expect a relapse, not to worry if they were anxious infrequently in the future, and to stammer and have a few butterflies in the next meeting to show that they were still nervous. "Make a point of showing your nervousness just to keep in touch with your feelings," the nurse leader said (predicting a relapse). One of the team members said, "I guess my problem about speaking up just cleared up by itself." The nurse leader explained the process of paradoxical intention to the group (demystifying or disengaging).

Choosing an Appropriate Change Model

There are many change models to choose from. Haffer (1986) suggested using an adaptation of Hersey and Blanchard's situational leadership styles (see Chapter 1) to choose the best change model for the group and the situation. This model shows the relationship between the amount of direction and support that the nurse leader provides and the designated team's willingness and ability to change.

Choose from one of the following nurse leader styles:

- *Telling* is useful when the team has a low ability and low willingness to change. For this type of situation, spell out clear directions, including what to do, when, and how. Power-coercive and rational models work best.
- *Selling* is for a low to moderate willingness and ability to change, take responsibility, and/or problem-solve. Spell out the models, and expect team members to be more willing to change if you provide a reason and some direction. Rational methods are more apt to succeed.
- *Participating* is for a moderate to high ability and willingness to change. Build confidence and motivation if you want change, and encourage collaboration. Use a supportive and nondirective style and encourage participants to mobilize local resources and use self-help methods.
- *Delegating* is for a high ability and high willingness to change. Team members are independent, consistent, and highly motivated to change. They need little direction or support. They determine their own direction, goals,

and motivation. If you tell or direct a team that operates at this level to do something, its members are apt to resist.

Dealing with Resistance to Change

You will not be successful in introducing change unless you are aware of the reasons for the resistance to change and find a way to deal with them.

Reasons for Resistance

According to Kotter and Schlesinger (1979), there are four reasons for resistance to change:

1. *Self-interest.* Some team members may be more concerned with the implication of the change for themselves and how it may affect their own interests rather than considering its effect on client care.
2. *Misunderstanding.* Communication problems and inadequate information can lead to a lack of understanding about change.
3. *Low tolerance to change.* Team members may like a feeling of stability and security and dislike the instability change brings.
4. *Different perspectives on the situation.* Not all team members may agree that change is needed and on the advantages and disadvantages of a particular change process.

Ford, Ford, and McNamara (2006) list other sources of resistance:

- *Complacency.* Complacent team members make comments such as "If it's not broken, don't fix it"; "Don't rock the boat"; and "Why mess with success?"
- *Resignation.* Resigned staff are used to failure; they do not expect any projects to work out. You may hear comments such as "My position doesn't give me any power" or "Why should we do this? It won't make any different anyway."
- *Cynicism.* In resignation, a person attributes failure to him- or herself; in cynicism, that same person attributes failure to other people and groups. Comments you may hear are "No one can make this work" and "I don't know why they bother. This won't work either." Conversations are apt to include comments about being let down, deceived, betrayed, or misled by powerful others.

Approaches to Dealing with Resistance

No matter what the source of resistance to change is, there are numerous ways to reduce it:

- *Communicate.* One of the best ways to reduce resistance is to provide accurate information about a change. By presenting information before the change, staff can see the logic of the change effort. This can reduce the number of unfounded rumors, and it's polite and respectful. Never just spring a change on staff.
- *Involve.* The more staff are involved in changes, the less likely they are to resist those changes.
- *Support.* By helping staff deal with their fears and anxieties during the transition period, you can provide a valuable service and reduce resistance to change.
- *Negotiate.* You can offer incentives to staff so they will not resist change or can allow team members who are resisting the change to veto certain threatening elements of the change.
- *Co-opt.* Co-opt with staff who resist change by bringing them into a change planning group and giving them a role that does not threaten the change effort.
- *Coerce.* Use coercion only when speed is essential and only as a last resort. You can force staff into accepting change by making it clear that resistance to change can lead to job losses, dismissals, transfers, and/or fewer promotions.

The best way to deal with complacent, resigned, and cynical staff may be through reinvention (Goss, Pascale, & Athos, 1993). Reinvention differs from change. Reinvention is about undoing what is and creating something new—a new context. Once the context is revealed, staff can take responsibility for creating a new order.

No matter what change model you choose, remember Schein's (1995) words: "To become motivated to change, we must accept the information and connect it to something we care about."

How do you help staff connect? Schein (1995) suggested that modeling how to handle change may not lead to positive results because the change procedures may not fit with staff personality or style or with the culture of the organization. Instead, he suggested the following procedures:

- Balance the amount of threat the change evokes with enough psychological safety to allow those involved to accept information, experience survival anxiety, and still be motivated to change.
- Get staff working in groups that can provide the safety and rewards they need.
- Devise parallel systems that allow some relief from day-to-day work pressures.
- Provide practice arenas in which errors are embraced as learning examples and not feared.

- Encourage staff to develop positive visions to encourage themselves and others: these could be demonstrated through shared symbols, colors, or words.
- Help staff break the change learning process into manageable steps.
- Provide online coaching to reduce anxiety and enhance motivation to learn and change.
- Instead of choosing words or symbols for a work group, provide a source of possible change solutions, and/or let group members choose from a list the solution that fits the culture within which they operate.
- Use Lewin's (1951) concept of action research to help staff learn about and change the system within which they work: choose a doable project focused on something that your nurses care about, that they are involved in, and that could make a real contribution to the organization; and encourage nurses to meet with other staff to report progress, share war stories and solutions, act as consultants for each other's change projects, and discuss how they can actually produce change that has an impact.

Leading Innovation

An **innovation** is the introduction of something new. Daphne Scordato, an RN and the director of patient services at Baptist Hospital in Pensacola, Florida, does not just think nurses should be innovative; she expects them to be innovative. Through Baptist Hospital's Bright Ideas program, all employees are required to submit three new ideas a year.

The Bright Ideas program has helped foster a spirit of unprecedented innovation and creativity. By providing a climate in which innovation and creativity are accepted, expected, and honored, Scordato has made it safe for nurses to innovate.

Research has demonstrated that for innovative behavior to emerge, professional nurses must have a high level of achievement motivation and work attitude, and they must work in a creative climate (Hengboriboonpong & Oumtanee, 2004). The Bright Ideas program is an example of how to begin to forge a creative climate.

Scordato believes that nurse leaders have a responsibility to model innovative behavior and encourage it in employees. Some questions to use to think of a new idea are:

- Why do we do it this way?
- Does it make the most sense to do things this way?
- Can you think of a different way to accomplish the same thing?

So far, the Bright Ideas program has generated ideas for education and communication, including developing a rapid response team, placing whiteboards at bedsides for staff communication, posting staff pictures and names to facilitate recognition by clients and coworkers, erecting a color-coded status board to allow nurses to signal their availability or need for assistance, and developing a database of notaries public to help finalize living wills (Federwisch, 2007).

One of the problems that innovators face is that most healthcare systems are not ready to support innovation. But that is changing, especially in nursing. Fortunately, the Robert Wood Johnson Foundation is leading the way to bolster safety, reliability, and a client-centered focus on medical-surgical units. This has led to the "one client, one nurse, one innovation a day" philosophy in a medical-surgical and orthopedics unit at Kaiser Permanente–Roseville in California. In this setting, Charles Meek, an RN and nurse manager, encourages bedside nurses to initiate better ways of providing care and to test those innovations out on a small scale (Federwisch, 2007).

Successful approaches undergo more wide-scale testing. Nurses keep track of the tests that are under way and the past successes on a whiteboard on the unit. One of the first tests was to try to lower the rate of non-ventilator-associated pneumonia because of aspiration. Working with a geriatric clinical nurse specialist, a nurse fellow identified some of the best practices in the literature and, from that, developed an oral care kit that was highly successful (Federwisch, 2007).

Other approaches include an innovation committee that gets together monthly to brainstorm and try to figure out how staff on four departments within surgical services can enhance communication with each other to improve client care (Federwisch, 2007).

Staff may protest that their workloads are increasing and that they don't have time to innovate. For them, starting small—one client at a time—may be the answer (Federwisch, 2007).

At least one healthcare provider has recognized the importance of innovation in nursing. The Kaiser Permanente Sidney R. Garfield Health Care Innovation Center has been building a team focused on identifying and assessing emerging clinical IT innovation. The center has advertised for a "clinical innovation leader for nursing" who will help shape the vision for and selection of new technologies for evaluation. This nurse will be involved in developing appropriate experiments for the center; providing leadership and expert consultation on the design, development, and implementation of experimental testing of new technologies; assisting in communicating experiment results; and providing leadership for subsequent live pilots (Kaiser Permanente, 2006).

Innovating in a Community Hospital

A significant part of your mission in a community hospital is to partner with community interests. You may need to commit to initiatives such as adult and child day care, free meeting space, hazardous waste disposal, forensic services, education, instruction in English as a second language, case management of the chronically ill, coordination of parish nursing programs, and providing low-cost or free bicycle helmets to kids (Joel, 1998).

Your community may require other services. To find out which ones it needs, you will have to search out the true community leaders and make them part of your inner circle. The survival of your healthcare organization may depend on being perceived as valuable to the community. Volunteer staff time may be an important component of being able to provide such value (Joel, 1998).

Summary

This chapter brought you information related to change and innovation, including theories and models for planned change, information about choosing an appropriate change model, approaches to dealing with change resistance, and advice on leading innovation.

Key Term Review

- The **change agent model** includes building a relationship of trust, diagnosing the problem through consensus, assessing resources, setting goals, selecting strategies, and reinforcing change.
- During the **change phase** of the change process model, the nurse leader encourages experimentation, provides a supportive climate and feedback, preserves confidentiality, energizes the group, and helps it return to freezing tactics when resistance arises.
- The **change process model** is divided into three phases: freezing, changing, and refreezing.
- An **innovation** is the introduction of something new.
- In the **normative model for planned change,** all members of the system are active participants in the change process, rationality is only one of the many factors that influence change, the system can resist or modify change, and education alone is not enough to implement change.
- In an **open systems framework,** change is possible in any work setting, and what happens in one part of the system will affect the whole system, including the nurse leader.
- The **power-coercive model** uses sources of power that are most available to the have-nots.
- Assumptions underlying the **rational model for planned change** are that people are logical and behave rationally; ignorance and superstition are the main roadblocks to change; and once people are informed, they will adopt a change willingly.
- The purpose of the **refreezing phase** is to make sure that the change becomes part of the system's everyday functioning.
- **Rogers's diffusion of innovation model** includes three steps: invention of the change, diffusion or communication of information about the change, and adoption or rejection of the change.
- The nurse leader **unfreezes the system** by using disconfirmation, guilt and anxiety, and psychological safety procedures.

Leadership Development Exercises

- **Leadership Development Exercise 14-1**
Explain the nature of change in nursing.

- **Leadership Development Exercise 14-2**
Discuss planned-change theories and their relevance to nursing.

- **Leadership Development Exercise 14-3**
  a. Try out different change theory measures discussed in this chapter.
  b. Share your results with at least three colleagues, and obtain feedback.

■ **Leadership Development Exercise 14-4**

   a. Choose at least two methods for dealing with resistance to change.

   b. Discuss the pros and cons of each method with at least three colleagues.

■ **Leadership Development Exercise 14-5**

   a. List innovation strategies.

   b. Choose two, and try them out.

   c. Discuss your findings with at least three colleagues, and obtain feedback.

Advanced Leadership Development Exercises

■ **Leadership Development Exercise 14-6**

   a. Find an acceptable teaching situation to teach peers or less experienced nurse leaders principles for introducing change. (One possible experiential exercise generates emotional responses to a merger, teaches about environmental turbulence and uncertainty, and allows participants to understand various change concepts, including bases of power and influence tactics. The exercise is available in K. S. McDonald & D. Mansour-Cole, Change requires intensive care: An experiential exercise for learners in university and corporate settings. *Journal of Management Education*, *24*[1], 127–148.)

   b. Teach the principles.

   c. Obtain feedback from the learners.

   d. Share your findings with at least three colleagues.

■ **Leadership Development Exercise 14-7**

   a. Design a problem statement to study change or innovation.

   b. Share your problem statement with at least three colleagues, and obtain feedback.

   c. Revise your problem statement, if needed.

■ **Leadership Development Exercise 14-8**

   a. Develop a research project to answer the problem statement you developed in Leadership Development Exercise 14-7.

   b. If possible, complete a pilot study.

   c. Share your findings with at least three colleagues.

References

Federwisch, A. (2007, May 7). What's the big idea? *Nursing Spectrum*, 38–39.

Ford, J. D., Ford, L. W., & McNamara, R. T. (2006). *Resistance and the background conversations of change.* Retrieved December 7, 2006, from http://www.12manage.com/methods_kotter_change_approaches.html

Goss, T., Pascale, R., & Athos, A. (1993). The reinvention roller coaster : Risking the present for a powerful future. *Harvard Business Review, 71(*6), 97–108.

Haffer, A. (1986). Facilitating change: Choosing the appropriate strategy. *Journal of Nursing Administration, 16*(4), 18–22.

Haley, J. (1973). *Uncommon therapy: The psychiatric techniques of Milton H. Erickson.* New York: Norton.

Havelock, R. (1973). *The change agent's guide to innovation in education.* Englewood Cliffs, NJ: Educational Technology Publications.

Hengboriboonpong, P., & Oumtanee, A. (2004, July). *Innovative behavior of professional nurses.* Paper presented at the 15th International Nursing Research Congress, Sigma Theta Tau International, Dublin, Ireland.

Joel, L. A. (1998). Absolutes and indefinites. *American Journal of Nursing, 98*(2), 7.

Kaiser Permanente. (2006). Clinical innovation leader for nursing. *Nursing Informatics Online.* Retrieved June 7, 2007, from http://www.informaticsnurse.com/forums/informatics-job-description-database/13719-clinical-innovation-leader-nursing-innovations-nurse.html

Kotter, J., & Schlesinger, C. (1979). Choosing strategies for change. *Harvard Business Review, 57*(2), 106–114.

Lewin, L. (1951). *Field theory in social science: Selected theoretical papers.* New York: Harper & Row.

Rich, V.L. (1998, January 26). Management perspectives: Back to basics. *The Nursing Spectrum,* pp. 4–5.

Rogers, E., & Shoemaker, F. (1971). *Communication of innovations* (2nd ed.). New York: Free Press.

Schein, E. (1995). Kurt Lewin's change theory in the field and in the classroom: Notes toward a model of managed learning. *Systems practice.* Retrieved June 8, 2007, from http://dspace.mit.edu/bitstream/1721.1/2576/1/SWP-3821-32761445.pdf

Schein, E., & Bennis, W. (1975). *Personal and organizational change through group method.* New York: Wiley.

Tappan, R. (1983). *Nursing leadership: Concepts and practice.* Philadelphia: Davis.

Watzlawick, P., Weakland, J., & Fisch, R. (1974). *Change: Principles of problem formation and problem resolution.* New York: Norton.

Using Information Technology

CHAPTER OBJECTIVES

After reading this chapter, answering the leadership challenges, and participating in the leadership development exercises, you will be able to:

- Describe the importance of information technology to the transformation of health care
- Discuss the relationship between evidence-based practice and nursing informatics
- Explain why clinician input is necessary for system selection and implementation
- Discuss the advantages of electronic health records
- Describe how to optimize clinical use of handheld technology
- Analyze seven strategies for managing technological change and involving staff in the process

Advanced nurses will be able to:

- Teach peers or less experienced nurse leaders how to use information technology
- Design a problem statement to study an informatics issue
- Develop a research project to study an informatics issue

Introduction

One of your roles as a nurse leader includes being engaged in evaluating and selecting clinical information systems that can help staff optimize their work (Kirkley & Rewick, 2003).

Information technology (IT) is the use of computerized systems to assist nurses and other healthcare workers to make good decisions and deliver safe care. **Nursing informatics** combines computer science, information science, and nursing science to assist nurses in their practice.

Nursing has used IT for many purposes, including to improve care; address the nursing shortage; improve the work experience of nurses; augment in-house nursing staff with remote support staff; identify staff schedule preferences; stay in real-time communication with colleagues; and, via hospital intranets, find procedures, standards of care, protocols, educational materials, and announcements (McBride, 2005).

This chapter examines the promise of IT, the use of innovative technology to decrease nursing demand and enhance client care, the relationship between evidence-based practice and informatics, the use of electronic health record systems, the prevention of medication and treatment errors with handheld technology, and the management of technological change.

LEADERSHIP IN ACTION

Angela was a new nurse leader who knew little about IT but was asked to investigate its possibilities for her geriatric nursing unit. She wasn't sure where to start.

LEADERSHIP CHALLENGE What advice do you have for Angela?

The Promise of IT

The government, employer groups, and consumers have called for the reduction of healthcare errors. As a result, measures have been taken to make health care safer. One measure has been to develop technology that supports the admission, discharge, and transfer of clients, as well as bed management and preregistration; checks drug interactions; handles billing; and verifies that payments were made (Priselac, 2003).

IT shows promise for nursing because of its ability to achieve safety, effectiveness, client/family-centeredness, timeliness, efficiency, equity, and global connectedness.

IT and Safety

IT enhances client safety by continuously monitoring healthcare settings and the information sharing that occurs when clinicians make decisions. Some nurses, such as those working in intensive care, have become accustomed to monitors that sound an alarm when clients' vital signs signify danger. Other monitors could be designed to alert nurses to drug contraindications and other problem predictors (McBride, 2005).

IT and Effectiveness

IT systems can improve effectiveness by disseminating standards and policies and making benchmarking possible. IT can allow quality improvement committees to track best practices by using a range of quality indicators (McBride, 2005).

IT and Client/Family-Centeredness

Several types of IT can provide information for clients and their families. Web sites can provide huge amounts of parent and family education, from supporting decision making to delivering client reminders. Smart technology can monitor changes in a client's activities of daily life at a distance, permitting seniors and others to stay at home without having to go to a clinic or practitioner's office.

Nurses and engineers worked on a client-centered **Nursebot** to identify needs of the elderly and develop personal robotic assistants for them. Funded by the National Science Foundation, this research and development initiative involved multidisciplinary collaboration between the University of Pittsburgh, Carnegie Mellon University, and the University of Michigan. The aim of the collaboration was to develop IT techniques that enable older adults at risk for institutionalization to sustain independent living. This project resulted in developing an initial user test of two prototype robotic devices for older adults: Pearl, a humanoid robot, and the IMP (Intelligent Mobility Platform), a robotic walker (Matthews, 2005).

> **KEY TERM**
>
> The **Nursebot Project** developed personal robotic assistants for older adults.

IT and Timeliness

IT makes possible continuous communication between clients and providers, eliminating routine clinic visits. Clients are seen only at the time they need care (Perlin & Roswell, 2004).

IT and Efficiency

IT can prevent people from asking the same questions or repeating unneeded lab tests. With IT, interventions are targeted. Healthcare organizations can customize outreach by zip code based on layering individual information over geographic information systems (Riner, Cunningham, & Johnson, 2004).

IT and Equity

IT can facilitate equitable access to health information. Telehospice is an example. Hospice care, including help with the dying process, is delivered directly into a client's home via videophone. Telehospice can be especially helpful in underserved rural and urban sites and for those with limited caregiver support (Whitten, Doolittle, Mackert, & Rush, 2004).

IT and Global Connectedness

IT permits a no-borders approach to health. Nurse practitioners handle emergencies at a distance and clients are able to "ask a nurse" their questions about their condition and its treatment across geographic borders (McBride, 2005).

LEADERSHIP CHALLENGE What would you tell Angela about IT that she may be able to use on her geriatrics unit?

KEY TERM

Evidence-based practice requires tracking the best evidence for a specific procedure.

Evidence-Based Practice and Nursing Informatics

Because the steps of **evidence-based practice** require tracking the best evidence for a specific procedure, nurses must understand the available resources and know how to find an answer to a clinical question; they must be computer literate (Pravikoff, Pierce, & Tanner, 2005). Beyond that, the American Nurses Association's *Scope and Standards of Nursing Informatics Practice* (2001) states that all nurses need informatics and computer competencies whether or not they specialize in informatics.

A recent nationwide investigation of 1,097 RNs examined their access to information resources and their perceived skills in using these resources (Pravikoff, Pierce, & Tanner, 2005). Key findings included:

- The most frequent source of information was a colleague or peer.
- Almost half were not familiar with the term *evidence-based practice*, although it has appeared in thousand of articles in nursing journals.
- More than half had never identified a researchable problem and did not believe that their colleagues used research findings in the practice environment.
- Most did not search appropriate information resources, such as Medline or the Cumulative Index to Nursing and Allied Health Literature database, to

gather practice information. Those who did search did not think that they were skilled at it.

- Only 27% of study participants ever received instruction in using electronic databases.

A little over half of the respondents had a medical or health science library where they work but may not have known where it was, may not have known how to access it, or may have believed that it was for physicians' use only.

LEADERSHIP TIP

Useful databases for healthcare information include the Cumulative Index to Nursing and Allied Health Literature and Medline (http://www.pubmed.com).

- Over 80% had Internet access in their facilities, and 60% had access in their nurses station; most of the respondents did search the Internet and felt successful while doing so.
- Almost half reported that print, electronic, and other resources were inadequate.
- Next to time, the greatest barrier to using information in practice was a "lack of value for research."
- The greatest barrier to using information in practice was the "presence of other goals with a higher priority."

These findings present serious implications for you as a nurse leader.

LEADERSHIP CHALLENGE What can you do as a nurse leader to make sure staff and clients use IT?

Some of the steps you can take as a nurse leader to help staff and clients understand and use the vast amount of information available on the Internet are to:

- Function as a role model and information champion and ask staff or clients to consider how they can use IT more efficiently and more often.
- Take staff or clients aside and ask how you can help them improve their search and evaluation skills and apply evidence to practice (or you could use a checklist of needed skills, ask staff and clients to respond to the items, and work from the answers they provide).
- Make journals, reviews, and Internet resources available to staff and clients.
- Demonstrate ways to search for evidence about a practice by using the search box on Internet Explorer and typing in a few relevant words (e.g., typing in "decubiti," results in more than 10 pages of relevant research materials).

LEADERSHIP TIP

Another way to zero in on research studies is to go to http://www.pubmed.com and type in a query in the box at the top of the page. Searching for "decubiti" resulted in a list of 7,240 studies.

Another way to zero in on research studies is to go to http://www.pubmed.com and type in a query in the box at the top of the page. Searching for "decubiti" resulted in a list of 7,240 studies.

LEADERSHIP CHALLENGE What would you tell Angela about using the Internet in her work?

Clinician Input for System Selection and Implementation

Nurses recognize and appreciate the important role technology plays in nursing care. They also recognize that technology systems may not be adequately designed or implemented. Most often, this occurs because nurses and other users have not been consulted during system development (Bradley, 2003).

In a *NurseWeek* study, only 24% of the nurses surveyed thought that training and education regarding new technology was very good to excellent. The study demonstrated that nurses do not think they are able to influence decisions about their workplace or client care (Bradley, 2003).

Nurse leaders can counter this trend by encouraging staff to exert control over their practice and improve their work environment by serving on technology planning committees or by offering to consult with technology designers. A small but growing number of healthcare settings are turning to nurses to help test, purchase, implement, and even design information systems. Vendors who bring products to hospitals often pay staff nurses to test products, fill out surveys, and make recommendations. Nurses often work hand in hand with technicians to redesign systems that have glitches. Some hospitals have nursing technology committees that evaluate and make recommendations for products that nurses will use. At Hackensack University Medical Center, 10 nurse informaticists evaluate IT for all clinical staff (Domrose, 2004).

Many hospitals have learned that if nurses do not like a specific technology or if it does not fit in their culture, the technology may not work. For example, despite numerous attempts to get nurses to document at the bedside using tablet computers, many nurses prefer to sit at the nurses station or in the nurses lounge to chart. Getting nurses involved in choosing and buying technology requires an investment in preparation, education, and evaluation time (Domrose, 2004).

LEADERSHIP TIP

As a nurse leader, if you want nurses to change their habits, you will need to show them the benefits of changing and reassure them of their value.

When machines such as automatic blood pressure and pulse machines were installed in hospitals, many nurses felt a loss of autonomy. To reduce loss of nurse autonomy it is important to help nurses understand that delegating tasks, such as taking blood pressure and pulse to technology, frees them to use their critical-thinking, assessment, and education skills with clients (Domrose, 2004).

See **Table 15-1** for examples of technology that are already in use by nurses across the country.

TABLE 15-1 ADVANTAGES AND DISADVANTAGES OF TECHNOLOGY IN USE NOW AND PROJECTED FOR THE FUTURE

Type of Technology	The Pluses	The Bugs	The Future
Vocera (communicator worn around the neck)	Easy to use and carry; eliminates playing phone tag; doesn't need to be connected to anything else	Nurses may have to adjust way of taking a call to preserve client privacy	Client call buttons will link to nurse-worn communicators to allow for direct communication
Ceiling lifts	Are stored in the ceiling; can prevent client falls and nurse back injuries	May be awkward to get clients into the sling	Disabled clients will use slingless lifts they can operate without help
Bar-coded client wristbands for meds	Nurses can be sure that they are giving the right medication to the right client; documentation is automatic	May take four to five swipes to register; client gets no meds when sleeping or out of the room	Nurses will use bar coding for blood tests and glucose screening
Handhelds and computers for charting; care plans; collecting data; and pulling up lab results, procedures, and insurance information	Saves hours of time; makes information easy to retrieve; leaves more time for clients	Not all systems are nurse-friendly; handhelds are too small, and tablet computers are hard to carry and break easily	Nurses will use smaller devices that are easy to carry and access, and that can be used for documentation, client entertainment, and education
Bedside computers for clients to check and send e-mail, play computer games, and do Internet research	Clients can stay in touch with work and family and make meal or room-change requests; they can watch videos on upcoming procedures or health issues, such as smoking cessation	There are charges for movies and Internet; some visitors may get more involved with the TV than with the client	Clients and families will use computers to access information about their condition and how to improve their health after discharge, dispense bar-coded meds, register vital signs, and show X-rays or pictures of clients' wounds

Source: Adapted from Domrose (2004).

LEADERSHIP CHALLENGE Which, if any, of the technologies in Table 15–1 might help Angela with her team?

Using Electronic Health Records

Electronic health records are now used by clients, nurses, and researchers to reduce the number of incorrect and unnecessary treatments and medications, to decrease treatment delays, and to allow for real-time communication and transmission of orders. By 2006, electronic health records were fully or partially implemented in 68% of US hospitals (Malloch, 2007).

The adoption of electronic health records, or "e-records," has resulted in numerous improvements that support client quality and safety. UPMC St. Margaret, part of the 19-hospital University of Pittsburgh Medical Center, served as a model for other community hospitals when it successfully converted to a comprehensive electronic health record system in 18 months, dramatically reducing the number of medication errors. The system:

- Simplified the process for medication administration
- Reduced the number of medication omissions by 77%
- Reduced the number of improper doses by 86%
- Reduced the number of unauthorized drugs or drugs given without an order by 46% (Zellner, 2006)

LEADERSHIP TIP

When planning to implement a computerized client record, it is important to start with a strategic vision. Evaluate the client information flow across systems, the capacity of hardware and software, the elements that can be upgraded to meet the additional data needs, and the elements to replace (Mooney, 1998b).

There are other ways that e-records can be used to improve client safety. Some possibilities include that with e-records, multiple variables involved in client errors can be analyzed, adequacy of pain management can be studied, alerts can be implemented earlier as an episode of care leading up to an error can be evaluated, real-time reports of client compliance can be generated, standards can be modified by identifying minor deviations in care, and data specific to cost of care and errors can be examined (Malloch, 2007).

Computerized client records can bridge the gap between costly emergency department visits and an urgent care center. Clients who visit an urgent care center can be given a magnetic swipe card (like a credit card) that identifies them in the system. The virtual room on the client computer allows them to touch the monitor screen and register, schedule an immediate appointment with a physician or nurse practitioner, and view a computerized introduction to their healthcare provider (Mooney,1998a).

Even with all the positives that e-records provide, there are still downsides, including the possibility of data entry errors, the need to develop an underlying organizational culture of safety, the possibility of documenting for the wrong client, the fact that caregivers can override alerts and rules, the fact that integrating clinical and management data systems is in its infancy, the fact that extracting data from electronic records to create reports still requires significant time, and the fact that developing fully integrated lifetime client records without errors is still a way off in the future (Malloch, 2007).

Preventing Medication and Treatment Errors with Handheld Technology

With nearly 300 drugs already carrying black box warnings and with thousands of Americans dying each year as a result of preventable medication errors, nurses—and especially nurse practitioners—must have access to voluminous amounts of clinically relevant information so they can ensure safe and effective client care. A **personal digital assistant** (PDA) may be the solution (Koeniger-Donohue, 2007).

> **KEY TERM**
>
> **Personal digital assistants** are handheld devices that are compact and powerful and make voluminous amounts of clinical information easily accessible.

Drug guides, references for specific practice areas, lab and diagnostic guides, formula-based calculators, and assessment and treatment guidelines are the most widely used applications. PDAs can also be used to check for potential drug interactions. Some clinical suites and drug guides are sold on a subscription basis. Users pay to download the program, and updates are available for the duration of the subscription (Koeniger-Donohue, 2007).

PDAs are supported by a laptop or desktop computer with a USB port, Internet access, and synchronization software. PDAs are backed up to an external memory card and should never store personally identifiable health information, such as client notes or dictation, that may contradict privacy and security provisions (Koeniger-Donohue, 2007).

Useful Web sites for PDAs include:

- General technology information and product reviews: http://www.cnet.com
- Online vendor for handheld clinical software: http://www.skyscape.com
- Miscellaneous Palm software and accessories: http://www.palmgear.com
- PDA resources for healthcare professionals, including software and a discussion forum: http://www.pdacortex.com

LEADERSHIP CHALLENGE Would Angela or her team have any use for PDAs? Give a rationale for your answer.

Seven Strategies for Managing Technological Change

Before Angela could make an accurate assessment of her team, she was informed that the hospital was implementing electronic health records. Angela wasn't sure how to break this change to the staff.

LEADERSHIP CHALLENGE What advice would you give Angela?

According to First (1990), it is nearly impossible to reap benefits from new technology until you've sold the staff and/or client on it. She presents seven strategies to make such transitions painless:

1. *Warm up the staff/client to the idea of a new system.* Make an effort not to make the change sound like an edict. Spend time selling the advantages of the change, and allow people to feel a sense of ownership by participating in the process of change. Set up situations for those involved in the new technology to figure out how they will work with the new changes.

2. *Make sure that middle managers get a new system going.* Managers will not want to do all the work, so they should make sure that their staff learn what is necessary.

3. *Pretest the system before using it.* Encountering frequent glitches can push even the most mild-mannered individual to the breaking point. Try out all technology before teaching staff or clients to use it.

4. *Decide on the best time to pull the plug on the old system.* Consulting with those who will use the new technology may be helpful.

5. *Avoid expecting perfection during the transition phase.* Build in sufficient practice time and prompts so learners can feel confident using the new system.

6. *Provide sufficient training with the new system.* Make sure that training is specific, not generic, and includes plenty of simulated practice with the system.

7. *Offer sufficient follow-up opportunities after training.* Develop a hotline or offer a suggestion box or e-mail address so users can ask questions and get fast answers. Make sure to answer any questions right away. If possible, appoint a person to whom users can go and ask questions.

Summary

This chapter has presented information on using IT, including the promise of IT, evidence-based practice and nursing informatics, clinician input for system selection and implementation, electronic health records, the prevention of medication and treatment errors with handheld technology, and seven strategies for managing technological change. The next part of this text focuses on the creative management of human resources.

Key Term Review

- **Electronic health records** have simplified the process of medication administration, reduced the number of incorrect or unnecessary medications, and decreased treatment delays.
- **Evidence-based practice** requires tracking the best evidence for a specific procedure.
- **Information technology** is the use of computerized systems to assist nurses and other healthcare workers in making good decisions and delivering safe care.
- The **Nursebot Project** developed personal robotic assistants for older adults.
- **Nursing informatics** combines computer science, information science, and nursing science to assist nurses in their practice.
- **Personal digital assistants** are handheld devices that are compact and powerful and make voluminous amounts of clinical information easily accessible.

Leadership Development Exercises

Leadership Development Exercise 15-1

Join with at least three other colleagues, and discuss the importance of IT to the transformation of health care. Include information from this chapter to provide a rationale for your statements.

Leadership Development Exercise 15-2

Join with at least three other colleagues to discuss the relationship between evidence-based practice and nursing informatics, and provide specific examples described in this chapter. Also go to the Web and Google "evidence-based practice and nursing informatics," and see what comes up.

Leadership Development Exercise 15-3

Join with at least three other colleagues to develop a plan for providing clinician input into one technology system and its implementation.

Leadership Development Exercise 15-4

Join with at least three other colleagues to discuss the advantages of electronic health records.

Optional: If a unit in your agency is using electronic health records, speak to at least two staff members and find out the glitches, the advantages, and the things that need to be changed in the system. If possible, share your findings with the class and/or a nurse leader in your agency.

Leadership Development Exercise 15-5

Join with at least three other colleagues to plan the purchase and use of handheld devices for your agency or hospital.

a. Decide (by volunteering or flipping a coin) who will visit each of the four Web sites that follow and bring back information:

- General technology information and product reviews: http://www.cnet.com
- Online vendor for handheld clinical software: http://www.skyscape.com
- Miscellaneous Palm software and accessories: http://www.palmgear.com
- PDA resources for healthcare professionals, including software and a discussion forum: http://www.pdacortex.com

b. Using the information obtained on the Web sites, decide which model to purchase based on price, usability, and staff and unit factors.

c. Report back to the class, or write a paper on what you learned.

■ Leadership Development Exercise 15-6

Choose one exercise from the list below:

a. Interview a nurse leader who has implemented a change. Be sure to cover the seven strategies for managing technology change and involving staff that appear in this chapter. If the nurse leader did not attend to all seven, inquire why he or she did not use a specific strategy. Report back your findings to the class or another group.

b. Join with two to three other colleagues, and devise a plan for implementing handheld technology or some other technology change not now in operation on a unit with which you are familiar. Be sure to be specific about exactly how the plan will be implemented. Present your findings to the class and/or to a nurse leader who is currently contemplating a technology change.

Advanced Leadership Development Exercises

■ Leadership Development Exercise 15-7

Teach about IT:

a. Plan a hypothetical in-class situation or a real situation to teach peers or less experienced learners about using one type of IT that's appropriate for their use.

b. Write up your findings.

c. Share your results with your colleagues, or submit a paper on your results for publication or as part of your course grade.

■ Leadership Development Exercise 15-8

Design a problem statement to study an informatics issue, and obtain feedback from a more seasoned nurse researcher or at least three colleagues about whether your problem statement can be tested. Revise your statement depending on that feedback.

■ **Leadership Development Exercise 15-9**

Develop a research project to study an informatics issue, and obtain feedback from a more seasoned nurse researcher or at least three colleagues about whether your design has flaws. Revise your research project depending on that feedback.

References

American Nurses Association. (2001). *Scope and standards of nursing informatics practice.* Washington, DC: Author.

Bradley, C. (2003). Technology as a catalyst to transforming nursing care. *Nursing Outlook, 51*, pp. S14–S15.

Domrose, C. (2004). Gadget gurus. *NurseWeek News.* Retrieved June 19, 2007, from http://www.nurseweek.com/news/Features/04-10/HiTech_print.html

First, S. E. (1990, April). All systems go: How to manage technological change. *Working Woman*, 47–48, 52.

Kirkley, D., & Rewick, D. (2003). Evaluating clinical information systems. *Journal of Nursing Administration, 33*, 643–651.

Koeniger-Donohue, R. (2007). Optimizing clinical use of handheld technology: PDAs for NPs. *American Journal for Nurse Practitioners, 11*, 22–33.

Malloch, K. (2007). The electronic health record: An essential tool for advancing patient safety. *Nursing Outlook, 55*, 159–161.

Matthews, J. (2005). *Research abstracts.* Retrieved November 15, 2007, from http://cre.nursing.pitt.edu/htmlabstracts/matthewsabs.html

McBride, A. (2005). Nursing and the informatics revolution. *Nursing Outlook, 53*, 183–191.

Mooney, S. (1998a). Computerized patient record bridges gap between costly ED visits and urgent care center. *Clinical Data Management, 5*(5), 7–8.

Mooney, S. (1998b). Focus on computerized patient records. *Clinical Data Management, 5*(5), 4–5.

Perlin, J. B., & Roswell, R. H. (2004). Why do we need technology for caregiving of older adults in the U.S.? *Public Policy and Aging Report, 14*, 22.

Pravikoff, D. S., Pierce, S. T., & Tanner, A. (2005). Evidence-based practice readiness study supported by academy nursing informatics expert panel. *Nursing Outlook, 55*, 49–50.

Priselac, T. M. (2003). Information technology's role in improving practice environments and patient safety. *Nursing Outlook, 51*, pp. S11–S13.

Riner, M. E., Cunningham, C. J., & Johnson, A. (2004). Public health education and practice using geographic information system technology. *Public Health Nursing, 21*, 57–65.

Whitten, P., Doolittle, G., Mackert, M., & Rush, T. (2004). Telehospice: End-of-life care over the lines. *Nursing Management, 34*, 36–39.

Zellner, W. L. (2006, November 29). *UPMC St. Margaret offers key lessons for community hospitals adopting electronic health records.* [Press release]. Pittsburgh, PA: University of Pittsburgh Health Sciences News Bureau.

Part IV

Creatively Managing Human Resources

Staffing and Nurse Retention

CHAPTER OBJECTIVES

After reading this chapter, answering the leadership challenges, and participating in the leadership development exercises, you will be able to:

- Describe the relationship between the nursing shortage and staffing
- Discuss the relationship between quality of care and staffing
- Debate the cost-effectiveness of staffing ratios
- Analyze the staffing needs of one unit
- Discuss critical issues in retaining nurses
- Discuss nursing theories that explain nurse retention

Advanced nurses will be able to:

- Teach peers or less experienced nurse leaders how to analyze staffing needs and retain nursing staff
- Design a problem statement to study a staffing issue
- Develop a research project to study a staffing issue

Introduction

The nurse shortage has placed a burden on every clinic, hospital unit, and community agency. Adequate nurse staffing is key to improving the quality of client care, to decreasing burnout, and, ultimately, to keeping nurses employed in settings where they are needed (Aiken, Clarke, & Sloane, 2002; Weverka, 2007).

LEADERSHIP IN ACTION

Karen, a new nurse leader, has been told that client care has to be improved and that costs, mortality rates, and infection rates have to be reduced. She has no idea how to make staffing cost-effective—let alone what to do about mortality or infection rates, how many nurses and assistants are needed on her unit, or what to do about staff who are threatening to quit because they have to work overtime several days a week.

LEADERSHIP CHALLENGE What advice would you give Karen?

The Relationship between Quality Care and Staffing

Using an international sample of hospitals, Aiken, Clarke, and Sloane (2002) examined the effects of nursing staffing and organizational support for nursing care on nurses' dissatisfaction with their jobs, burnout, and reports of quality of client care. There were 10,319 medical-surgical nurse participants. Reports of low-quality care were three times as likely in hospitals with low staffing and low support for nurses as in hospitals with high staffing and support.

Adequate staffing is not linked only to staff reports; client infections and whether clients live or die are also important. Nijssen et al. (2003) found that nursing workload was inversely associated with nurses' adherence to hand hygiene, the best safety precaution against infection. Multiple studies have identified reduced nurse-to-client ratios as a risk factor for the transmission of nosocomial pathogens and even for client outcome. When staffing ratios are high, nurses may not think that they have time to wash their hands.

Grundmann, Hori, Winter, Taria, and Austin (2002) found that exposure to relative staff deficit was the *only* variable significantly associated with clustered cases of methicillin-resistant staphylococcus aureus (MRSA) colonization. Fridkin, Pear, Williamson, Galgiani, and Jarvis (1996) identified a high client-to-nurse ratio as an independent risk factor for central venous catheter-associated bloodstream infections occurring in a surgical ICU. Needleman, Buerhaus, Mattke, Stewart, and Zelevinsky (2002) found a positive association between the proportion of total daily hours of nursing care by registered nurses and six outcomes

LEADERSHIP TIP

To reduce MRSA and other infections in the workplace, reassure nurses they have time to wash their hands between clients and encourage them to do so.

in medical clients (length of stay, rates of urinary tract infections, upper gastrointestinal bleeding, hospital-acquired pneumonia, shock, and cardiac arrest).

LEADERSHIP CHALLENGE **What advice would you give Karen about reducing infection?**

> **LEADERSHIP TIP**
>
> Adequate staffing may very well be the key to quality care. Nurse leaders must know how to analyze staffing needs and find a way to show the administration that they need an adequate number of RNs to reduce the added costs of infection and mortality.

Cost-Effectiveness of Staffing Ratios

Responding to research confirming the link between nurse staffing and client outcomes, 14 states have introduced legislation to limit client-to-nurse ratios. One study compared client-to-nurse ratios ranging from 8:1 to 4:1. Client mortality and length-of-stay data for different ratios were based on two large hospital-level studies, and cost estimates were drawn from the Bureau of Labor Statistics. Incremental cost-effectiveness was calculated for each ratio with general medical and surgical clients. Eight clients per nurse was the least expensive ratio but was associated with the highest client mortality rate. Decreasing the number of clients per nurse improved mortality and increased costs, but even at a ratio of 1:4, it did not exceed $449,000 per life saved. The researchers concluded that the 4:1 ratio was reasonably cost-effective and in the range of other commonly accepted interventions (Rothberg, Abraham, Lindenauer, & Rose, 2005).

> **LEADERSHIP TIP**
>
> Nurse-to-client ratios are most expensive at 1:4, but they are the safest (i.e., associated with the lowest client mortality rate), are reasonably cost-effective, and are in the range of other commonly accepted interventions.

Determining Staffing Needs

To formulate a staffing schedule, identify your client needs, determine the ideal staffing level, and strive toward that goal. Schedule the right combination of nurses and assistants for each shift, and deploy staff so that you neither overextend nor waste resources.

Some steps to follow when quantifying staffing requirements were discussed by Weverka (2007):

- *Use census estimates.* **Census estimates** focus on the number of clients on the unit and how much care each one requires. To compute the estimate, multiply the number of clients (CL) by the average amount of time (T) that each requires to estimate the hours of care (HOC). The results provide an estimate of how many work hours are needed per shift.

> **KEY TERM**
>
> A **census estimate** includes the number of clients on a unit multiplied by the amount of care required.

$$HOC = CL \times T$$

KEY TERM

Acuity levels refer to the level of care clients need and can be used to determine staffing schedules.

KEY TERM

Determining a **mix of skills** includes maintaining a profile of each staff member, including their qualifications, certifications, general skills, language skills, and background.

KEY TERM

A **standard scheduling process** includes formulating policies for choosing vacation times, selecting shifts, and exchanging shifts.

- *Determine client acuity.* The level of care clients need is called the **acuity level,** and it can be very high in the ICU. Some nurse managers use acuity ratings to help determine staffing requirements.
- *Determine a **mix of skills.*** To meet the needs of a unit, each shift requires staff with the correct mix of qualifications. A nurse manager must assemble a team that's capable of meeting the clients' needs on a particular unit and maintain a profile of all staff members that includes their qualifications, certifications, general skills, language skills, and background.

Staffing is always a matter of compromise and accommodation. Staff have favored days and times to work, and developing a reasonable work schedule may not always be easy. It is important to schedule around employees' needs while still guaranteeing that staffing meets clients' needs. Some ways to achieve this goal are to:

- *Devise a **standard scheduling process.*** Formulate policies for choosing vacation times, selecting shifts, and exchanging shifts. Ask staff members to submit their work preferences to you in advance, and tell them that the sooner they let you know their needs, the more apt you will be able to accommodate those needs. Explain that the process used to devise the schedule, and make sure that staff know it applies to everyone. Such measures will eliminate any arguing about the schedule, although you may have to repeat the policies several times. Whenever possible, post a draft schedule that is open to revisions from management and staff.
- *Schedule in advance.* By scheduling in advance, nurses have a chance to look ahead and sign up for unassigned shifts. As a result, you will have to make fewer calls to nurses to ask them to fill in for other staff at the last moment.
- *Keep the budget in mind.* It is important to keep an eye on overtime, making sure costs do not exceed the budget. Recruiting a set of temporary and part-time nurses, rather than hiring more expensive agency nurses and per diem staff, can save money.

Critical Issues in Retaining Staff

Staff retention is vital to solving the nursing shortage. A host of factors—including job satisfaction, supervision, the work environment, and personal factors—affect whether staff remain in their jobs or resign.

Job Satisfaction

Job satisfaction plays an important role in retention. See Box 16-1 for factors that are significantly related to hospital staff nurses' job satisfaction.

Heavy client loads, the mental and physical demands of the job, excessive paperwork, and an inability to make decisions (i.e., a lack of autonomy) can frustrate nurses and lead them to resign. Low staffing levels and low salaries can also lead to dissatisfaction (Beech, 1995; Strachota, Normandin, O'Brien, Clary, & Krukow, 2003).

Supervision

Nurses tend to stay on the job longer when nurse leaders use a participative leadership model and encourage staff to participate in decisions (Fisher, Hinson, & Deets, 1994). Units with leaders who have a large number of staff reporting to them have higher levels of staff turnover. Units with managers who use a positive leadership style have lower levels of staff turnover. Having a large number of staff reporting to managers reduces any positive effect of positive leadership (like transformational and transactional leadership styles) on staff satisfaction and increases the effect of negative leadership (like laissez-faire styles; see Chapter 1) on staff satisfaction.

> **BOX 16-1   FACTORS SIGNIFICANTLY RELATED TO NURSES' JOB SATISFACTION**
>
> - Autonomy (Carter, 2004)
> - In very good health (as opposed to being in just good health)
> - White (as opposed to being black)
> - Educated in the United States (as opposed to being educated elsewhere)
> - Career oriented
> - Supported and encouraged by their supervisors
> - In a cohesive and friendly work group
> - Rewarded for their work
> - In a setting that does not interfere with their work
> - In a job that does not conflict with family responsibilities
> - Given lighter workloads (Lewis, 2007)

The Work Environment

Incivility or a lack of mutual respect pervades the workplace (Hutton, 2006). Negative, nonsupportive, unpleasant, and uncooperative peers and coworkers are key impediments to finding joy at work (Manion, 2003). Teams that work together, support one another, and resolve conflicts are critical to staff nurse retention (Anthony et al., 2005); employee friendliness and cooperation are critical reasons why nurses stay with their jobs (Fisher, Hinson, & Deets, 1994; Kangas, Kee, & McKee-Waddle, 1999; MacRobert, Schmele, & Henson, 1993).

In one study, between 60% and 70% of nurses agreed that due to understaffing and heavy workloads, finding enough time to provide quality care was difficult, frustrating and stressful (Aiken, Clarke & Sloane, 2001).

> **LEADERSHIP TIP**
>
> To reduce nurse uncertainty and prevent burnout and resignations, communicate about organizational changes that accompany new work environments.

Crowded client rooms that allow for little personal space and privacy can influence client attitudes and satisfaction levels. These frustrations are often directed toward the nursing staff, which, in turn, lowers nurses' satisfaction with their work (Beech, 1995).

When healthcare organizations restructure, downsize, or merge, nurses' stress levels rise. Nurse leaders and administrators must not ignore this factor for the sake of cost containment and efficiency (Leveck & Jones, 1996). Changing from a primary nursing model to a client-centered managed model can be very stressful. Few nurses anticipate the emotional exhaustion and depersonalization that can result. Nurse leaders who communicate about the organizational changes that accompany new work environments can reduce nurse uncertainty and prevent burnout and resignations (Miller & Apker, 2002).

Personal Factors

Even when nurses are somewhat satisfied with their work situation, they may still leave for personal reasons.

Age is a major factor that influences retention. Older nurses who are nearing retirement may stay to obtain benefits, but younger nurses may want a variety of experiences and may leave if the situation becomes intolerable.

More educated nurses will often stay because they are able to actualize their professional role and have more autonomy (MacRobert, Schmele, & Henson, 1993). Nurses in their first nursing job are often more dissatisfied than experienced nurses (Shader, Broome, West, & Nash, 2001).

RNs who felt their job did not conflict with their family life were more satisfied than those who perceived that their job conflicted with family life (Lewis, 2007). Family and kinship responsibilities, such as caretaking others, can affect absences and turnover (Borda & Norman, 1997).

If nurse leaders hope to resolve the nursing shortage, they must deal with all the factors that lead to retention.

LEADERSHIP CHALLENGE What would you tell Karen about retaining staff who are complaining about working conditions?

Better Retention through Nursing Theory

To increase retention, it is important to keep staff satisfied and healthy. The **modeling and role-modeling theory** uses Maslow's hierarchy of needs, which assumes that as basic physiological and safety needs are met, nurses can move to seeking social belongingness, self-esteem, self-actualization, and transcendence (Benson & Dundis, 2003).

Without adequate wages, staff cannot provide shelter, food, water, heat, and clothing for their families. If wages are adequate and physiological needs are met, the next human need to consider is safety. For staff to progress to the belongingness phase, benefits, training, and adequate supplies and precautions to guard against infections and exposure to harmful agents must be in place, and there must be a lack of workplace violence, discrimination, sexual harassment, and stress (Arruda, 2005).

> **KEY TERM**
>
> The **modeling and role-modeling theory** uses Maslow's hierarchy of needs, which assumes that as basic physiological and safety needs are met, nurses can move to seeking social belongingness, self-esteem, self-actualization, and transcendence.

For staff to feel that they belong and are able to work well in a team, they must perceive their relationships with nurse leaders as being collaborative and respectful. At least one study has shown that nurse leaders tend to perceive their leadership style's effectiveness as significantly more effective than their RN staff do (McElhaney, 2006).

Once staff have conquered belongingness needs, they are ready to move on to self-esteem. This step includes the desire to achieve, be competent, and gain recognition for a job well done. To provide what staff need at this point, offer timely feedback, especially performance evaluations (see Chapter 20); share governance (see Chapter 19); and give them autonomy. It is highly important never to reverse decisions made by the group, which can reduce self-esteem (Benson & Dundis, 2003).

> **LEADERSHIP TIP**
>
> To enhance your relationship with staff, query team members to elicit their perceptions, and then be sure to bolster your own leadership skills to meet their expectations.

The next level is self-actualization. Staff development efforts (see Chapter 19) can help nurses prepare for advancement opportunities (see Chapter 22).

The final stage in Maslow's hierarchy is transcendence. Employees can transcend their level of self-actualization by mentoring other staff (see Chapter 21).

When using this theory, it is important to foster an environment where staff members feel comfortable expressing their concerns, desires, questions, and needs. Appreciating staff members and listening to what they have to say are key to success (Arruda, 2005).

Summary

This chapter focused on staffing and retaining staff, including the relationship between quality of care and staffing, the cost-effectiveness of staffing ratios, determining staffing needs, critical issues in retaining staff, and achieving better retention through nursing theory. The next chapter presents critical information about recruiting and interviewing.

Key Term Review

- **Acuity levels** refer to the level of care clients need and can be used to determine staffing schedules.
- A **census estimate** includes the number of clients on a unit multiplied by the amount of care required.
- Determining a **mix of skills** includes maintaining a profile of each staff member, including their qualifications, certifications, general skills, language skills, and background.
- The **modeling and role-modeling theory** uses Maslow's hierarchy of needs, which assumes that as basic physiological and safety needs are met, nurses can move to seeking social belongingness, self-esteem, self-actualization, and transcendence.
- A **standard scheduling process** includes formulating policies for choosing vacation times, selecting shifts, and exchanging shifts.

Leadership Development Exercises

- **Leadership Development Exercise 16-1**

Describe the nursing shortage's impact on staffing to at least three colleagues.

- **Leadership Development Exercise 16-2**

Discuss the relationship between job satisfaction and staffing.

- **Leadership Development Exercise 16-3**

Debate the cost-effectiveness of safe nurse staffing with at least one other colleague.

- **Leadership Development Exercise 16-4**

  a. Analyze staffing needs for one real or hypothetical unit using the information in this chapter.
  b. Devise a plan to show administration that your staffing plan is cost-effective.

- **Leadership Development Exercise 16-5**

Discuss critical issues in retaining nursing staff with at least three other colleagues.

- **Leadership Development Exercise 16-6**

Discuss with at least three colleagues how to use the modeling and role-modeling theory to retain staff.

Advanced Leadership Development Exercises

■ Leadership Development Exercise 16-7

Teach peers or less experienced nurse leaders how to analyze staffing needs and retain nursing staff.

■ Leadership Development Exercise 16-8

Design a problem statement to study a staffing issue. Obtain feedback from at least three colleagues with research knowledge. Ask them if your problem statement is researchable. If it isn't, ask for suggestions about how to specify the problem statement. Revise your problem statement based on that feedback.

■ Leadership Development Exercise 16-9

Develop a research project to study a staffing issue. Obtain feedback from at least three colleagues with research experience in undertaking nursing studies. Ask these nursing colleagues whether your design will answer your problem statement. If not, revise your project based on that feedback.

References

Aiken, L. H., Clarke, S. P., & Sloane, D. M. (2001). Nurses' reports on hospital care in five countries. *Health Affairs (Millwood)*, *20*(1), 45–52.

Aiken, L. H., Clarke, S. P., & Sloane, D. M. (2002). Hospital staffing, organization, and quality of care: Cross-national findings. *Nursing Outlook*, *50*, 187–194.

Anthony, M., Standing, T., Glick, J., Duffy, M., Paschall, F., Sauer, M.R., et al. (2005). Leadership and nurse retention. *Journal of Nursing Administration*, *35*, 146–155.

Arruda, E. H. (2005, April). Better retention through nursing theory. *Nursing Management*, 16–17.

Beech, B. M. (1995). *Patient satisfaction and nursing staff work satisfaction in an urban public teaching hospital.* Unpublished dissertation, University of Texas HSC at Houston School of Public Health.

Benson, S., & Dundis, S. (2003). Understanding and motivating health care employees: Integrating Maslow's hierarchy of needs, training and technology. *Journal of Nursing Administration*, *11*, 315–320.

Borda, R. G., & Norman, I. J. (1997). Factors influencing satisfaction and anticipated turnover for nurses in an academic medical center. *Journal of Nursing Administration*, *34*(6), 385–394.

Carter, J. K. (2004). *Leadership styles of nurse managers and the effects on work satisfaction and intent to stay of staff nurses.* Midwest Nursing Research Society. Retrieved November 26, 2007, from http://www.nursinglibrary.org/Portal/main.aspx?pageid=4040&PID=5914

Doran, D., McCutcheon, A. S., Evans, M. G., MacMillan, K., Hall, L. M., Pringle, D., et al. (2004). *Impact of the manager's span of control on leadership and performance.* Retrieved November 26, 2007, from http://www.chsrf.ca/final_research/ogc/pdf/doran2_e.pdf

Fisher, M. I., Hinson, N., & Deets, C. (1994). Selected predictors of registered nurses' intent to stay. *Journal of Advanced Nursing*, *20*(5), 950–957.

Fridkin, S. K., Pear, S. M., Williamson, T. H., Galgiani, J. N., & Jarvis, W. R. (1996). The role of understaffing in central venous catheter-associated bloodstream infections. *Infection Control in the Hospital, 17*(3), 150–158.

Grundmann, H., Hori, S., Winter, B., Taria, A., & Austin, D. J. (2002). Risk factors for the transmission of methicillin-resistant staphylococcus aureus in an adult intensive care unit: Fitting a model to the data. *Journal of Infectious Diseases, 185*(4), 481–488.

Hutton, S. (2006). Workplace incivility: State of the science. *Journal of Nursing Administration, 36,* 22–27.

Kangas, S., Kee, C. C., & McKee-Waddle, R. (1999). Organizational factors, nurses' job satisfaction, and patient satisfaction with nursing care. *Journal of Nursing Administration, 29*(1), 32–42.

Leveck, M. I., & Jones, C. B. (1996). The nursing practice environment, staff retention and quality of care. *Research in Nursing and Health, 19*(4), 331–343.

Lewis, D. (2007). Multiple factors affect job satisfaction of hospital RNs. *RWKF Research Highlight, 22,* 1–2.

MacRobert, M., Schmele, J. A., & Henson, R. (1993). An analysis of job morale factors of community health nurses who report a low turnover rate. *Journal of Nursing Administration, 23*(6), 22–28.

Manion, J. (2003). Joy at work? *Journal of Nursing Administration, 33,* 652–659.

McElhaney, R. (2006). *Perceptions of nurse managers' leadership style by nurse managers and RN staff.* Retrieved April 6, 2007, from http://www.nursinglibrary.org/Portal/main .aspx?pageid=9760

Miller, K. I., & Apker, J. (2002). On the front lines of managed care: Professional changes and communicative dilemmas of hospital nurses. *Nursing Outlook, 50,* 154–159.

Needleman, J., Buerhaus, P., Mattke, S., Stewart, M., & Zelevinsky, K. (2002). Nurse-staffing levels and the quality of care in hospitals. *New England Journal of Medicine, 346*(22), 1715–1722.

Nijssen, S., Bonten, M., Franklin, C., Verhoef, J., Hoepelman, A., & Weinstein, R. (2003). The relative risk of physicians and nurses to transmit pathogens in a medical intensive care unit. *Archives of Internal Medicine, 163,* 2785–2786.

Rothberg, M. B., Abraham, I., Lindenauer, P. K., & Rose, D. N. (2005). Improving nurse-to-patient staffing ratios as a cost-effective safety intervention. *Medical Care, 43*(8), 785–791.

Shader, K., Broome, M. E., West, M. E., & Nash, M. (2001). Factors influencing satisfaction and anticipated turnover for nurses at an academic medical center. *Journal of Nursing Administration, 31*(4), 210–216.

Strachota, E., Normandin, P., O'Brien, N., Clary, M., & Krukow, B. (2003). Reasons registered nurses leave or change employment status. *Journal of Nursing Administration, 33*(2), 111–117.

Weverka, P. (2007). *Schedule nursing staff.* Retrieved November 26, 2007, from http:// office.microsoft.com/en-us/workessentials/HA011924881033.aspx

Recruiting and Interviewing

CHAPTER OBJECTIVES

After reading this chapter, answering the leadership challenges, and participating in the leadership development exercises, you will be able to:

- Describe the process of recruitment
- Discuss the practice of conducting regular employee satisfaction surveys as a recruitment approach
- Debate the use of staff nurses' cars for recruitment
- Discuss steps in recruiting and retaining top-level staff
- Describe basic measures used to judge recruitment efforts
- Analyze the interview process

Advanced nurses will be able to:

- Teach peers or less experienced nurse leaders about recruitment and interviewing practices
- Design a problem statement to study a recruitment or interviewing issue
- Develop a research project to study a recruitment or interviewing issue

Introduction

For recruitment to be successful, recruiters, managers, nurse leaders, and nurse administrators must collaborate and agree on an overall strategy. Recruitment should be part of job interviews and provide potential employees with job descriptions and other relevant information.

LEADERSHIP IN ACTION

Karen, a new nurse leader, was asked to work on the recruitment committee. She wanted to be prepared for the first meeting but was not sure where to go to find out what she wanted to know.

LEADERSHIP CHALLENGE What advice would you give Karen?

Collaborating with Other Departments

As a nurse leader, you may partner with your marketing department in your recruitment efforts. The marketing staff builds and promotes your organization's services and brand, and by talking with them, you can find out how to use their connections and information to assist with recruitment efforts.

Collaboration may be as simple as adding career or recruitment information to the organization's Web site. Ensure that the recruitment section of the Web site is intriguing. Does it provide the basics (physical address, phone number, fax number, and e-mail addresses) and link to the benefits program, local real estate agents, public schools, and facts about the organization's location? Be sure to include a message from nursing leadership to prospective nurses. This is a chance to promote leader vision, set the tone for a great employment experience, and reach out to candidates (Christmas, 2007).

Think through the positions for which you are recruiting. Labor and delivery positions, for example, can be as different as night and day: one might be a family birthing center with 500 births a month and another can be a high-risk center with 5,000 deliveries a month.

Some questions to ask when assessing the adequacy of Web recruitment are:

- How many clicks does it take to get to job postings?
- Do the postings truly describe each unit's unique work environment?
- Do postings include the types of clients treated and the pace of the workload?
- Do online videos provide virtual tours of the unit, offer testimonials from current staff, and highlight the most positive aspects of the unit?

- Does the site offer online chat sessions with recruiters or even employees?
- Are exceptional opportunities—such as specialized equipment, low nurse-to-client ratios, outstanding continuing education, or tuition reimbursement—emphasized?
- Can potential candidates picture themselves practicing in your environment based on what they see on your Web site?

LEADERSHIP CHALLENGE Would any of this information be of use to Karen for her first recruitment meeting? Give a rationale for your answer.

To build an effective recruitment program, relationships with marketing must be ongoing. It takes time to build such relationships, but the results can be well worth the effort (Christmas, 2007).

Strengthening Recruitment in the Community

In addition to recruiters, managers, nurse leaders, and nurse administrators, staff nurses can play a vital role as recruiters in their communities. Staff nurses often network with local or regional specialty associations and with colleagues and friends at social events (Christmas, 2007).

For this reason, you should be aware of any issues (e.g., a lack of equipment, a negative work environment, ineffective managers) that could be discussed during these conversations. Preparing staff nurses to be effective recruiters includes helping them identify the positive aspects of working in their organization.

LEADERSHIP CHALLENGE What steps would you suggest for a nurse leader to take to help prepare staff nurses to be effective recruiters?

Creating Survey Programs

More and more, employers conduct employee satisfaction surveys with nurses to gauge their involvement and attitude. Because nurses interact with clients far more than any other employees, low nurse satisfaction could point to trouble.

This approach can backfire if the nursing staff share their opinions with management and their concerns are not addressed. The most successful organizations have a budget for marketing and act on the information they receive, making the necessary changes to improve their employees' work environment (Christmas, 2007).

LEADERSHIP CHALLENGE Before Karen goes to her first recruitment meeting, should she find out whether her organization conducts employee satisfaction surveys with nurses? Considering the pros and cons, give a rationale for your answer.

Using Ambassador Cards to Recruit Nurses

KEY TERM

Ambassador cards are like business cards and are provided to staff nurses to make it easy for them to invite outstanding colleagues to join the organization. The cards include recruitment phone numbers, the appropriate Web site address, and a space for nurses to insert their names and titles.

If the nurses in your organization are satisfied with their workplace, ambassador programs can extend the reach of recruitment. **Ambassador cards** are like business cards. They are provided to staff nurses to make it easy for them to invite outstanding colleagues to join the organization. The cards include recruitment phone numbers, the appropriate Web site address, and a space for nurses to insert their names and titles. The company may print information about nursing culture, values, or work environment as a further enticement.

Encourage staff to distribute ambassador cards to peers at conferences and even at chance meetings in the grocery line or at church. This ambassador program not only assists the company in recruiting new nurses, but it can be used to recognize nurse contributions to recruitment efforts (Christmas, 2007).

LEADERSHIP CHALLENGE Karen thinks that ambassador cards are a good idea. Should she bring up the idea at the recruitment meeting if her organization does not use ambassador cards, or should she just listen and then talk to nurse leaders individually? Give a rationale for your answer.

Deploying Staff Vehicles as Roving Recruitment Billboards

Some metropolitan hospitals and medical centers pay nurses to use their cars to recruit more nurses. Such programs use easily removable billboards that do not scratch paint surfaces. The boards carry recruitment messages on them, along with the appropriate Web site address and/or contact phone numbers.

LEADERSHIP CHALLENGE Is paying nurses to use their cars to recruit more nurses a good or a bad idea? Give a rationale for your answer.

Recruiting and Interviewing Top-Level Staff

To attract and keep the top talent in the nursing market, it is important to follow a few basic steps.

Define the Job Description

Clearly define job responsibilities, including a list of mandatory skills, and how candidates will fit into and grow within the organizational structure.

Determine an Appropriate Strategy

Decide whether the position will be filled internally or whether your unit's budget is better spent on searching outside the organization. When searching outside the organization, advertise in nursing journals, in association publications, and on the Web sites of various nursing organizations. When potential candidates submit résumés, make an initial telephone contact, and arrange for on-site interviews.

Set Interviewing and Selection Processes

Be prepared to take immediate action on the most viable applicants before they take other positions. To get a better sense of applicants, ask each candidate to bring a professional portfolio that includes certificates of attendance for continuing education programs, diplomas for formal education, letters of appreciation for contributions to a committee or board, copies of protocol or procedures for clinical pathways, client education plans they've developed, a personal philosophy of nursing, annual evaluations, completed skills checklists, presentations they've given or written materials they've developed, copies of articles they've published, copies of brochures indicating poster presentations, abstracts of studies they've completed, letters indicating grants they've received, self-assessments of career goals and achievements, and an evaluation of progress toward goals (Dennison, 2007).

To enlist an ideal team from the ground up, use a positive process:

- Recruit the first team member yourself based on his or her leadership skills and your ability to work together. Consider setting up a role-playing or simulation situation to see how your potential employee handles important events.
- Once you have selected that team member, the two of you should select the next member, choosing someone with experience in similar challenges.
- Once you two have selected the third team member, all three should choose the next employee, basing your selection on specific skills that are aligned with the tasks of the job.
- Continue on, and have the staff choose the next members of the team.

Although this process takes longer than one-on-one recruiting, you'll assemble a highly skilled group with a much greater likelihood of working well together than if only one person had selected the team (Sanders, 1999).

If you already have a partial team, enlist them all to help narrow down applicants to a group of five strong potential new hires for each available position. Bring each applicant back for a follow-up interview. Especially for top positions, pick the two top candidates, and bring each one back for a day to talk to staff members, shadow one, and get a feel for the organization.

LEADERSHIP TIP

Examples of incentives you could offer include flextime, more autonomy, specialized training, telecommuting, job sharing, an enhanced job title, child care, elder care, tying job goals directly to compensation, tying a financial incentive to completing a specific project, and offering a percentage of realized savings from innovative prevention programs (Mooney, 1998).

KEY TERM

Tailored incentives such as flextime, more autonomy, specialized training, telecommuting, job sharing, an enhanced job title, child care, elder care, tying job goals directly to compensation, tying a financial incentive to completing a specific project, and offering a percentage of realized savings from innovative prevention programs can be offered to entice top staff to accept employment.

KEY TERM

The **Equal Employment Opportunity Commission** protects applicants from discrimination.

Offer Tailored Incentives to Attract Top Staff

While interviewing candidates, watch and listen for clues that tell you what could make your organization attractive to the potential employee. Small organizations may not have the budgets to provide higher salaries, but you may be able to develop creative incentive and compensation packages.

Examples of incentives you could offer include flextime, more autonomy, specialized training, telecommuting, job sharing, an enhanced job title, child care, elder care, tying job goals directly to compensation, tying a financial incentive to completing a specific project, and offering a percentage of realized savings from innovative prevention programs (Mooney, 1998).

Always be upfront with candidates. Ask, "What is most important to you—salary, autonomy, location, or something else?" While gathering information, offer facts about the organization so potential employees can make a sound decision (Mooney, 1998).

Posing Legal Inquiries When Interviewing Applicants

When interviewing applicants, be sure to use only legal inquiries.

The **Equal Employment Opportunity Commission** protects applicants from discrimination. Because of this protection, you cannot ask questions when interviewing that pertain to relatives, marital status, residence, pregnancy, physical health, family, name, sex/gender, photographs, age, education, citizenship, origin/ancestry, race or color, religion, organizational affiliations, military service, height and weight, and arrests and convictions. For specific questions that you can and cannot ask during a job interview, see **Table 17-1**.

TABLE 17-1 QUESTIONS TO ASK WHEN INTERVIEWING APPLICANTS

Subject	Unlawful Inquiries	Lawful Inquiries
Relatives/marital status	"Are you married?" "What are the names of your relatives?" "How old are your children?"	"What are the names of your relatives who work for this company [or our competitor]?"
Residence	"Do you live nearby?" "Do you own or rent?" "With whom do you live?"	"What is your contact address?" (A post office box is a valid address.) "Will you have problems getting to work on time?"
Pregnancy	All questions relating to a pregnancy and its medical history.	"Do you foresee any long-term absences in the future?"
Physical health	"Do you have any handicaps?" "What caused your condition?" "What is the prognosis?" "Have you ever had any serious illnesses?" "Do you have any physical disabilities?"	"Can you lift 40 pounds?" "Do you need any special accommodations to perform the job?" "How many days of work [or school] did you miss in the past year?"
Family	Anything concerning a spouse, children, dependents, or child care arrangements.	"Can you work overtime?" "Is there any reason you can't be on the job on time?"
Name	Any inquiries about the interviewee's name that divulges marital status, lineage, ancestry, national origin, or descent: for example, "If your name has been legally changed, what was your former name?"	Whether the applicant worked for a competitor under a different name: for example, "What name are you known to the reference you provided us?"
Sex/gender	Any inquiry.	None.
Photographs	A request for a photo before being hired.	A request for a photo after being hired that's for identification purposes.
Age	Any questions that can identify applicants as being age 40 or above.	"If hired, can you furnish proof of age?"

(continues)

TABLE 17-1 QUESTIONS TO ASK WHEN INTERVIEWING APPLICANTS *(continued)*

Subject	Unlawful Inquiries	Lawful Inquiries
Education	Any question about a school's nationality, racial affiliation, or religious affiliation.	All questions related to the academic, vocational, or professional education of the applicant; the names of schools attended; the degrees or diplomas received; the dates of graduation; and the course of study.
Citizenship	Whether the applicant is a citizen requiring a birth certificate, naturalization, or baptismal certificate and any inquiry into citizenship that would tend to divulge the applicant's lineage, descent, etc.	Whether the applicant is prevented from being lawfully employed in this country because of visa or immigration requirements and whether the applicant can provide proof of citizenship (e.g., a passport), a visa, or an alien registration number after being hired.
National origin/ancestry	"What is your nationality?" "How did you acquire the ability to speak, read, or write a foreign language?" "How did you acquire familiarity with a foreign country?" "What language is spoken in your home?" "What is your mother tongue?"	"What languages do you speak, read, or write fluently?" (This is legal only when the inquiry is based on a job requirement.)
Race or color	Any question that relates directly or indirectly to race or color.	None.
Religion	Any question that relates directly or indirectly to a religion: for example, "What religious holidays do you observe?"	None, except "Can you work on Saturdays?" (and then only if relevant to the job).

TABLE 17-1 QUESTIONS TO ASK WHEN INTERVIEWING APPLICANTS *(continued)*

Subject	Unlawful Inquiries	Lawful Inquiries
Organizational affiliations	"To what organizations, clubs, societies, or lodges do you belong?"	"To what professional organizations do you belong?" (except any whose names or character indicates the race, religious creed, color, national origin, or ancestry of its members).
Military service	Any question related to the type or condition of an applicant's military discharge or experience in a military other than the US armed forces; any request for discharge papers.	Inquiries concerning education, training, or work experience in the US armed forces.
Height and weight	Any inquiries not based on actual job requirements.	Inquiries about the ability to perform a job (being a specific height or weight cannot be considered a job requirement unless the employer can show that no employee with an ineligible height and weight could do the work).
Arrests and convictions	All inquiries relating to arrests: for example, "Have you ever been arrested?" (Note: arrests are not the same as convictions; an innocent man can be arrested.)	"Have you ever been convicted of any crime? If so, when, where, and what was the disposition of the case?" "Have you been convicted under criminal law within the past 5 years, excluding minor traffic violations?" (It is permissible to inquire about convictions for acts of dishonesty or breach of trust.)

These guidelines, called the Fair Inquiry Guidelines, were established by the Equal Employment Opportunity Commission to provide specific protection from discrimination in hiring certain protected classes. For more information, go to http://www.eeoc.gov

Choosing a Candidate

It is not always easy to choose one candidate. What are some things to watch for while interviewing that may help you decide? Borgatti (2007) offers tips for interviewees that can also provide clues for interviewers.

Watch for the candidate who:

> **LEADERSHIP TIP**
>
> Prior to interviewing a candidate for a position, be sure to prepare some typical clinical, teaching, research, and/or leadership situations and questions to ask candidates about how they would handle each one.

- Impresses from the get-go with a professional cover letter, résumé, and telephone reply or message
- Has a handshake that is warm and firm and held for 3–4 seconds, makes good eye contact, smiles, avoids chewing gum or sucking on lozenges, and sits still during the interview
- Is dressed appropriately in a classic tailored suit in a neutral color that is not too tight, too loose, or too short and wears plain jewelry and a simple hairstyle
- Anticipates questions and is poised and prepared when answering
- Is able to provide examples of how to handle specific situations
- Asks intelligent questions about the facility and position
- Sends a thank-you note after the interview, spells interviewers' names correctly, and uses the opportunity to reiterate his or her assets

Measuring Recruitment Efforts

As healthcare budgets shrink, nurse leaders must make recruitment efforts effective and cost-efficient. Tracking pertinent data can provide useful information for future recruiting. Basic measures that may be of benefit include:

- The average age of staff members by nursing unit and for the department overall can help in the development of recruitment plans.
- The average age of retirement, based on organizational history, can also be helpful. Consider whether labor-saving devices, job modification, or new recruits are the answer for older RNs who are thinking of retiring, or for encouraging them to stay.
- Turnover and vacancy rates by unit or department, by key positions, and by transfer to and from units determines negative and positive turnover. Transfer to another unit in the same organization is not negative.
- Posthire and interim interviews, exit interviews, and interviews with accepted and rejected applicants can provide valuable recruitment data.
- Cost-per-hire data can help identify hard-to-fill positions. Recruiters' competency, the number of nursing schools in the area, and the organization's location may also influence how quickly a position is filled.

- Interview-to-hire ratios pinpoint ineffective interviewing or selection processes that can waste money and/or time. Training in interviewing applicants and selecting hires may be necessary.
- To identify the most important recruitment strategies, rank the effectiveness of hiring sources, including employee referrals and capture rates from clinical rotations, e-mails, advertising, hiring or career fairs, and national conferences.
- Contract labor costs provide valuable information when compared to other recruitment and retention data. (Haeberle & Christmas, 2006)

LEADERSHIP CHALLENGE How can Karen obtain numbers for this recruitment data?

Summary

This chapter presented information that's important to recruiting and interviewing potential candidates, including collaborating with other departments, strengthening recruitment in the community, creating survey programs, using ambassador cards to recruit nurses, deploying staff vehicles as roving recruitment billboards, recruiting and interviewing top-level staff, posing legal inquiries when interviewing applicants, choosing a candidate, and measuring recruitment efforts. The next chapter provides important information on establishing a healthy environment.

Key Term Review

- **Ambassador cards** are like business cards and are provided to staff nurses to make it easy for them to invite outstanding colleagues to join the organization. The cards include recruitment phone numbers, the appropriate Web site address, and a space for nurses to insert their names and titles.
- The **Equal Employment Opportunity Commission** protects job applicants from discrimination.
- **Tailored incentives** such as flextime, more autonomy, specialized training, telecommuting, job sharing, an enhanced job title, child care, elder care, tying job goals directly to compensation, tying a financial incentive to completing a specific project, and offering a percentage of realized savings from innovative prevention programs can be offered to entice top staff to accept employment.

Leadership Development Exercises

■ Leadership Development Exercise 17-1

Develop questions you'd like to ask a member of your marketing department about how nursing and marketing can collaborate. If possible, ask the questions of someone in the marketing department or role-play it with at least one other colleague and then analyze the results.

■ Leadership Development Exercise 17-2

Develop an interview schedule for potential applicants. If possible, conduct an in-person, online, or phone interview with a marketing person or a colleague, using your interview schedule. Evaluate the results and obtain further practice if necessary.

■ Leadership Development Exercise 17-3

Evaluate the adequacy of your organization's Web recruitment efforts. If your organization doesn't have a Web site, go online and evaluate another organization's site using information available in this chapter.

■ Leadership Development Exercise 17-4

Make a list of 10 ways you can strengthen recruitment in your community. Discuss your list with at least three other colleagues. Obtain feedback, and revise your list as needed.

Optional: Collaborate with your colleagues, and share the best ideas with a nurse leader.

■ **Leadership Development Exercise 17-5**

Compose questions that you would use to survey nurses about their job satisfaction. Try them out with at least two other nurses, and obtain feedback. Revise your questions as needed. Compare your survey with other nurse satisfaction surveys in the nursing literature.

Optional: Interview at least two other nurses, and write up your results.

■ **Leadership Development Exercise 17-6**

Debate with a colleague whether using staff nurses' cars for recruitment is a good idea or not. Flip a coin to see which side of the debate you will take. When you're finished, switch sides and debate again. Write up what you learned from this exercise.

■ **Leadership Development Exercise 17-7**

Write your ideal job description.

■ **Leadership Development Exercise 17-8**

Write an advertisement to hire a nurse leader for your organization. Obtain feedback from two or more colleagues.

■ **Leadership Development Exercise 17-9**

Develop a professional portfolio for yourself. Share your completed portfolio with at least two other colleagues, and obtain feedback. Revise, if necessary.

■ **Leadership Development Exercise 17-10**

Work with two other colleagues to analyze the recruitment process.

   a. Role-play a job interview with a colleague.
   b. Using Table 17-1, have another colleague observe and make sure that the interviewer asks no discriminatory questions. Ask this observer to critique the mock interview.
   c. Repeat this process two more times, each time with a different person in the roles of applicant, interviewer, and observer.
   d. Write up your results, and share them with the class.

Optional: Complete the role-playing in front of the class, and ask your classmates to observe for discrimination and to analyze the process.

■ **Leadership Development Exercise 17-11**

Interview a nurse recruiter in person, on the phone, or online to find out how his or her organization measures recruitment efforts. Report your findings to at least two colleagues.

Advanced Leadership Development Exercises

■ **Leadership Development Exercise 17-11**

Teach peers or less experienced nurse leaders about recruitment and interviewing practices. Obtain feedback from learners.

Optional: Write up your results, and share them with at least two other colleagues.

■ **Leadership Development Exercise 17-12**

Design a problem statement to study a recruitment or interviewing issue. Obtain feedback from at least two other colleagues. Revise your problem statements as necessary.

■ **Leadership Development Exercise 17-13**

Develop a research project to study a recruitment or interviewing issue. Obtain feedback from at least two other colleagues. Revise as necessary.

References

Borgatti, J. (2007, January). Ace that interview. *American Nurse Today*, 50–51.

Christmas, K. (2007, January). Forging relationships to strengthen recruitment. *Nursing Economics*, *25*, 37–39.

Dennison, R. D. (2007, January). Advance your nursing career with a professional portfolio. *American Nurse Today*, 42–43.

Haeberle, S., & Christmas, K. (2006). Recruitment and retention metrics: Implications for leadership. *Nursing Economics*, *24*(6), 328–330.

Mooney, S. E. (1998). Recruiting and retaining top-level IT staff. *Clinical Data Management*, *5*(5), 11–12.

Sanders, D. (1999, February). Recruiting your health promotion dream team. *Health Promotion Practitioner*, 8.

Establishing a Healthy Environment

CHAPTER OBJECTIVES

After reading this chapter, answering the leadership challenges, and participating in the leadership development exercises, you will be able to:

- Describe physical factors that make for a healthy environment
- Discuss the hallmarks of a healthy, professional nursing practice environment
- Describe how authentic leaders create a healthy work environment
- Analyze how employee engagement relates to a healthy working environment

Advanced nurses will be able to:

- Teach peers or less experienced nurse leaders how to build a healthy environment
- Design a problem statement to study an aspect of a healthy environment
- Develop a research project to study an aspect of a healthy environment

Introduction

This chapter explores factors that make for a healthy environment (including physical, psychological, and social ones), the negative effects of urban sprawl, and how to establish a working culture that includes a sense of belonging, engagement, and empowerment.

LEADERSHIP IN ACTION

Constance, a nurse leader, just returned from a conference on healthy nurse environments. She'd heard about hospital-acquired infections, evidence-based design, urban sprawl's potential effect on clients, work environments' support of professional nursing practice, and nurse leaders' responsibility to engage staff and create a healthy work environment. She also heard that if all that fails, nurses themselves can learn to promote self-caring and healing in their workplaces. Now that she is back, she is unsure of how to put all her learning into action.

Factors That Make for a Healthy Environment

Some factors discussed in this section that can make for a healthy environment include reducing hospital infection rates, designing the environment for peak healing, and using the "look, think, and act" model.

Reducing Hospital Infection Rates

Hospital-acquired infections continue to rise at an alarming rate. Urgent steps are needed to reduce infections in the work environment and to avoid compromising the health of clients and staff. Although nurses may not be directly affected by the rise of hospital-acquired infection, their workload increases as clients get sicker.

In one study, factors associated with hospital-acquired infections included hospital beds being placed too close together, hospital staff working while having communicable symptoms, and the use of high-flow oxygen therapy and positive-pressure ventilation. Although this study focused on SARS, the senior author, Joseph Sung, MD, PhD, concluded that the findings are relevant for other infections transmitted by droplets. Providing hand-washing, showering, and changing facilities can also reduce the risk ("Study Identifies Risk Factors for Spread of Respiratory Infections in Hospitals," 2007).

Fortunately, recent nursing research has identified another solution. Simple hand-washing videos can reduce hospital infection rates. See Box 18-1 for the details.

LEADERSHIP CHALLENGE How could Constance and the unit on which you work use hand-washing videos or posters with clients? Should videos and posters also be used for staff? Give a rationale for your answers.

BOX 18-1   REDUCING HOSPITAL-ACQUIRED INFECTIONS

Summary. The nurse researchers compared two simple, cost-effective measures to see how they could improve hygiene and reduce hospital-acquired infections like methicillin-resistant staphylococcus aureus (MRSA) in a pediatric intensive care unit. While this kind of infection occurs in about 10 percent of adults in general hospital wards, children in pediatric intensive care units have a 20% to 30% chance of becoming infected, according to Dr. Li-Chi Chiang from the China Medical University in Taiwan.

Sample. The sample included parents, grandparents, aunts, and uncles with similar profiles and education levels from 123 families who visited their children in a pediatric intensive care unit in Taiwan.

Method. For the first 2 months, 62 families were shown posters illustrating hand-washing techniques and discussed with staff the 10 key steps to avoiding the spread of infection. Family members were observed during subsequent visits to see if they washed their hands as suggested.

During the second 2 months, 61 different families were shown a hand-washing video and took part in the same discussions with staff and were observed.

Findings. Both groups' compliance increased during each of the five visits after they saw posters or watched a video and discussed effective techniques with staff. Both groups significantly improved their hand-washing behavior, but the video initiative proved to be much more effective.

Recommendations. Dr. Chiang suggested that the video be shown repeatedly in such areas as intensive care unit waiting rooms and that staff should be trained to reinforce the information in the video when interacting with family members.

(Chen & Chiang, 2007)

Designing the Work Environment for Peak Healing

Client milieus affect both client and nurse satisfaction and, ultimately, RN retention. A boon in hospital construction has led to evidenced-based design concepts to create environments that enhance client outcomes and staff efficiency, increase comfort, and reduce stress, thereby speeding client recovery and improving nurse job satisfaction. For example, researchers found that clients in rooms facing the sunniest exposures recovered the fastest, used less pain medication, and were more satisfied with their hospital experience than clients in other rooms.

Architects include more private rooms, noise-reduction measures, calming gardens, separate hallways for service and delivery carts, and small nursing stations outside client rooms to reduce RNs' travel time and fatigue. The nation's military health systems will incorporate healing design features at outdated facilities, including Walter Reed Army Medical Center in Washington, DC ("Healing Designs Gain Popularity," 2007).

For more information on healthcare design, visit http://www.healthdesign .org. While there, sign up for the newsletter, which will keep you updated about new information on evidence-based building design.

LEADERSHIP CHALLENGE What advice would you give Constance for finding out more about healing milieus and to start implementing them?

Other Ways to Promote Self-Care and Healing in the Workplace

Even in tense, hectic, and noisy surroundings, you can be a nurse leader and help improve your staff's comfort and peace of mind. The way to start this process is to evaluate the environment, using the **"look, think, and act" model,** a problem-solving action research process (Brown, 2006; Stringer & Genat, 2003).

The first step is to assess your environment:

- Are the colors pleasing?
- Is the space cluttered?
- Is there any privacy?
- Is the space clean and orderly?
- Is the noise level tolerable?

The next step is to think about the findings:

- Is the space healing and peaceful for you and others?
- Do you come to work rested and ready for work?
- Do you add to the sense of peace or bring more tension?
- What would make the space more peaceful?
- Would a plant, a picture of a calming mountain or seashore setting, soothing music, a pleasant aromatherapy spray, a written guided imagery situation or affirmation, a statue or model, an inspiring poem, or some other calming addition bring peace?

The next step is to take action:

- Decide on what small part of your work environment to turn into an oasis of peace and comfort for others.
- Find a small bulletin board, a tiny corner, a desktop or table, a basket, or some other small but symbolic place.
- Encourage others in the environment to collaborate with you to make the space more peaceful.

- Ask each person to contribute an item or idea.
- Prepare the space, and try it out for a few days or a week.
- Consider adding an item to your desk or locker that signals healing and relaxation to you.

The next step is to evaluate your action:

- How do you and others react to the healing environment you've created?
- Should you add something to the space or keep it as is?

LEADERSHIP CHALLENGE **What can Constance do to enhance self-care and healing on her unit? Give a rationale for your answer.**

Urban Sprawl

Since the time of Florence Nightingale, nurses have been involved in the environmental aspects of health promotion. One of the most difficult issues facing the professional workforce today is obesity. It used to be thought that if nurses counseled clients to eat better and exercise, those clients would lose weight. Changing behavior is often more complex than that, especially when the environment in which the behavior occurs contributes to the problem.

The nation's worsening obesity epidemic underscores the importance of the environment we've built for ourselves. **Urban sprawl** is a development pattern in cities that is characterized by decentralized, automobile-dependent neighborhoods. Its health implications include obesity, stress, mental health issues, and physical inactivity (Lopez & Welker-Hood, 2007).

Living in a neighborhood with unsafe streets or parks (which make exercising difficult) and with only fast-food restaurants (which offer options that contain too much fat and sugar and not enough fruits and vegetables) can lead to a life of obesity.

Community-oriented and health-promotion-oriented nurse leaders must play a critical role in combating urban sprawl's effects by helping clients eat the nutritious foods they need to stay well. If this obesity-disease cycle goes uninterrupted, clients will continue to be ill and have to reenter hospitals for related conditions (such as diabetes, heart disease, and gallbladder disease) that can be prevented, or at least well controlled, by following a healthy eating regime and regularly exercising.

KEY TERM

Urban sprawl is a development pattern in cities that is characterized by decentralized, automobile-dependent neighborhoods. Its health implications include obesity, stress, mental health issues, and physical inactivity.

LEADERSHIP TIP

To promote health, nurses need to better understand how neighborhoods and their constraints contribute to obesity and lower physical activity for nurses and clients (Lopez & Welker-Hood, 2007).

Urban sprawl affects nurses in other ways besides increased client workload because of hospital reentry. Working long hours while eating an improper diet and not taking sufficient time for exercise can lead to fatigue and practicing at less than full potential.

Some actions nurses can take themselves and help clients address include:

- Working shorter hours
- Scheduling breaks in the workday to seek out healthy meals and to take a short walk or exercise at a work-sponsored gym
- Carpooling with coworkers to decrease the stress of commuting
- Bargaining for a housing allowance in employment contracts and living closer to the job (Lopez & Welker-Hood, 2007)

LEADERSHIP CHALLENGE **How could Constance use this information with her staff and herself? Give a rationale for your answer.**

Developing Environments to Support Professional Nursing Practice

Many changes have occurred in the healthcare arena as a result of economic constraints, including reimbursement for care, rapid advances in clinical technologies and care modalities, and corporatization of healthcare systems (American Association of Colleges of Nursing [AACN], 2002).

Despite these problems, nurse leaders can take action to develop work environments that support professional nursing practice.

KEY TERM

The **Magnet Recognition Program** does nothing to improve staffing ratios, but it does provide a framework to recognize excellence in client care.

Magnet Recognition Program

Although the **Magnet Recognition Program** does nothing to improve staffing ratios (Massachusetts Nurses Association, 2004), the program does provide a framework to recognize excellence in:

- Nursing services management, philosophy, and practices
- Adherence to standards for improving the quality of client care
- Leadership of the chief nurse executive and competence of nursing staff
- Attention to the cultural and ethnic diversity of clients, their significant others, and care providers in the healthcare system (AACN, 2002)

Preceptorships and Residencies

Preceptorships provide opportunities for nursing students to work closely with staff nurses to gain role socialization and to increase clinical skills, knowledge, competence, and confidence. Preceptorships can also decrease the cost of lengthy orientation programs and reduce turnover rates (AACN, 2002).

> **KEY TERM**
>
> **Preceptorships** provide opportunities for nursing students to work closely with staff nurses to gain role socialization and to increase clinical skills, knowledge, competence, and confidence.

LEADERSHIP CHALLENGE How can Constance use preceptorships and/or residencies to provide a more positive work environment?

Residencies or **internships** help new graduates transition into the practice arena. Residency experiences also facilitate recruitment, increase retention, and increase commitment to the organization (AACN, 2002).

> **KEY TERM**
>
> **Residencies** or **internships** help new graduates transition into the practice arena; they also facilitate recruitment, increase retention, and increase commitment to the organization.

Differentiated Nursing Practice

Differentiated practice models differentiate nurses by level of education, expected clinical skills or competencies, job descriptions, pay scales, and participation in decision making.

Differentiated practice models foster positive outcomes for job satisfaction, staffing costs, nurse turnover rates, adverse events, nursing roles, and client interventions and outcomes. This model allows nurses to capitalize on their education and experience. This model is often supported by a **clinical ladder,** or defined steps for advancement within the organization based on experience, additional education, specialty certification, or other indicators of excellence (AACN, 2002).

> **KEY TERM**
>
> **Differentiated practice models** differentiate nurses by level of education, expected clinical skills or competencies, job descriptions, pay scales, and participation in decision making.

LEADERSHIP CHALLENGE Should Constance try to initiate a clinical–ladder approach? Give a rationale for your answer.

> **KEY TERM**
>
> A **clinical ladder** includes defined steps for advancement within the organization based on experience, additional education, specialty certification, or other indicators of excellence.

Interdisciplinary Collaboration

The report "To Err Is Human: Building a Safer Health System" (Kohn, Corrigan, & Donaldson, 1999) summarized client safety problems in the United States and recommended increasing interdisciplinary collaboration to reduce errors. As a result, many professional education programs for medical, nursing, and allied health students now require curricula that support interdisciplinary practice in a variety of clinical settings.

These programs emphasize teamwork, conflict resolution, and the use of informatics to promote collaboration in client care (Wakefield & O'Grady, 2000). Such an integrated health delivery system can evolve toward a model of interdisciplinary teamwork that delivers care to complex clients. Studies of environments that support collaboration provide evidence of improved outcomes for both acute and chronically ill clients (Pew Health Professions Commission, 1998).

LEADERSHIP CHALLENGE What might be a first step for Constance to establish interdisciplinary teamwork?

Hallmarks of a Professional Nursing Practice Environment

Characteristics of the practice setting that best support professional nursing practice and allow nurses to practice to their full potential include:

- A philosophy of clinical care with nursing input that emphasizes quality, safety, interdisciplinary collaboration, continuity of care, professional accountability, and adequate staffing patterns that speak to the complexity of care
- Differentiated nurse practice roles that are based on educational preparation, certification, and advanced preparation and that compensates and rewards role distinctions between staff nurses and other expert nurses based on those criteria
- Executive-level nursing leadership that promotes nurse participation in the governing body; reports to the high-level operations or corporate officer; has the authority and accountability for all nursing care delivery, financial resources, and personnel; and is supported by adequate managerial and support staff
- Empowered nurse participation in clinical decision making and the organization of clinical care systems by including nurses in systemwide committees and communication structures, giving them leadership roles to improve performance, involving them in reviews of clinical care errors and client safety concerns, and giving them the authority to develop and execute nursing care orders and actions to control their practice
- Clinical advancement programs, including financial rewards for clinical advancement and education; opportunities for promotion based on

education, clinical expertise, and professional contributions; annual (or more often) peer review, client, collegial, and managerial input for performance evaluation; and alignment between nurse leaders' education and credentials and their roles and responsibilities

- Support for nursing that is demonstrated through resource support for advanced education in nursing; preceptorships; refresher programs; residency programs; internships; incentive programs for registered nurse education; long-term career support targeted at older, home care, and operating room nurses and those from diverse ethnic backgrounds; specialty certification and advanced credentials that are encouraged, promoted, and recognized; advanced practice nurses, nurse researchers, and nurse educators who are employed and used in leadership roles to support clinical nursing practice; and linkages between healthcare institutions and schools of nursing to provide support for continuing education, collaborative research, and clinical educational affiliations
- Collaborative relationships that are supported by members of the healthcare provider teams
- Technological advances that are used in clinical care and information systems (AACN, 2002)

LEADERSHIP CHALLENGE Which of these hallmarks do you think Constance should try to implement? What advice would you give to help her? Give a rationale for your answer.

Developing an Engaged Nursing Workforce

The Health Resources and Services Administration (2002) estimates a shortage of more than 1 million nurses by 2020. The nursing workforce is aging, and client volume continues to grow as baby boomers demand more services.

As a nurse leader, you can play a critical role in creating and sustaining a culture of excellence in your healthcare facility. Research confirms that an employee's relationship with an immediate supervisor is a primary determinant of his or her job satisfaction and willingness to stay at the job (Hayes et al., 2006).

Rosabeth Moss Kanter's (1993) model of organizational empowerment offers a framework for creating a positive work culture. Kanter argues that when employees have access to "power tools"—such as information, support, resources, and the opportunity to learn and grow—they are motivated and more engaged than those without this access.

LEADERSHIP CHALLENGE How would you use Kanter's model of organizational empowerment to create a positive work culture? Be specific.

Laschinger and Finegan (2005) found that nurses felt empowered when managers treated them with concern for their well-being in relation to organizational decisions and provided them with explanations to justify these decisions. Such empowerment led nurses to trust the organization, enjoy greater job satisfaction, and display a stronger commitment to the organization.

Building and sustaining a culture of excellence takes time and effort. There is a growing interest in moving beyond satisfying nurses to engaging them in the organization's work. Nurses who are more engaged use their energy to drive an organization to top performance, which can impact absenteeism and client satisfaction, outcomes, and safety (Wagner, 2006).

The Healthcare Association of New York State received a grant from the New York State Department of Health to help hospitals develop the skills to engage nurses. The association surveyed 500 organizations, asking nurses in each hospital to complete a Web-based series of questions. According to this survey, the common factors of highly engaged nurses include:

- Feeling valued
- Believing that the organization practices what it preaches
- Willing to recommend the organization to others
- Feeling included in decision making
- Knowing that there are safe and effective ways to communicate complaints
- Trusting upper management to listen to employee ideas and opinions
- Believing that supervisors understand key issues in their departments
- Believing that the organization encourages and supports innovation
- Believing that their supervisor is an effective leader

When asked what engaged nurses, survey respondents commented that developing close relationships and mutual support with coworkers, deriving meaning and satisfaction from interacting with clients, receiving flexible work schedules, and having good working relationships with their nurse managers were important (Wagner, 2006).

In the most successful organizations, leaders believe that people matter. Nurse leaders who commit to seeing a change through to the desired results are a critical factor in engaging nurses. Leaders who help their teams manage daily work pressures; provide perspective, rationale, and encouragement for change; and are willing to make a difference are a critical component to successful change (Wagner, 2006).

LEADERSHIP CHALLENGE What advice do you have for Constance about empowering and engaging her staff? Give a rationale for your answer.

Summary

This chapter presented some environmental issues nurse leaders can address, including factors that make for a healthy environment and urban sprawl. It also provided information on fostering environments that support professional nursing and creating an engaged nursing workforce. The next chapter examines staff development and governance.

Key Term Review

■ A **clinical ladder** includes defined steps for advancement within the organization based on experience, additional education, specialty certification, or other indicators of excellence.

■ **Differentiated practice models** differentiate nurses by level of education, expected clinical skills or competencies, job descriptions, pay scales, and participation in decision making.

■ The **"look, think, and act" model** is a problem-solving action research process.

■ The **Magnet Recognition Program** does nothing to improve staffing ratios, but it does provide a framework to recognize excellence in healthcare provision.

■ **Preceptorships** provide opportunities for nursing students to work closely with staff nurses to gain role socialization and to increase clinical skills, knowledge, competence, and confidence.

■ **Residencies** or **internships** help new graduates transition into the practice arena; they also facilitate recruitment, increase retention, and increase commitment to the organization.

■ **Urban sprawl** is a development pattern in cities that is characterized by decentralized, automobile-dependent neighborhoods. Its health implications include obesity, stress, mental health issues, and physical inactivity.

Leadership Development Exercises

■ **Leadership Development Exercise 18-1**

   a. Survey your work environment to see the measures it follows to prevent hospital-acquired infections.
   b. Develop a protocol for reducing hospital-acquired infections with at least two other colleagues.
   c. Present your solutions to a group of colleagues.
   d. Ask for suggestions for implementing your recommendations.
   e. **Optional:** If possible, present your findings to a nurse leader or nurse executive.

■ **Leadership Development Exercise 18-2**

   a. Design a model nursing unit, including a blueprint and self-healing measures.
   b. Share your design with at least two other colleagues, and obtain feedback.
   c. Adjust your design as needed.

■ **Leadership Development Exercise 18-3**

   a. Observe a neighborhood for factors that contribute to obesity and other unhealthy conditions.

b. Share your findings with at least two other colleagues.

c. Come up with a way to use what you found to benefit clients or the neighborhood.

■ **Leadership Development Exercise 18-4**

a. Develop a clinical ladder for nurse advancement within an organization.

b. Share your ladder with at least two colleagues.

c. Obtain feedback.

d. Revise your ladder as necessary.

■ **Leadership Development Exercise 18-5**

a. Use the information in "Hallmarks of a Professional Nursing Practice Environment" to evaluate at least one healthcare organization or unit. Interview a nurse leader on the phone, in person, or online, if possible.

b. Present your findings to at least two colleagues.

■ **Leadership Development Exercise 18-6**

a. Use the information in "Other Ways to Promote Self-Care and Healing in the Workplace" to evaluate your work environment.

b. Decide on a way to make your personal space more of a peaceful oasis for you.

c. Collaborate with at least two colleagues to make that area more peaceful.

d. Evaluate the effect on your peace of mind.

e. Share your findings with your colleagues.

Advanced Leadership Development Exercises

■ **Leadership Development Exercise 18-7**

a. Teach less advanced nurse leaders about one aspect of a healthy nursing environment.

b. Obtain feedback from learners.

c. Write up your results, and share them with at least two colleagues.

■ **Leadership Development Exercise 18-8**

a. Develop a problem statement for a research study focused on establishing a healthy environment.

b. Obtain feedback from at least one other seasoned nurse researcher about whether the statement can be researched as stated.

■ **Leadership Development Exercise 18-9**

a. Develop a research project for your problem statement.
b. Obtain feedback from a more seasoned nurse researcher about your design.
c. Revise your research project as needed.

References

American Association of Colleges of Nursing. (2002). *Hallmarks of the professional nursing practice environment.* Retrieved June 29, 2007, from http://www.aacm.nche.edu /Publications/positions/hallmarks.htm

Brown, C. J. (2006, December). Promoting self-caring and healing in your workplace. *American Nurse Today,* 54–55.

Chen, Y.-C., & Chiang, L.-C. (2007). Effectiveness of hand-washing teaching programmes for families of children in paediatric intensive care units. *Journal of Clinical Nursing, 16,* 1173–1179.

Hayes, L. J., O'Brien-Palles, L., Duffield, C., Shamian, J., Bachan, J., Hughes, F., et al. (2006). Nurse turnover: A literature review. *International Journal of Nursing Studies, 43,* 237–263.

Healing design gains popularity. (2007). *Nurse Practitioner World News, 12*(6), 9.

Health Resources and Services Administration. (2002). Projected supply, demand and shortage of registered nurses: 2000–2020. Retrieved October 17, 2007, from http:// bhpr.hrsa.gov/ bhpr/workforce/rnsupplyanddemand2002.pdf

Kanter, R. M. (1993). *Men and women of the corporation.* New York: Basic Books.

Kohn, L. T., Corrigan, J. M., & Donaldson, M. S. (Eds.). (1999). *To err is human: Building a safer health system.* Washington, DC: National Academies Press.

Laschinger, H. K. S., & Finegan, J. (2005). Using empowerment to build trust and respect in the workplace: A strategy for addressing the nursing shortage. *Nursing Economics, 23*(1), 6–13.

Lopez, R., & Welker-Hood, K. (2007, January). Environment, health, and safety: Urban sprawl and the built environment. *American Nurse Today,* 56.

Massachusetts Nurses Association. (2004). *Position statement on the "Magnet Recognition Program for Nursing Services in Hospitals" and other consultant-driven quality improvement projects that claim to improve care.* Retrieved June 29, 2007, from http://www .massnurses.org/pubs/positions/magnet.htm

Pew Health Professions Commission. (1998). *Recreating health professional practice for a new century.* San Francisco: Author.

Stringer, E., & Genat, W. (2003). *Action research in health.* Columbus, OH: Pearson Merrill Prentice Hall.

Study identifies risk factors for spread of respiratory infections in hospitals. (2007, March 16). *Science Daily.* Retrieved November 27, 2007, from http://www.sciencedaily.com/ releases/2007/03/070315160857.htm

Wagner, S. E. (2006). Staff retention: From "satisfied" to "engaged." *Nursing Management, 37*(3), 24–29.

Wakefield, M., & O'Grady, E. (2000). Putting patients first: Improving patient safety through collaborative education. In Health Resources and Services Administration (HRSA), *Collaborative education to ensure patient safety* (pp. 19–32). Washington, DC: HRSA.

Developing Staff

CHAPTER OBJECTIVES

After reading this chapter, answering the leadership challenges, and participating in the leadership development exercises, you will be able to:

- Describe the elements in developing effective learning systems
- Discuss the developmental needs of new RNs
- Describe how a novice leader program develops new RNs
- Discuss research that details how nurse executives prepare new nurse leaders
- Analyze why training in computers and electronic resources should be part of staff development efforts
- Discuss the importance of developing nurse practitioners' leadership skills
- Describe the LEAD Project for minority nurses
- Discuss the work of leadership development coordinators
- Analyze failure disclosure as a way to develop leaders

Advanced nurses will be able to:

- Teach less skilled nurse leaders about staff development
- Develop a problem statement for a research study focused on staff development
- Develop a research project for a problem statement focused on staff development

Introduction

According to the Magnet hospital studies (Scott, Sochalski, & Aiken, 1999), what nurses want in their leaders is someone who (1) is visionary and enthusiastic, (2) is supportive and knowledgeable, (3) maintains high standards and high staff expectations, (4) provides values education and professional development to all nurses within the organization, (5) is highly visible to staff nurses, (6) is responsive and maintains open lines of communication, and (7) is actively involved in state and national organizations.

The question is, how can organizations educate nurses to produce these qualities? This chapter attempts to answer that question by examining aspects of staff development that can help foster leadership.

LEADERSHIP IN ACTION

Georgette had been asked to develop a new leadership training program for nurses. She wasn't sure how to begin or where to look. Her first action was to do a search on the Internet.

LEADERSHIP CHALLENGE **What other sources of information would you suggest to Georgette?**

Designing Effective Learning Systems

Designing effective learning systems requires knowledge of learning theory, learning systems, and the learner. It also includes skills in writing behavioral objectives and learning contracts. Because people at all levels of management and all leaders have a responsibility to improve employee performance, they must be familiar with effective learning methods and the theory underlying those methods.

Social Cognitive Learning Theory

KEY TERM

Self-efficacy is the belief in one's ability to perform adequately and has proved to be a more consistent predictor of behavioral outcomes than other motivational constructs.

Bandura (1977, 1986, 1997, 2001) developed a social cognitive theory that has been widely used and accepted (Graham & Weiner, 1996). Bandura (1986) wrote that individuals possess beliefs about themselves that enable them to exercise control over their thoughts, feelings, and actions.

Self-efficacy, or the belief in one's ability to perform adequately, has proved to be a more consistent predictor of behavioral outcomes than other motivational constructs (Graham & Weiner, 1996). Learners with high self-efficacy expect higher grades and put forth the effort to get them. These learners approach difficult tasks as challenges, rather than as situations to be avoided.

Certain environmental characteristics can cause even highly self-efficacious and well-skilled learners not to behave in concert with their beliefs and abilities. This includes times when they:

- Lack the incentive
- Lack the necessary resources
- Perceive social constraints

Bandura (1977) wrote that learning would be laborious and hazardous if learners had to rely only on themselves. Luckily, learners have nurse leaders to model appropriate behavior for them. This vicarious learning permits individuals to learn novel behaviors without going through the arduous task of trial-and-error learning.

Bandura (1977) emphasized the importance of modeling behaviors, attitudes, and emotional reactions. He believed that it was the human capability to symbolize that allowed learners to:

- Extract meaning from the environment
- Construct guides for action
- Solve problems cognitively
- Support well-thought-out courses of action
- Gain new knowledge by reflective thought
- Communicate with others at any distance in time and space
- Use self-reflection to make sense of their experiences
- Engage in self-evaluation and alter their thinking and behavior accordingly (Bandura, 1986)

LEADERSHIP CHALLENGE **Based on what you know about Bandura's theory, what is the role of staff development in relation to leaders?**

Learning Systems

A **learning system** consists of:

- A learner
- A learning goal
- A procedure for achieving the goal

KEY TERM

A **learning system** consists of a learner, a learning goal, and a procedure for achieving the goal.

By this definition, self-paced or individualized materials, programmed instructional materials, and small-group exercises used by learners according to specified instructions are learning systems.

A learning system need not include an educator except in its design, but some learning systems do include visibly present educators or facilitators. A group of learners who have been given a learning goal and then hear a lecture compose one type of learning system. Many learning systems added together constitute a curriculum.

In the past, memorization of predigested amounts of information often composed the content of leadership courses. Now the process goals that are necessary to develop leaders—such as creativity, inquiry, and inductive thinking—require that objectives be tied to the curriculum, teaching/learning strategies, and learner needs (Joyce, Weil, & Calhoun, 2004; Kizlik, 2006).

Teaching/learning methods are chosen based on the purpose of instruction:

- If objectives such as learning to learn and the learner's responsibility for learning are the focus, self-paced materials are appropriate.
- If learning objectives include prepractice in a safe environment and an integrated cognitive, affective, and perceptual-motor approach, simulations and simulation games are appropriate.
- When receiving immediate feedback and making presentations in front of others are important, audiotape, videotape, and videoconferencing methods can be used.
- When content can be broken down into small, sequential bits of knowledge and when learners learn individually, programmed materials are useful.
- When learning focuses on values, moral development or ethics, perceptual exercises, journal writing, and/or value clarification can be used.
- Peer supervision or small-group methods are helpful if processing input, collaborating with peers, and learning leadership qualities are essential objectives.

The Learner-Centered Syllabus

According to Diamond (1998), a **learner-centered syllabus** can help you when you're trying to develop your staff. The syllabus should:

- Define learner responsibilities and help manage time by providing a clear idea of learning goals and a time frame for accomplishing them
- Improve learner note-taking and studying skills by providing a detailed outline, essential diagrams and tables, and copies of overhead transparencies, case studies, and so forth
- Reduce learner anxiety by providing sample review questions, readings that may be difficult to obtain, and important handouts

- Improve learner efficiency by including detailed descriptions of major ideas and behaviors with samples of expected responses

Possible content for a learner-centered syllabus includes:

- The title and date of the course
- A welcome letter to the learner that describes the course's intent, purpose, and overall goals
- A table of contents
- The purpose of the learner manual and how to use it
- An introduction, including how the course fits in the general program and for whom it was designed, general directions for learners, and where notices and related items will be posted
- A list of the personnel involved in the course, including their contact information, office hours, and e-mail addresses
- An overview of the course, including a course outline, a module outline, options, and course objectives
- Evaluation procedures (e.g., evaluation systems, scales, or forms)
- A list of textbooks or handouts, including where and how to get them and how to use them
- A calendar that includes topics by class meeting, projects, deadlines, and so forth
- A list of the facilities that will be used
- A checklist for assignment due dates
- Self-tests for learners to evaluate their ability to meet course objectives
- Additional information on using the library and computing center
- For online segments, a description of how to log on to the course, how to contact the help desk, how to use the e-mail system, the nurse educator's e-mail address, where to find online postings of the class syllabus and schedule, and other information (such as details about forums, online exams, etc.)

Learning Contracts

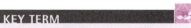

The design of a learning system is influenced by the quantity of staff development and learner input. A major issue in instructional procedures is the **educator/learner contract**.

There are a number of basic contracts:

- *The educator-made and educator-assigned contract.* In this kind of contract, the teacher makes all the decisions concerning the content and sequence of learning activities. This contract is most commonly used in individualized instruction approaches.

- *The educator-made and learner-assigned contract.* Learners are able to select a contract based on their own choices and preferences. The educator prepares a number of contracts, and learners choose those that appeal to them.
- *The learner-made and learner-assigned contract.* This contract is based on areas identified by learners as those in which they are academically weak or in which they have a special interest. Learners begin to learn to assess their own instructional needs and areas of interest or nursing specialty. Such a contract has implied objectives and potential for learning to learn and life-long learning.
- *The jointly written contract.* This kind of contract is developed between the educator and learner during a series of meetings. The content of the contract and the procedures surrounding it are discussed and forged through discussion. This type of contract has potential for teaching cooperative and collaborative skills, for working through two-person teaching/learning difficulties, and for developing mentor or sponsor relationships where educators and learners are on a more equal level than in traditional learning situations. A jointly written learning contract includes:

  - An initial description of the learner's work
  - The specific goals, purposes, and time frame for the work
  - A description of learning activities and resources
  - The criteria that will be used to evaluate the attainment of the learning goals

Age Differences in Learning

A leader's needs may differ by his or her age. For example, **Generation X learners** (born between 1965 and 1976) tend to:

KEY TERM

Generation X learners are highly independent, challenge authority, problem-solve, and multitask.

- Be highly independent
- Challenge authority often
- Solve problems independently
- Multitask

Generation Y learners (who began entering college in 2000):

KEY TERM

Generation Y learners are culturally diverse, are self-reliant, question things, are technologically advanced, expect others to earn respect, and are addicted to visual media.

- Are the most culturally diverse group of all time
- Are self-reliant
- Question things
- Are technologically advanced
- Expect others to earn respect
- Are addicted to visual media

Leaders must ensure that learning methods align with the expectations, values, and needs of these learners (Walker et al., 2006).

Active Learning Processes

Active learning procedures are more apt to promote critical thinking. Active learning systems that enhance critical thinking include:

- Structured role-play
- Simulations and simulation games
- Peer supervision
- Self-paced learning materials
- Programmed instructional materials
- Audiovisual and computer methods of learning
- Perceptual exercises
- Journal writing, value clarification, and small-group methods
- Other novel strategies that work well even with large groups of learners

A Novice Leader Program to Develop New RNs

Research on the experience of new graduates reports the need for specialized transition programs. One study found that 30% of new nurses left within a year and that 57% quit within 2 years. Its authors cited unsafe nurse-to-client ratios as the most frequent reason why nurses left (Bowles & Candela, 2005).

Florida Atlantic University's Christine E. Lynn College of Nursing in Boca Raton developed the Novice Nurse Leadership Institute. The program smooths the transition to full-time practice while nourishing leadership talent. About two dozen nurses participate in the yearlong leadership institute, which has them attending all-day educational sessions every 2 weeks, completing an evidence-based research project, and working with preceptors from their originating facilities (Wood, 2007).

The program includes:

- A self-assessment using the Myers-Briggs personality type test to help participants understand how their personality and their fit with their organizations affect their learning style
- Three credits toward either a BSN or MSN, depending on participants' current degree
- Opportunities to share stories and support each other
- Teaching learners how to lead without holding a position of authority
- Cultural sensitivity training
- The business of health care and the economics of nursing
- The role of research, ethics, strategic thinking, working with other disciplines, horizontal violence, and advocacy to affect local, regional, and national policy

LEADERSHIP CHALLENGE How could Georgette use this information to help develop staff? Give a rationale for your answer.

Research on How Nurse Executives Prepare New Nurse Leaders

In a survey, one-third of nurse managers reported that they expected to add nursing manager roles in the future. Six in 10 did not expect to add nursing manager roles (Denning & Associates, 2004).

When nurse executives were asked how they prepared new nurse managers, they mentioned:

- Planned orientation (scheduled meetings with agendas with their colleagues)
- A nursing leadership academy
- A manager mentoring program

Almost all nurse executives in the study reported that they prepared their new nurse leaders with on-the-job training. More than four-fifths reported using workshops, and almost two-thirds used continuing education classes (Denning & Associates, 2004).

When asked whether their organization had sufficient resources available to help prepare new nurse managers, nearly one-third of the nurse executives reported that they had enough resources to help them prepare new nurse managers and nurse leaders. More than 6 in 10 reported that there were not enough resources.

Nurse executives reported they would like to see the following added to their organizations:

- Ways to produce effective work environments with an emphasis on leadership development, especially transitioning from a clinical to a supervisory role, as well as ongoing professional information, resources, and support.
- A program that is accessible, affordable, flexible, able to meet a diverse audience (e.g., rural and urban learners, novice and expert learners), and culturally sensitive.
- Programming to accomplish enhanced leaderships can be curriculum based on on-site support, speakers bureaus, study guides, and/or Web-based formats. (Denning & Associates, 2004)

LEADERSHIP CHALLENGE Which, if any, of this information could Georgette use to help develop staff? How, specifically, could she use this information? Give a rationale for your answer.

The Importance of Training in Computers and Electronic Resources

Nursing administrators and leaders should be aware of the large number of nurses who were educated before the Internet was such an important part of daily life. These nurses may be uncomfortable with, or may not even be familiar with, electronic searching processes.

Healthcare organizations should train employees on the use of computers and electronic resources. The increasing use of electronic healthcare records will make such training mandatory.

The amount of training necessary to increase nurses' comfort levels with computers varies from nurse to nurse. One question nurse leaders can ask is, "What kinds of interventions can we develop to improve nurses' search skills, research evaluation skills, and ability to apply evidence to practice?" There are many tools—including journals, reviews, and commentaries on research—to facilitate the use of evidence (Pravikoff, Pierce, & Tanner, 2005).

LEADERSHIP CHALLENGE How should Georgette use this information on training in computers and electronic resources to help develop her staff? Give a rationale for your answer.

Leadership Skills Development for Nurse Practitioners

Leadership skills are an increasingly important part of the nurse practitioner (NP) role. NPs must use leadership skills not only to provide optimal health care but also to navigate the healthcare system, advocate for sound policies, and guide multidisciplinary teams (Judkins & Friedrich-Cuntz, 2007).

An exploratory study evaluated NPs' leadership skills before and after participating in a continuing education leadership training institute (LTI) program offered by the Center for Leadership in Nursing and Health Care at the School of Nursing at the University of Texas at Arlington. Researchers asked 225 NPs in northern Texas to describe their leadership skill needs. Participants identified conflict management, business management, negotiation, strategic planning, change management, and human resource management as essential to effective leadership. Based on these topics, the institute developed a 2.5-day program.

The researchers used the Nurse Practitioner Leadership Questionnaire, a 37-item Likert-type (1=always/quite often; 5 = never) questionnaire to measure leadership. Paired *t*-tests showed immediate improvement in leadership skills. Statistically significant (P = <.05) changes were noted in actively exercising a leadership role, overcoming difficulties in achieving organizational objectives, and demonstrating creative problem solving.

Participants also reported taking new leadership roles (e.g., director of a clinic, serving on an influential committee, or becoming the NP liaison to a neonatal intensive care service). More than 70% of the NPs also expressed an understanding of the importance of networking. Although networking was not a planned topic, participants repeatedly mentioned the value of networking with other NPs when asked to evaluate the overall program.

Based on the findings, the researchers suggested that leadership development should be included as part of the NP curriculum by using a training format like the one described in their study (Judkins & Friedrich-Cuntz, 2007).

LEADERSHIP CHALLENGE **Explain how Georgette could use this information to help develop her staff. Give a rationale for your answer.**

The LEAD Project for Minority Nurses

Minority nurses are underrepresented in leadership positions (Schmieding, 2000). Bessent and Fleming (2003) developed the **Leadership Enhancement and Development (LEAD) Project** for minority nurses based on a pilot project on leadership and race (which interviewed minority nurses on the faculty of a majority university and others from a historically black university in a collaborative relationship with a majority university) and a search of the literature.

Bessent and Fleming (2003) identified the following five essentials elements for the leadership model:

1. *Knowledge of self.* Black female nurses' full leadership potential has gone untapped; their experiences have focused on others' needs and not on trying to understand themselves.

2. *Integrity.* Minority nurses may have learned not to share their feelings, which can lead to not expressing what they really believe is pertinent to solving problems and handling issues.

3. *Vision.* Minority nurses think strategically but do not feel that they get credit for the information they provide.
4. *Communication.* Assisting minority nurses in communicating effectively is a challenge because many feel that they are not listened to in certain contexts.
5. *Collaboration.* Minority nurses may not be used to having power shared with them, but sharing power is an important skill to learn.

Bessent and Fleming (2003) suggested that this model has potential for research and service as well as for helping educate future leaders.

LEADERSHIP CHALLENGE How can Georgette use this information to help develop her staff? Give a rationale for your answer.

Shared Governance

In a **shared governance model,** decisions are made at the point of service, and the nurses involved in care are part of the decision-making process and communication flow within an organization. In this philosophy, the nurse leader and staff address issues together. The focus is always on improving care.

A first step in putting this philosophy into action is to initiate staff meetings that include discussions of unit operations. During the discussions, each staff member should be asked for suggestions for improvement. As discussions proceed, natural leaders on each unit will emerge and set an example for others to follow (Anderson & Paden, 1998).

Nursing Leadership Development Coordinators

Some hospital administrators recognize the need for authentic leadership that fosters true collaboration and participatory decision making. Florida Hospital hired Sandy Swearingen, RN, PhD, as a **leadership development coordinator** to help clinically competent nurses acquire the leadership skills they need to reduce errors, maximize client outcomes, and increase job satisfaction.

LEADERSHIP TIP
Use the shared governance model to empower staff to make changes, enhancing the likelihood of success.

KEY TERM

In a **shared governance model**, decisions are made at the point of service, and the nurses involved in care are part of the decision-making process and communication flow within an organization.

KEY TERM

A **leadership development coordinator** is hired by an organization to help clinically competent nurses acquire the leadership skills they need to reduce errors, maximize client outcomes, and increase job satisfaction.

Swearingen is accountable for developing and implementing a nursing leadership curriculum on Florida Hospital's seven campuses called Journey to Leadership. Much of the up to 200 hours of content (depending on individual needs) is taught by her, but external and internal experts are responsible for lessons on critical thinking, assertiveness, conflict resolution, and creating a culture of engagement. It is Swearingen's belief that the vision of the organization can be best implemented when staff support one another and focus on delivering high-quality care.

The biggest challenge for the program is to change the top-down management style, in which top executives make decisions, to participative leadership, in which all nurses help decide the issues that affect them (Alfaro-LeFevre, 2006).

Failure Disclosure as Leadership Development

LEADERSHIP TIP

Failure is inevitable and can even be useful in helping staff develop leadership skills.

KEY TERM

Failure disclosure means admitting failure to employees, clients, and families.

Everyone makes mistakes, but not everyone wants to admit them. Leaders especially may want to hide their errors, believing that the people they supervise may respect them less because of those errors.

Leaders who remain silent and refuse to take responsibility for their mistakes can be perceived as lacking integrity. Leaders who handle failure by openly admitting mistakes and offering an apology will most often be perceived as human and of high integrity.

Failure disclosure means admitting failure to employees, clients, and families. Leaders' failures can be categorized into three areas:

1. *Failure of omission* occurs when leaders know about a situation, like a difficult employee or a toxic environment, but fail to speak up or intervene because they fear the consequences.
2. *Failure by commission* occurs when leaders do not hold the line against an unsafe staffing ratio: client results include death or another serious consequence.
3. *Failure by being accountable* occurs when employees give the wrong medication or disclose confidential client records; these are behaviors for which leaders must take responsibility even though they are not directly involved. (Kerfoot, 2006)

Kerfoot (2006) urges leaders to take the lead from clinical practice and move from an era of cover-up and nondisclosure to a culture where errors can be discussed openly and resolved. Saying "I'm sorry" opens up the door to mend relationship breakdowns and has amazing healing properties. Attorneys, insurance companies, and hospital administrators often ask nurses and other clinicians to avoid apologizing for medical mishaps. Yet, silence can lead to anger, hurt, and a sense of betrayal; and an apology returns respect and dignity, decreases anger, and promotes dialogue (Sparkman, 2005).

Apologies have a great power in the legal arena as well. Studies have shown that apologies encourage the settlement of grievances and avoid litigation (Vincent, Young, & Phillips, 1994). More lawyers are recommending apologies, too (Duffy, 2005).

In a study involving the Veterans Administration Medical Center in Lexington, Kentucky, administrators adopted a disclosure policy that included:

- Identifying an instance of an accident, possible negligence, or malpractice
- Notifying the client that there was a "problem" with the care they received
- Holding a face-to-face meeting to disclose all aspects of the event
- Offering continuing assistance to the client while he or she was obtaining compensation

Summary

This chapter focused on developing staff for leadership positions. Topics addressed included designing effective learning systems, developing a novice leader program, research on how nurse executives prepare new nurse leaders, the importance of training in computers and electronic resources, developing leadership skills in nurse practitioners, the LEAD Project for minority nurses, shared governance, the role of nursing leadership development coordinators, and failure disclosure as a way to develop leaders. The next chapter focuses on evaluating staff performance and quality assurance.

Key Term Review

■ **Educator/learner contracts** can be educator or learner assigned or made.

■ **Failure disclosure** means admitting failure to employees, clients, and families.

■ **Generation X learners** are highly independent, challenge authority, problem-solve, and multitask.

■ **Generation Y learners** are culturally diverse, are self-reliant, question things, are technologically advanced, expect others to earn respect, and are addicted to visual media.

■ A **leadership development coordinator** is hired by an organization to help clinically competent nurses acquire the leadership skills they need to reduce errors, maximize client outcomes, and increase job satisfaction.

■ The **LEAD Project** for minority nurses was based on a pilot project on leadership and race.

■ A **learner-centered syllabus** defines learner responsibilities, provides detailed course outlines and essential written materials, includes sample review questions and detailed descriptions of major ideas and sample expected responses.

■ A **learning system** consists of a learner, a learning goal, and a procedure for achieving the goal.

■ **Self-efficacy** is the belief in one's ability to perform adequately and has proved to be a more consistent predictor of behavioral outcomes than other motivational constructs.

■ In a **shared governance model,** decisions are made at the point of service, and the nurses involved in care are part of the decision-making process and communication flow within an organization.

Leadership Development Exercises

■ **Leadership Development Exercise 19-1**

Analyze a learning system for its effectiveness for nurse leaders.

■ **Leadership Development Exercise 19-2**

  a. Gather with a group of colleagues, and conduct a survey of new RN leadership needs.
  b. Share your findings with the class.
  c. **Optional:** Write up your findings, and present them to the staff development department or use the information in some other creative way.

■ **Leadership Development Exercise 19-3**

Plan a novice leader program based on the information in this chapter.

■ **Leadership Development Exercise 19-4**

Take a poll of staff on one unit to determine their computer and Internet skills.

■ **Leadership Development Exercise 19-5**

Interview at least two nurse practitioners, and find out which leadership skills they possess and which skills they believe they need to develop.

■ **Leadership Development Exercise 19-6**

Interview several minority nurses to see what they think of the LEAD Project and whether they agree with the essential five elements discussed in this chapter.

■ **Leadership Development Exercise 19-7**

Talk to at least one person in staff development at a hospital or medical center. Discuss the idea of a leader development coordinator covered in this chapter and whether the role might be beneficial in that hospital or medical center.

Advanced Leadership Development Exercises

■ **Leadership Development Exercise 19-8**

a. Teach a group of less skilled nurse leaders about staff development.
b. Obtain feedback from your learners.
c. Report your results to at least two colleagues.

■ **Leadership Development Exercise 19-9**

a. Develop a problem statement for a question related to staff development.
b. Obtain feedback on your problem statement from at least two colleagues with research know-how.
c. Revise your statement, if necessary.

■ **Leadership Development Exercise 19-10**

a. Prepare a research project to answer your problem statement/research question.
b. Obtain feedback from more skilled nurse researchers.
c. Revise your design, if necessary.

References

Alfaro-Lefevre, R. (2006, July 3). Sandy Swearingen, RN, MSN, on helping clinically competent nurses develop as leaders. *Nursing Spectrum*, 24.

Anderson, B., & Paden, K. K. (1998, March 9). Management perspectives. *Nursing Spectrum*, 4–5.

Bandura, A. (1977). *Social learning theory*. New York: General Learning Press.

Bandura, A. (1986). *Social foundation of thought and action: A social cognitive theory*. Englewood Cliffs, NJ: Prentice Hall.

Bandura, A. (1997). *Self-efficacy: The exercise of control*. New York: W. H. Freeman.

Bandura, A. (2001). Social cognitive theory: An agentic perspective. *Annual Review of Psychology, 52*, 1–26.

Bessent, H., & Fleming, J.W. (2003). The Leadership Enhancement and Development (LEAD) project for minority nurses in the New Millenium Model. *Nursing Outlook, 51*, 255–260.

Bowles, C., & Candela, L. (2005). First job experiences of recent RN graduates: Improving the work environment. *Journal of Nursing Administration, 35*(3), 130–137.

Denning, D. R., & Associates. (2004). *Nurse executive/nurse manager survey, evaluation results*. Retrieved January 9, 2007, from http://www.moln.org/files/NurseSurvey Revised4-29-2004.ppt

Diamond, R. M. (1998). *Designing and assessing courses and curricula: A practical guide*. San Francisco: Jossey-Bass.

Duffy, T. (2005, June 21). More lawyers recommend apologies in med-mal cases. *Missouri Medical Law Report*, 2.

Graham, S., & Weiner, B. (1996). Theories and principles of motivation. In D. C. Berliner & R. C. Calfee (Eds.), *Handbook of educational psychology*. New York: Simon & Schuster/Macmillan.

Joyce, B. R., Weil, M., & Calhoun, E. (2004). *Models of teaching* (7th ed.). Boston, MA: Allyn & Bacon.

Judkins, S., & Friedrich-Cuntz, A-G. (2007). Leadership skills development among nurse practitioners. *American Journal of Nurse Practitioners, 11*(5), 49–57.

Kerfoot, K. (2006). The art of truth telling: Handling failure with disclosure. *Nursing Econonmics, 24*(4), 216–217

Kizlik, R. (2006). *Common mistakes in writing lesson plans (and what to do about them)*. Retrieved November 27, 2007, from http://www.adprima.com/mistakes.htm

Pravikoff, D. S., Pierce, S. T., & Tanner, A. (2005). Evidence-based practice readiness study supported by academy nursing informatics expert panel. *Nursing Outlook, 53*(1), 49–50.

Schmieding, J. (2000). Minority nurses in leadership positions: A call for action. *Nursing Outlook, 48*, 124.

Scott, J. G., Sochalski, J., & Aiken, L. H. (1999). Review of Magnet hospital research: Findings and implications for professional nursing practice. *Journal of Nursing Administration, 29*(1), 9–19.

Sparkman, C. A. G. (2005). Legislating apology in the context of medical mistakes. *AORN Journal, 82*(2), 263–264, 266, 269–272.

Vincent, C., Young, M., & Phillips, A. (1994). Why do people sue doctors? A study of patients and relatives taking legal action. *Lancet, 343*, 1609–1613.

Walker, K. (2007). Fast-trac for fast times: Catching and keeping Generation Y in the nursing workforce. *Nurse Recruitment and Retention 24*, 147–158.

Wood, D. A. (2007, April 9). Novice leader program aims to retain new grads. *Nursing Spectrum*, 10–11.

Evaluating Staff Performance and Ensuring Quality

CHAPTER OBJECTIVES

After reading this chapter, answering the leadership challenges, and participating in the leadership development exercises, you will be able to:

- Try out performance appraisal approaches
- Discuss the use of simulations to improve performance leadership
- Describe a clinical practice development model to measure nursing practice
- Analyze nursing situations that can affect quality of care

Advanced nurses will be able to:

- Teach less skilled nurse leaders about evaluating performance and improving quality of care
- Develop a problem statement for a research study focused on evaluating performance and improving quality of care
- Develop a research project for a problem statement focused on staff performance and quality of care

Introduction

As a nurse leader, you may be expected to evaluate other employees or to help evaluate them. If the work setting includes teams, they may be able to help evaluate individuals' underlying traits, such as flexibility, adaptability, and the ability to get along with others—all of which are so critical to the job (Gross, 1995).

Quality care goes hand in hand with excellent performance. This chapter examines both and the relationship between them.

LEADERSHIP IN ACTION

Henry, a new clinical leader, was asked to participate in performance appraisals. He had mixed feelings about performance appraisals and was not sure exactly how to conduct this semiannual review at his agency.

LEADERSHIP CHALLENGE **What advice would you give Henry? Give a rationale for your answer.**

KEY TERM

Performance appraisals are semiannual or annual evaluations of employee accomplishments and are often tied to rewards.

Performance Appraisals

Performance appraisals were first used annually or semiannually to identify the best-performing employees (who were usually rewarded with promotions and bonuses) and the worst-performing employees (who were counseled to perform better and, in extreme cases, demoted or docked pay). Today, a development approach is often used that helps employees meet organizational objectives; employees are recognized as individuals who can participate in the goal-setting and evaluation process.

Performance Appraisal Requisites

Some of the qualities needed to perform performance appraisals in an effective way are:

- Translating the organization's goals into individual job objectives
- Communicating the organization's expectations regarding employee performance to the employee
- Providing feedback to the employee about job performance
- Diagnosing employee strengths and weaknesses without prejudice
- Collaborating to determine developmental activities that will help employees perform better or meet their objectives

Performance Criteria

Major criteria for measuring the performance of individuals or teams include behavioral competencies, demonstration of skills and knowledge, achievement of specific objectives, and results (Gross, 1995).

Hospitals and agencies may develop a list of behavioral competencies, skills, and knowledge based on job descriptions, or that may be left to the manager or leader to develop. Management by objectives, now somewhat out of vogue, can be a highly efficient approach to evaluating an employee's performance. Objectives can be short range, long range, related to routine tasks, organizationally developed, problem oriented (such as reducing medical errors), innovative (i.e., to stimulate creativity), or developmental (Gross, 1995).

Results may appear to be the best choice for evaluating performance, but they are not always within the employee's control. Many other factors contribute to whether a person obtains the required result (Gross, 1995).

The Performance Appraisal Process

There are four steps to the performance appraisal process:

1. *Perform an assessment of the employee using a performance appraisal form.* Depending on the institution, the evaluator and/or the employee may complete an assessment. Peers may also be asked to provide an evaluation, especially for the purposes of advancement.
2. *Share evaluation materials with the employee.* Meet in a private area with the employee. Establish a common understanding about expectations, the work accomplished by the employee, and how that work is evaluated. Draw out the employee, asking for reactions to the items being evaluated, and then listen to responses without becoming defensive.
3. *Discuss the evaluation materials, and devise a developmental plan.* The employee usually has the right to respond to the evaluation in writing. To provide the best experience, the leader asks for input from the employee, and they agree on a plan to enhance the employee's work. This plan often includes new objectives, timelines for meeting the objectives, and other ideas for enhancing the employee's work.
4. *Set up a follow-up meeting.* Conduct this meeting in about a month to discuss what the employee has accomplished. It is important to find a way to praise any movement toward the objectives and express confidence in the employee.

Performance Appraisal Techniques

Numerous performance appraisal techniques exist, including essays, rating scales, forced-choice ratings, critical incident reviews, and employee collaboration.

Essays

Essays by evaluators include information about the employee's strengths, weaknesses, and potential. Although an essay may provide more valid information than other methods, a big drawback is that it is difficult to compare essays because one evaluator may report observations that other evaluators have not witnessed. The essays' length and content may also vary greatly, making it difficult to compare them.

Rating Scales

Rating scales can be more consistent; thus, they are more reliable than essay methods. Through this approach, an employee's quality and quantity of effort can be assessed, as can his or her personal traits, such as reliability and willingness to cooperate. This method takes less time and effort than writing an essay.

A rating scale usually has four levels of performance:

1. Exceptional performance
2. Fully meets expectations for performance goals and competencies
3. Does not meet standard
4. Not measurable/not observed

Behaviors are weighted, giving more points to the more complex actions (Gross, 1995).

Forced-Choice Ratings

Forced-choice ratings may be less biased than rating scales or essays. In this method, raters are asked to choose from among groups of statements those that best fit and least fit the individual employee. The statements are then scored.

Critical Incident Reviews

Critical incident reviews are based on factual incidents. Supervisors or leaders keep a record for each employee and record actual incidents of positive and negative behavior. During a performance appraisal, the discussion with the employee focuses on actual behavior, not on traits or personality, and on ways to perform differently to receive a higher rating next time.

Employee Collaboration

Employees can be asked to assess their work, provide evidence of their accomplishments, and devise their own work objectives based on their job description. This method encourages leadership behavior in employees and respects their opinions.

Roadblocks When Using Performance Appraisals

Nurse leaders must be aware of the following obstacles when trying to implement an effective appraisal system:

- Personal bias can interfere with appraisals, and less competent employees may get preferential treatment.
- Appraisers may not have good communication skills and may not inform employees that they are being judged and why.

- Negative feedback to employees can result in lower morale and lack of motivation.
- Performance appraisals can be viewed as inconsistent by employees in an organization that claims to use participative management.

Overcoming Difficulties with Performance Appraisals

Adding space on evaluation forms for specific examples and asking for written input from employees on their behavior can help make the appraisal a more collaborative effort. This one action alone may help overcome many of the obstacles that performance appraisals present.

Simulation is a learning technique that can provide practice in a safe learning environment. To gain practice in helping employees align their goals and behavior with the organization's strategic goals, see Rachman-Moore and Kenett (2006).

A Model to Measure Nursing Practice

Performance appraisal is not the only method of evaluating nursing performance. Clinical narratives and nursing theory can provide solutions.

> **KEY TERM**
>
> **Clinical narratives** are stories nurses tell in evaluation conferences about their level of expertise.

At St. Luke's Medical Center in Milwaukee, nurses use their own **clinical narratives** to describe individual nursing practices as evaluation and promotion procedures.

LEADERSHIP CHALLENGE Is there a way for Henry to use clinical narratives at his work site? Give a rationale for your answer.

Nursing theory can also provide a base for evaluating staff. In addition to using Benner's (1984) Novice to Expert theoretical framework (Nedd, Nah, Galindo-Ciocon, & Belgrave, 2006) to recognize the level of nursing expertise, Haag-Heitman and Kramer (1998) also used three recurring domains of practice along Benner's five-stage continuum (novice, advanced beginner, competent, proficient, and expert) including caring, clinical knowledge and decision making, and collaboration.

> **KEY TERM**
>
> The **caring domain** includes developing trust, understanding, and a healing environment.

The **caring domain** includes:

- Establishing trust with the client and family based on being with them, not doing something for them
- Demonstrating to the client and family a deep understanding of health and disease

■ Providing a healing environment of hope and trust

The **clinical knowledge domain** includes:

■ Recognizing patterns and similarities in problems and avoiding unfruitful possibilities
■ Anticipating problems and intervening
■ Acting to obtain a timely response from physicians
■ Prioritizing and adjusting strategies in unpredictable situations
■ Applying technology that matches the client's response

The **collaboration domain** includes:

■ Coordinating resources with team members
■ Providing support for colleagues
■ Encouraging teamwork

Both the level of nursing expertise and the domains of practice can affect the next topic discussed here: quality of care.

Quality of Care

Nursing actions shown to contribute to quality of care include staffing ratios, nurse-specific outcome measures, evidence-based practice, facial photo capture, nursing home processes, appropriate use of technology, discharge planning, results-driven rounding, and providing support and helping clients navigate the healthcare system.

LEADERSHIP IN ACTION

Samantha, a nurse leader, worked in a nursing home and was asked by her boss to help improve the quality of care. She went right to the Internet and searched for "quality of care." She wasn't surprised to find that staffing ratios affected quality of care because she'd seen increased errors when nurses were assigned too many clients.

Staffing Ratios

A study examining the effects of nurse staffing and organizational support on nurse reports of quality of client care focused on an international sample of more than 10,000 nurses working in US, Canadian, English, and Scottish hospitals. Nurse reports of low-quality care were three times as likely in hospitals with low staffing and support for nurses as they were in hospitals with high staffing and support.

The researchers concluded that adequate nurse staffing and organizational/managerial support for nursing are key to improving the quality of care (Aiken, Clarke, & Sloane, 2002). Recent surveys of consumers reporting on their most recent hospitalizations found substantial public dissatisfaction with the quality of health care (Donelan, Blendon, Schoen, Davis, & Binns, 1999; Donelan et al., 2000). Physicians concur that the quality of hospital care was threatened by a shortages of nurses (Blendon, Schoen, & Donelan, 2001). Based on this finding, perhaps nurses and physicians should rally together to increase nurse ratios.

LEADERSHIP CHALLENGE How could Samantha use the information from this study to enhance the quality of care? Give a rationale for your answer.

Nurse-Specific Outcome Measures

The Joint Commission is in the final phase of selecting hospitals to evaluate 15 nurse-specific measures endorsed by the National Quality Forum (NQF), a non-profit membership organization created to develop and implement a national strategy for healthcare quality measurement and reporting (Leighty, 2007). (Additional information about the NQF appears at http://www.qualityforum.org.) The Joint Commission will likely validate nursing-specific measures as important standards for hospitals to use in improving client care.

Mary Blegen, RN, PhD, FAAN, is the director of the Center for Patient Safety at the University of California, San Francisco School of Nursing. She won a Robert Wood Johnson Foundation grant to examine how nurse staffing levels in client care units affect client-centered measures. The results of Blegen's and the other grantees' nursing studies can provide consumers a broader view of a hospital's quality of care (Leighty, 2007).

Because nursing services are not billed, figures estimating nursing costs are not available for examining quality performance. Perhaps Blegen's research (as well as the research of other nurse grantees at universities, colleges, and clinics across the country) will provide hospitals the impetus to use nursing outcomes in quality-of-care data.

LEADERSHIP CHALLENGE How could Samantha use this information to improve the quality of care? Give a rationale for your answer.

Evidence-Based Practice

Interest in quality care has led hospitals to focus on evidence-of-practice variability, to identify best practices, and to apply those best practices to improve client outcomes. **Evidence-based practice** means integrating a clinical approach with the best available research findings. One way evidence-based practice has been introduced into care is through **clinical practice guidelines**, which set out appropriate health procedures for specific clinical situations.

Problems remain with clinical practice guidelines. Practitioner adherence with practice guideline recommendations is inconsistent and highly variable (Mor, et al., 2000; Roghmann & Sexton, 1999; Srinivasan & Fisher, 2000; Taylor, Auble, Calhoun, & Mosesso, 1999). Another problem with practice guidelines is that most have been developed to measure physician and primary care provider attitudes, adherence, and practice. Studies of practice guideline use often contain confounding variables. Dykes (2003) suggested sound measures of adherence and impact and methods of controlling for confounding variables be addressed. She also pointed out that questions remain about the most useful format for practice guidelines. Until these are developed, it may be difficult to measure adherence to practice guidelines and determine quality of care.

LEADERSHIP CHALLENGE How can Samantha use this information about practice guidelines to improve the quality of care? Give a rationale for your answer.

Facial Photo Capture

Electronic bar codes and radio-frequency microchips are being used to prevent medical errors and increase the quality of care. Researchers with the MedStar Health network are experimenting with software that can pick human faces out of photo images. Nurses can permanently tie a client's face to the corresponding electronic health record with just one click. The software can associate the right face to any medication order or blood product before it goes into a client. Anyone who approaches a MedStar triage desk is photographed. To help with privacy issues, the system quickly erases images that a nurse does not attach to a medical record (Zwillich, 2007).

LEADERSHIP CHALLENGE How could Samantha use this information to enhance the quality of care? Give a rationale for your answer.

Nursing Home Processes

Health services research findings have demonstrated the critical importance of having RNs on the staff of nursing homes to improve the quality of care (Harrington, 2005).

Most nursing homes show widespread quality-of-care problems, including inadequate assistance with eating (an average of 3 minutes to 7 minutes of assistance per meal); little verbal interactions during mealtime (18% to 25% of the time); false charting; inadequate toileting assistance and turning of residents; residents who are left in bed most of the day; little walking assistance; untreated pain; and untreated depression (Cadogan, Schnelle, Yamamoto-Mitani, Cabrera, & Simmons, 2004; Schnelle, Bates-Jensen, Chu, & Simmons, 2004; Schnelle, Simmons, et al., 2004; Simmons et al., 2004).

A study funded by the Centers for Medicare and Medicaid Services (CMS) found that high staffing levels for short-stay nursing home residents led to fewer rehospitalizations for avoidable diagnoses, including congestive heart failure, electrolyte imbalances, respiratory infections, urinary tract infections, and sepsis (CMS, 2001).

As in other settings, staff turnover rates can affect the quality of care in nursing homes. A study of 1,100 nursing homes in California showed that high turnover is associated with low staffing levels and low wages (Harrington & Swan, 2003).

Other factors that can reduce the quality of care in nursing homes include inadequate education and training and the use of registry personnel (CMS, 2001; Institute of Medicine, 2003; Wunderlich, Sloane, & Davis, 1996). One study found that residents in nursing homes with more LVNs than RNs were at a greater risk for hospitalization (Carter & Porell, 2003). Experts also point to the poor management of nurses and their lack of adequate training to supervise care in nursing homes (Institute of Medicine, 2003; Wunderlich, Sloane, & Davis, 1996).

Not all the problems occurring in nursing homes may be identified because Medicaid uses resource utilization groups. This system is based on a uniform nursing home resident report called the Minimum Data Set, or MDS, that seriously understates certain clinical problems, such as pain and depression (Cadogan et al., 2004; Schnelle, Simmons, Harrington, Cadogan, Garcia, & Bates-Hensen, 2004; Simmons et al., 2001).

Some nursing home residents wonder why nursing homes exist. Corbet (2007) points out that the residents are there because they need temporary or permanent care but that in-home help could provide quality care and save taxpayer money. Since the 1999 Supreme Court decision in *Olmstead v. L.C.*, the law has recognized that disability services should be in the "most integrated setting," yet the distribution of federal money continues to be heavily biased in favor of institutional services. Until that money is redirected, nursing homes may be the only option for many Americans. A resource to share with clients to help them choose a nursing home appears at http://www.aarpmagazine.org.

LEADERSHIP CHALLENGE How can Samantha use this information? Provide a rationale for your answer.

Appropriate Use of Technology

Healthcare settings are in dire need of technology to help nurses manage the tasks and activities that disrupt direct client care. Some activities that could be handled by new technology include reporting on the change of shifts or new client admissions, verifying medication orders, preparing medications, completing charting and other paperwork, following up via telephone on test results or orders, confirming dietary orders, scheduling procedures, transporting clients, housekeeping, ordering and restocking supplies, retrieving critical items needed on the unit, planning discharges, offering education, providing competency training and certification, and communicating with family members, visitors, and multidisciplinary teams (Sipe, Marthinsen, Baker, Harris, & Opperman, 2003).

LEADERSHIP CHALLENGE How could Samantha use this information to improve the quality of care? Give a rationale for your answer.

Discharge Planning

Despite the importance of discharge planning (Collier & Harrington, 2005), several studies have shown faulty discharge planning and case management in hospitals. In one study, discharge planners overrated their adequacy in providing information, and family members and clients believed they had been given little or no information, were not meaningfully involved in the planning process, and were pressured, forced, badgered, or bullied to opt for nursing home placement (Clemens, 1995).

A similar study found caregivers had often been required to make decisions about a nursing home within a short time period. The authors suggested that the use of Web-based resources can help family and caregivers make satisfactory decisions (Travis & McAuley, 1998).

LEADERSHIP CHALLENGE How could Henry use this information at his work site? Give a rationale for your answer.

Results-Driven Rounding

Results-driven rounding allows nurses to spend less time answering call lights, freeing them for other tasks. A growing number of hospitals across the country are involved in following the protocol. Results include less stress for nurses,

more productive shifts, and higher client safety and satisfaction scores. Checking on hospitalized client needs reduces call light use by 18%, falls by 50%, and cases of skin breakdown by 14%.

Initiating hourly rounds for clients is like adding one full-time RN to the staff for a week because nurses' time is not used answering call lights. Clients stop leaning on their call lights because they know a nurse will be there to give them special attention every hour.

Nurses use the three *P*s on their rounds:

1. *Positioning.* Make sure the client is comfortable, and assess for pressure ulcers.
2. *Personal needs.* Schedule trips to the bathroom to avoid falls.
3. *Pain.* Ask clients to describe their pain level on a scale of 0 to 10, and then take action accordingly. (Leighty, 2006)

Providing Support and Helping Clients Navigate the Healthcare System

Nurses are among the most verbal advocates for the quality of care. Mary Macklin, MSN, ARNP, related how staff refused to answer questions, would not let her accompany her friend during procedures or be an overnight guest (even though the Patient Bill of Rights allows it), discussed their weekend plans, and complained about their jobs in front of her (Macklin, 2007).

Another nurse, who asked to have her name withheld, recounted the events of a hospitalization and reported that she was not given a breakfast she could eat; she was not listened to when she told the nurse that the arm being used for blood pressure checks was injured; the nurse would not discuss her medications with her; every time an aide answered her call light and told her that a nurse would be informed, no nurse ever responded; and her discharge instructions had the wrong doses of medication ("Hospital Stay a Nightmare," 2007).

These are only two instances, but they underline some of the problems nurses face if clients are to receive quality care. Although problems do exist, some organizations are working to fix the communication problems like those in the two previous examples.

The responses to a survey completed by parents who experienced the death of a child in a pediatric ICU at Children's Hospital Boston about what helped them most while their children were dying show the way for nurses to offer spiritual comfort to grieving mothers and fathers. Comfort includes being fully present in the moment, listening carefully (even to angry words and affirming what they are feeling, e.g., "You're feeling angry now"), being comfortable with long silences, not providing explanations unless asked for information, offering to help if a parent wants to wash an unconscious child's hair or shave her legs, and noticing cues about when and if to inform the parents of resources (Wilder, 2006).

A study of older women with breast cancer showed that community-based nurse case managers improved quality of care by helping manage coexisting medical conditions, providing support and education, assisting with the activities of daily living, and helping navigate the healthcare system (Jennings-Sanders & Anderson, 2003).

Summary

This chapter focused on evaluating staff performance and ensuring quality and covered such topics as performance appraisals, measuring nursing practice, and measuring quality of care. The next chapter provides information on coaching and mentoring staff.

Key Term Review

- The **caring domain** includes developing trust, understanding, and a healing environment. The **clinical knowledge domain** includes recognizing patterns, anticipating problems, obtaining a timely response from physicians, prioritizing and adjusting strategies, and applying appropriate technology.
- **Clinical narratives** are stories nurses tell in evaluation conferences about their level of expertise.
- **Clinical practice guidelines** set out appropriate health procedures for specific clinical situations.
- The **collaboration domain** includes coordinating resources, supporting colleagues, and encouraging teamwork.
- **Evidence-based practice** integrates a clinical approach with the best available research findings.
- **Performance appraisals** are semiannual or annual evaluations of employee accomplishments and are often tied to rewards.
- **Results-driven rounding** allows nurses to spend less time answering call lights, freeing them for other tasks.

Leadership Development Exercises

- **Leadership Development Exercise 20-1**

  a. Pair off with a colleague.
  b. Flip a coin to see which of you will conduct a performance appraisal of the other, using information in this chapter.
  c. Discuss your findings.
  d. Replay the performance appraisal, using whatever you learned from the first role-play.

- **Leadership Development Exercise 20-2**

Enhance your performance management skills by using Rachman-Moore and Kenett's (2006) performance management simulation.

- **Leadership Development Exercise 20-3**

Analyze nursing situations that can affect quality of care.

  a. Go to a nursing home, and observe for assistance with eating, verbal interactions during mealtimes, toileting assistance and turning of residents, walking assistance, and untreated pain and depression.
  b. Compare your findings with what you read in this chapter.
  c. Share your findings with at least two other colleagues.
  d. Brainstorm a way to share your findings with the public and/or improve the quality of care.
  e. If possible, implement one or more of your ideas.

■ **Leadership Development Exercise 20-4**

a. Brainstorm with a group of at least two other colleagues to develop ideas for technological answers to reducing time nurses spend:

- Reporting on the change of shifts or new client admissions
- Verifying medication orders
- Preparing medications
- Completing charting
- Doing paperwork
- Following up via telephone on orders and test results
- Making dietary orders
- Scheduling procedures
- Transporting clients
- Housekeeping
- Ordering and restocking supplies
- Retrieving critical items
- Planning discharges
- Providing education, competency training, and certification
- Communicating with the interdisciplinary team, family members, and visitors

b. Share your findings with at least two colleagues.
c. Write up your findings.
d. Talk to a technology expert about putting your ideas into action.
e. **Optional:** Publish your findings.

■ **Leadership Development Exercise 20-5**

Work with a group of colleagues to develop information for a Web site related to quality indicators for nursing homes and the nursing home decision. Use http://www.calnhs.org as a template.

■ **Leadership Development Exercise 20-6**

a. Role-play being physically present with a mother whose child has died. Use the suggestions for listening, waiting out silences, and not explaining that are discussed in this chapter.
b. Role-play helping a woman with breast cancer who is having difficulty making an appointment to see her oncologist.

Advanced Leadership Development Exercises

■ **Leadership Development Exercise 20-7**

a. Teach a group of less experienced nurse leaders about some aspect of quality of care.

   b. Obtain feedback.

   c. Write up your results.

■ **Leadership Development Exercise 20-8**

   a. Write a problem statement for some aspect of quality care.

   b. Share your statement with a nurse researcher, and obtain feedback about whether your statement is doable or needs refinement.

   c. Revise your problem statement as needed.

■ **Leadership Development Exercise 20-9**

   a. Design a research study to answer your problem statement.

   b. Obtain feedback on your project from a more experienced nurse researcher.

   c. Revise your project as necessary.

References

Aiken, L. H., Clarke, S. P., & Sloane, D. M. (2002). Hospital staffing, organization, and quality of care: Cross-national findings. *Nursing Outlook, 50*, 187–194.

Blendon, R. J., Schoen, C., & Donelan, K. (2001). Physicians' views on quality of care: A five-country comparison. *Health Affairs, 6*, 233–243.

Cadogan, M. P., Schnelle, J. F., Yamamoto-Mitani, N., Cabrera, G., & Simmons, S. F. (2004). A minimum data set prevalence of pain quality indicator: Is it accurate and does it reflect differences in care processes? *Journal of Gerontology, 59A*, 281–285.

Carter, M. W., & Porell, F. W. (2003). Variations in hospitalization rates among nursing home residents: The role of facility and market attributes. *Gerontologist, 32*, 175–191.

Centers for Medicare and Medicaid Services. (2001). *Report to Congress: Appropriateness of minimum nurse staffing ratios in nursing homes.* Washington, DC: Author.

Clemens, E. (1995). Multiple perceptions of discharge planning in one urban hospital. *Health and Social Work, 20*, 254–261.

Collier, E. J., & Harrington, C. (2005). Discharge planning, nursing home placement, and the Internet. *Nursing Outlook, 53*, 95–103.

Corbet, B. (2007, January/February). Embedded. *AARP,* 79–80, 84, 86–87, 91, 100.

Donelan, K., Blendon, R. J., Schoen, C., Binns, K., Osborn, R., & Davis, K. (2000). The elderly in five nations: The importance of universal coverage. *Health Affairs, 19,* 226–235.

Donelan, K., Blendon, R. J., Schoen, C., Davis, K., & Binns, K. (1999). The cost of health system change: Public discontent in five nations. *Health Affairs, 19,* 206–216.

Dykes, P. C. (2003). Practice guidelines and measurement: State-of-the-science. *Nursing Outlook, 51*, 65–69.

Gross, S. E. (1995). The role of performance appraisal. *Compensation for teams.* New York: American Management Association.

Haag-Heitman, B., & Kramer, A. (1998). Creating a clinical practice development model. *American Journal of Nursing, 98*(8), 39–43.

Harrington, C. (2005). Quality of care in nursing home organizations: Establishing a health services research agenda. *Nursing Outlook, 53*, 300–304.

Harrington, C., & Swan, J. H. (2003). Nurse home staffing, turnover, and case mix. *Medical Care Research Review, 60*, 366–392.

Hospital stay a nightmare [Letter to the Editor]. (2007). *Nursing Spectrum, 17*(7), 4.

Jennings-Sanders, A., & Anderson, E. T. (2003). Older women with breast cancer: Perceptions of the effectiveness of nurse case managers. *Nursing Outlook, 51*, 108–114.

Leighty, J. (2006, December 4). Let there be less light. *Nursing Spectrum (Florida)*, 12–13.

Leighty, J. (2007, May 7). Nursing gets chance to shine on quality care measures. *Nursing Spectrum (Florida)*, 21.

Macklin, M. (2007). Margie, medicine, and memories. *Clinician Reviews, 17*(2), 76.

Mor, V., Laliberte, L. L., Petrisek, A. C., Intrator, I., Wachtel, T., Maddock, P., et al. (2000). Impact of breast cancer treatment guidelines on surgeon practice patterns: Results of a hospital-based intervention. *Surgery, 128*, 847–861.

Rachman-Moore, D., & Kenett, R. S. (2006). The use of simulation to improve the effectiveness of training in performance management. *Journal of Management Education, 30*(3), 455–476.

Roghmann, M. C., & Sexton, M. (1999). Adherence to asthma guidelines in general practice. *Journal of Asthma, 36*, 381–387.

Schnelle, J. F., Bates-Jensen, B., Chu, L., & Simmons, S. F. (2004). Accuracy of nursing home medical record information about care process delivery; implications for staff management and improvement. *Journal of the American Geriatric Society, 52*, 1395–1398.

Schnelle, J. F., Simmons, S. F., Harrington, C., Cadogan, M., Garcia, E., & Bates-Hensen, B. (2004). Relationship of nursing home staffing to quality of care. *Health Services Research, 39*, 225–250.

Simmons, S. F., Cadogan, M. P., Cabrera, G. R., Al-Samarrai, N. R., Jorge, J. S., Levy-Sipe, M., et al. (2001). Using technology to improve patient care. *Nursing Outlook, 51*, S35–S36.

Sipe, M., Marthinsen, J., Baker, J., Harris, J., & Opperman, J. (2003). Using technology to improve patient care. *Nursing Outlook, 51,* S35–S36.

Srinivasan, R., & Fisher, R. S. (2000). Early initiation of post PEG feedings: Do published recommendations affect clinical practice? *Digestive Diseases & Sciences, 45*, 2065–2068.

Taylor, D. M., Auble, T. E., Calhoun, W. J., & Mosesso, V. N., Jr. (1999). Current outpatient management of asthma shows poor compliance with International Consensus Guidelines. *Chest, 116*, 1638–1645.

Travis, S., & McAuley, W. (1998). Searches for a nursing home: Personal and situational factors. *Journal of Applied Gerontology, 17*, 352–371.

Wilder, J. (2006, December 4). Being present in the present: Nurses' presence alone can help bereaved parents. *Nursing Spectrum (Florida)*, 29.

Wunderlich, G., Sloane, F., & Davis, C. (1996). *Nursing staff in hospitals and nursing homes: Is it adequate?* Institute of Medicine. Washington, DC: National Academies Press.

Zwillich, T. (2007, January). Facial photo capture could prevent errors. *Clinical Psychiatry News*, 58.

Resource

Storms, L., Osterweill, D., & Schnelle, J. F. (2004). The minimum data set depression quality indicator: Does it reflect differences in the care process? *Gerontologist, 44*, 554–564.

Coaching and Mentoring

CHAPTER OBJECTIVES

After reading this chapter, answering the leadership challenges, and participating in the leadership development exercises, you will be able to:

- Discuss the difference between coaching and mentoring
- Describe coaching interventions with staff nurses
- Discuss Kramer's reality shock theory and its relationship to coaching and mentoring

Advanced nurses will be able to:

- Teach less skilled nurse leaders about coaching and mentoring
- Develop a problem statement for a research study focused on coaching or mentoring
- Develop a research project for a problem statement focused on coaching or mentoring

Introduction

Nurse leaders have been identified by staff nurses as a crucial link in creating an environment of improved quality of care, safety, performance, and nurse retention. Coaching and mentoring are ways to help staff nurses develop their potential.

As a nurse leader, you may be expected to coach and/or mentor staff nurses, so you will need to know the difference and the process for each. This chapter focuses on coaching and mentoring staff nurses and provides a theory, research findings, and specific steps to take as a coach or mentor.

LEADERSHIP IN ACTION

Alice, a clinical leader, had been observing the staff for several weeks. She noticed that several nurses might be able to benefit from coaching and/or mentoring. She wasn't exactly sure of the difference between the two interventions, so she consulted with a clinical specialist who provided coaching to several nurses on another unit.

LEADERSHIP CHALLENGE What do you think the clinical specialist told Alice about coaching and mentoring?

KEY TERM

Mentoring is an exclusive long-term relationship, with someone other than one's direct supervisor, that is oriented toward nurses who are focused on learning complex thinking and problem-solving skills and want to move forward in nursing administration or advanced clinical education.

KEY TERM

Coaching gives staff nurses the sense of being valued, heard, and encouraged as they develop clinical, teamwork, and leadership skills and prepare to take on increased responsibility.

Coaching versus Mentoring

Mentoring is an exclusive long-term relationship oriented toward nurses who are focused on moving forward in nursing administration or advanced clinical education. Mentoring focuses less on tasks and more on learning more complex ways of thinking and problem solving. In most cases, the mentor is not the nurse's immediate supervisor (Yoder, 2007).

Coaching is geared to all nursing staff and focuses on enhancing immediate professional development. Coaching is an ongoing two-way process in which an immediate supervisor or manager shares knowledge and experience to help the staff nurse achieve agreed-upon goals (Yoder, 2007).

Coaching can have more wide-ranging effects for a team or organization because it affects more nurses. Coaching is also an essential link to ongoing development because the employee is guided in a positive, encouraging environment, which is more apt to lead to growth in the staff nurse and more engagement with the manager or leader (Yoder, 2007). The overall goal of coaching is to achieve measurable change or improved development in staff nurses' skill development, teamwork, leadership, and preparation for increased responsibility. Because the coach takes the time to listen and to provide support and helpful information, staff nurses start to feel valued and heard. Staff will also be more loyal to a leader who takes the time to help them grow (Hill, 2007).

LEADERSHIP IN ACTION

Alice overheard Delilah complaining that no one on the team ever helps her even though she's always helping them. Alice wasn't sure whether to intercede or wait for Delilah to bring up her problem later.

LEADERSHIP CHALLENGE What would you tell Alice? Give a rationale for your answer.

The Teachable Moment

Teachable moments are times when a nurse leader recognizes that employees are open to receiving developmental feedback (Yoder, 2007). Teachable situations include when staff nurses ask for feedback, express puzzlement or concern about an outcome, ask directly or indirectly for information about a new position, experience a poor job fit, or want to talk about a promotion.

It is not necessary to wait for a teachable moment. Clinical nursing specialists (CNSs) often schedule individual 10-minute coaching sessions with each nurse on a unit. To initiate a plan, each staff nurse is asked to identify areas that need improvement. Later sessions focus on priorities for the unit, including evidence-based practice (Ervin, 2005).

To create an environment for self-learning, staff nurses are asked to set aside a half hour each week to scan current journals, or their nurse leader can provide study abstracts for them based on client assignments (Ervin, 2005).

Because not all information in journals is accurate, current, or meant to be translated into practice, CNSs encourage staff nurses to discuss and debate which studies provide the best evidence. CNSs can also conduct unit-level in-service programs that use case studies and other activities that encourage staff nurses to actively analyze and synthesize literature. CNSs may conduct group coaching, using listening exercises and assertiveness training, and writing workshops and may provide critiques of written work to assist staff nurses in developing their writing skills (Ervin, 2005).

KEY TERM

Teachable moments are times when a nurse leader recognizes that employees are open to receiving developmental feedback.

LEADERSHIP TIP

Clinical coaching covers knowledge of current literature and effective communication skills, evidence-based procedures, protocols, and clinical guidelines.

Coaching Behaviors

Coaching follows a predictable process:

- *Observing.* Observing a staff nurse provides information about how coaching may be helpful. Observe behavior both informally (e.g., during a report or a staff meeting) and formally (e.g., while the nurse is performing a nursing procedure). While observing, ask yourself, "What is the nurse doing or not doing effectively? What impact does his or her action have on team, organizational, or individual goals?" If you're unsure of how to answer those questions, observe the nurse some more.

- *Examining coach motives.* When coaching someone you believe might not be performing effectively, ask yourself, "Am I expecting too much? Is my anger or frustration with this person interfering with my observation and analysis? Have I made several attempts to listen actively to this person? Have I remembered to give this person positive feedback often enough so I'm not contributing to a problem behavior or attitude? Do I model excellent listening skills?" Become aware of your own development needs by doing a reality check with a trusted peer. It will help you become a better leader and coach (Hill, 2007).

- *Creating a discussion plan for the coaching session.* Think about what you will discuss, including the following questions: What is the purpose of the session? What outcomes do I desire? What potential difficulties might arise, and how would I handle them? Share your plan with the nurse you're coaching, and ask for input and other suggestions. Treat coaching as a partnership (Hill, 2007).

- *Initiating.* Keep the tone positive and focused on personal development. Emphasize your wish to be helpful. Discuss your observations with the nurse (e.g., "This is what I observed. If I were in that team member's shoes, I might think . . ."). Be sure to describe the behavior and its impact in a truthful and straightforward way that is both calm and supportive. Make good eye contact, listen first and evaluate later, avoid interrupting the other person except to ask questions for clarification, repeat back to the person what you heard, and ask, "Here's what I heard; is it correct?" or "How might you handle that differently in the future?" You can also suggest, "Let's role-play that and see what we can come up with." Avoid planning your responses in advance. Use open-ended questions to explore alternatives ("What would happen if . . . ?"), to uncover attitudes or needs ("How do you evaluate your progress to date?"), and to establish priorities ("What do you think are the major issues?" or "What can I help you with?"). Include a timetable and an agreed-upon measure of success (Hill, 2007).

- *Providing and eliciting feedback.* Present your ideas and advice in a clear and balanced way. Define or express the desired behavior in specifics (e.g., "I'm going to work with you to help reduce medication errors [improve your charting, set limits with other staff, work together as a team, etc.]"). Use initiating comments such as ("You sound interested in that; I'd like to suggest you give an in-service program on that topic") or ("I saw a video on that topic; I'll get the information for you to watch"). Make the observations behind your suggestions explicit ("I observed you interrupting Jerry three times during our last staff meeting"; "The support you gave Mrs. Johnson was effective"). Encourage the nurse you're coaching to provide feedback ("What did I do that made you think that?" "How were my suggestions helpful to you?" or "Give me an example of that") (Hill, 2007; Yodor, 2007).

- *Follow-up meeting.* Be sure to meet at specific checkpoints to evaluate progress. Ask what is going well and what requires more assistance. Share your observations, emphasizing progress toward the goals; identify possible modifications in the plan; and obtain feedback on what was helpful in the coaching session (Hill, 2007; Tudor, 2007).

LEADERSHIP CHALLENGE How can Alice use this information to coach her staff? Give a rationale for your answers.

Studies Demonstrating the Positive Effects of Coaching

Two studies set in business settings demonstrated positive individual and organizational outcomes because of coaching (Ellinger, 1999; Patton, 2001). Evidence that coaching can improve employee and customer satisfaction and retention and the success and financial performance of the organization has also been presented (Kepler & Morgan, 2005). Coaching has been related to increased individual and team performance and to enhanced employee autonomy and organizational performance (Savage, 2001). Research completed in Magnet hospitals supports the idea of coaching by showing that ongoing organizational support improves quality of nursing care, job satisfaction, and retention (Kramer & Schmalenberg, 2004).

Kramer's Reality Shock Theory

In her book *Reality Shock: Why Nurses Leave Nursing*, Marlene Kramer (1974) coined the phrase "**reality shock**" to explain why new nursing graduates leave the profession. She studied the way new graduates adapted to the professional role after they discovered the difference between nursing school ideals and the reality of working as a nurse.

> **KEY TERM**
>
> **Reality shock** is the conflict new graduates face when presented with the differences between nursing school ideals and the realities of professional nursing.

She identified four phases that all new graduates experience as they try to adapt to being a professional nurse:

1. *The honeymoon phase.* New graduates are excited, idealistic, and enthusiastic about being nurses.
2. *The shock phase.* With the realization that nursing is not what they expected, new graduates experience anger, frustration, disappointment, and negativism, and they may show signs of depression and fatigue.
3. *The recovery phase.* New graduates begin to realize there may be more than one perspective on the nursing profession, and their sense of humor and enthusiasm for nursing may return.
4. *The resolution phase.* New graduates may adapt to their current job, seek employment elsewhere, quit nursing, go back to school, develop full-fledged burnout, or integrate the two conflicting value systems of school and work into a successful framework for practice.

LEADERSHIP CHALLENGE What advice would you give nurse coaches to help new nurses bypass reality shock?

Mentor Programs

Mentor programs can help reduce the chance of reality shock. Developing a relationship with an experienced nurse mentor who is not evaluating performance can help new nursing graduates glimpse a broader perspective on what it means to be a nurse and can offer a venue for expressing feelings, venting frustration, and exploring career options (Pesut, 2004).

It's not just new nurses who need mentoring: mentoring relationships offer support and professional development for nurses at all levels of practice (Kanaskie, 2006). But different generations may require different types of coaching and mentoring.

Coaching and Mentoring Different Generations

Different generations have had unique experiences that can affect their coaching and mentoring needs and preferences. Veteran nurses (born 1925–1945) may be more comfortable with one-on-one coaching and mentoring. They value seniority and experience in a coach and may want handwritten notes, plaques, and pictures of them with the chief nursing officer to recognize their achievements (Duchscher & Cowin, 2004; Weston, 2001).

Baby boomer nurses (born 1946–1964) enjoy collegiality and participation and prefer being coached by peers. They like to reach consensus. Boomers are optimistic and tend to think big. They like to feel empowered in the work setting and to be asked for their feedback. Baby boomers value lifelong learning and are interested in participating in situations that improve their performance. They are motivated by public recognition for jobs well done and perks, such as employee parking spaces, newsletter recognition, and professional award nominations (Duchscher & Cowin, 2004; Halfer, 2004; Siela, 2006; Weston, 2001).

Generation X staff (born 1965–1980) prefer opportunities to demonstrate their expertise when learning and prefer not to be micromanaged or to attend meetings. They want to see rapid progress toward their goals and think that career advancement and recognition ought to be based on merit. Xers are flexible and informal. Give them freedom in setting their schedules, and offer them the latest tech tools. They should be valued for their innovative ideas and creative approaches to unit issues. They are often instrumental in designing new approaches to nursing care delivery. When selecting a coach or mentor, avoid putting an Xer and boomer together; they are apt to clash. When rewarded, Xers value paid time off, cash awards, or a part in cutting-edge projects (Karp, Fuller, & Sirias, 2002; Sherman, 2006; Siela, 2006).

The Millennial generation (born 1981–2000), sometimes called Nexters or Generation Y, accepts multiculturalism, terrorism, violence, drugs, and cell phones as a way of life. They were raised by parents who nurtured and structured their lives and expect more coaching and mentoring than any other generation. Specifically, they want structure, guidance, and extensive orientation, coaching, and mentoring. They value internships and formalized clinical coaching and mentoring (Halfer, 2004), but they may turn down a last-minute request to cover an extra shift. Millennials like quick personal feedback and flexible scheduling. They also enjoy teamwork and team meetings as a forum for communication, and they do not appreciate reading policies and procedures. E-mails and chat rooms are good ways to provide coaching and mentoring to them. Ensure that coaches and mentors learn about the Millennials' goals and are able to provide close support. If Millennials' needs are not met, expect high staff turnover (Clausing, Kurtz, Prendeville, & Walt, 2003; Howe & Strauss, 2000; Siela, 2006).

A nurse is not a nurse is not a nurse. All nurses have individual talents. Instead of trying to fix a nurse's weaknesses, focus on helping individuals cultivate their talents and empower them to be who they have the potential to become. This may require you to (1) overcome your own fears about nurturing nurses who may become better nursing professionals than you are and (2) to move away from training nurses to obey rules and follow instructions so that their creativity and innovation can thrive.

Encourage nurses to set challenging goals and strive for what they believe in. To do that, you must foster a climate of

LEADERSHIP TIP

Whether coaching or mentoring, it is important to recognize talent. Nurses with ideas and imagination must be nourished.

trust, one that allows nurses to try out their talents and skills and provides them with coaching and mentorship opportunities that broaden their perspectives and abilities (Tan, 2006).

Summary

This chapter focused on coaching and mentoring. It provided information about the difference between coaching and mentoring, teachable moments, coaching behaviors, studies demonstrating the positive effects of coaching, Kramer's reality shock theory, and mentoring programs. The next chapter focuses on workplace violence.

Key Term Review

- **Coaching** gives staff nurses the sense of being valued, heard, and encouraged as they develop clinical, teamwork, and leadership skills and prepare to take on increased responsibility.
- **Mentoring** is an exclusive long-term relationship, with someone other than one's direct supervisor, that is oriented toward nurses who are focused on learning complex thinking and problem-solving skills and want to move forward in nursing administration or advanced clinical education.
- **Reality shock** is the conflict new graduates face when presented with the differences between nursing school ideals and the realities of professional nursing.
- **Teachable moments** are times when a nurse leader recognizes that employees are open to receiving developmental feedback.

Leadership Development Exercises

- **Leadership Development Exercise 21-1**

Find a nursing coach, and speak together in person, on the phone, or via e-mail or fax.

  a. Ask how that person coaches nurses, find out whether he or she uses teachable moments or some other method, and obtain any other information about coaching you can.
  b. Write up your findings (take notes during the interview if possible, unless you fax or e-mail).
  c. Share your findings with at least two other colleagues.

- **Leadership Development Exercise 21-2**

  a. Identify a mentor, and interview him or her in person, on the phone, or via e-mail or fax.
  b. Find out what specific things the mentor does to help other nurses.
  c. Ask him or her for examples of how mentorship helps nurses.
  d. Write up your findings.
  e. Share your findings with at least two other colleagues.

- **Leadership Development Exercise 21-3**

Obtain permission to shadow a nurse for at least 3 hours, and if possible, provide feedback to that person.

  a. Answer as many questions as you can from the section in this chapter entitled "Coaching Behaviors."
  b. What did you observe?

   c. What else did you find out about coaching?

   d. What feedback would you, or did you, give the person you shadowed?

■ **Leadership Development Exercise 21-4**

Talk to several nurses in each of Kramer's reality shock stages.

   a. How did you know which stage each was in?

   b. Share your findings with at least two other colleagues.

■ **Leadership Development Exercise 21-5**

Speak with a nurse from each of the different generations mentioned in this chapter.

   a. Using the categories mentioned in this chapter, compose a questionnaire.

   b. Using the specific questions on your questionnaire, ask your participants how they prefer to be coached or mentored.

   c. Tally your findings.

   d. Explain any discrepancies from the behaviors mentioned for each generation in this chapter.

   e. Share your findings with at least two colleagues.

   f. **Optional:** Speak to four nurses, and see whether you can identify which generation they belong to from their answers.

Advanced Leadership Development Exercises

■ **Leadership Development Exercise 21-6**

   a. Provide a brief in-service or in-class teaching session on some aspect of coaching or mentoring.

   b. Obtain feedback from your learners.

   c. Share your findings with at least two colleagues.

■ **Leadership Development Exercise 21-7**

   a. Develop a problem statement suitable to test some aspect of coaching or mentoring.

   b. Share your problem statement with at least one more experienced nurse researcher, and obtain feedback on whether your statement is feasible.

   c. Revise your problem statement as needed.

■ **Leadership Development Exercise 21-8**

   a. Develop a research project to test your problem statement.

b. Consult with a more seasoned nurse researcher about your research project.
c. Revise your project.
d. Share your findings with at least two colleagues.

References

Clausing, S. L., Kurtz, D. L., Prendeville, J., & Walt, J. L. (2003). Generational diversity: The Nexters. *AORN Journal, 78*(3), 373–379.

Duchscher, J. E., & Cowin, L. (2004). Multigenerational nurses in the workplace. *Journal of Nursing Administration, 34*(11), 493–501.

Ellinger, A. D. (1999). Antecedents and consequences of coaching behavior. *Performance Improvement Quarterly, 12*(4), 45–70.

Ervin, N. (2005). Clinical coaching: A strategy for enhancing evidence-based nursing practice. *Clinical Nurse Specialist, 19*(6), 296–301.

Halfer, D. (2004, April 21). *Developing a multigenerational workforce. Paper presented at the annual meeting of the American Organization of Nurse Executives*, Phoenix, AZ.

Hill, L. A. (2007). *Coaching.* Retrieved November 27, 2007, from http://www.harvardman agementor.com/demo/plusdemo/coach/index.htm

Howe, N., & Strauss, W. (2000). *Millennials rising: The next great generation.* New York: Vintage.

Kanaskie, M. L. (2006). Mentoring: A staff retention tool. *Critical Care Nursing Quarterly, 29*(3), 248–252.

Karp, H., Fuller, C., & Sirias, D. (2002). *Bridging the boomer-Xer gap.* Palo Alto, CA: Davies-Black.

Kepler, A. D., & Morgan, F. T. (2005). The leader as coach. In H. Morgan, P. Harkins, & M. Goldsmith (Eds.), *The art and practice of leadership: Coaching.* Hoboken, NJ: John Wiley.

Kramer, M. (1974). *Reality shock: Why nurses leave nursing.* New York: C. V. Mosby.

Kramer, M., & Schmalenberg, C. (2004). Magnet hospitals: What makes nurses stay? *Nursing 2004, 34*(6), 50–54.

Patton, C. (2001). Rating the returns. *Human Resources Executive, 15*(5), 40–43.

Pesut, D. J. (2004). *The reality shock of nursing.* Retrieved June 26, 2007, from http://www .nursingsociety.org/youbelonghere/YBH_V3_8.html

Savage, C. M. (2001). Executive coaching: Professional self-care for nursing. *Nursing Economics, 19*(4), 178–182.

Sherman, R. O. (2006). Leading a multigenerational nursing workforce: Issues, challenges and strategies. *Online Journal of Issues in Nursing, 11*(2). Retrieved March 27, 2007, from http://www.medscape.com/viewarticle/536480

Siela, D. (2006, December). Managing the multigenerational nursing staff. *American Nurse Today*, 47–49.

Tan, P. (2006). Nurturing nursing leadership: Beyond the horizon. *Singapore Nursing Journal, 33*(1), 33–38.

Weston, M. (2001). Coaching generations in the workplace. *Nursing Administration Quarterly, 25*(2), 11–21.

Yoder, L. H. (2007, May 7). Coaching makes nurses' careers grow. *Nursing Spectrum (Florida)*, 16–18.

Reducing Workplace Violence

CHAPTER OBJECTIVES

After reading this chapter, answering the leadership challenges, and participating in the leadership development exercises, you will be able to:

- Discuss the statistics on workplace violence
- Describe environmental designs that can reduce workplace violence
- Analyze administrative controls to reduce workplace violence
- Discuss how to respond to an immediate threat of workplace violence
- Describe suggested ways to deal with the consequences of workplace violence
- Discuss measures nurses can use and teach staff to use to reduce workplace violence

Advanced nurses will be able to:

- Teach less advanced nurse leaders about workplace violence
- Design a problem statement focused on workplace violence
- Prepare a research project focused on some aspect of workplace violence

Introduction

Physical violence often starts when individuals do not have the words to express their negative emotions. They must learn how to identify and give name to their feelings and learn to listen.

A careful analysis of violent behavior reveals that violent episodes are often the culmination of long-standing identifiable problems, conflicts, disputes, and failures. When materialism reigns, product is more important than people, distancing individuals from their feelings. To reduce workplace violence, policies must be based on employee-employer collaboration and communication, or they will result in scapegoating, denial, and even violence (Braverman, 1999).

LEADERSHIP IN ACTION

Wanda, a nurse leader, had noticed staff arguing and drugs missing since the board of directors of the hospital had voted to downsize and restructure. Wanda wasn't sure what to do about her observations, but she did find out that the hospital had no violence prevention program.

LEADERSHIP CHALLENGE What would you tell Wanda to do? Give a rationale for your answer.

Facts and Statistics about Violence

The causes and nature of violence are complex, but social and environmental factors play major roles. Every day in the United States, three children die of abuse and neglect. An estimated 3 million to 4 million women are abused by their partners annually (Capaldo & Lindner, 1999). And 25% to 40% of all women in the United States have been physically assaulted by a spouse or male partner (Abner, 1995), and battering or abuse during pregnancy is a widespread problem (Campbell, 1998, 1999).

Two out of every five American households with children contain guns, and 15% of those guns are either loaded or unlocked. It's not surprising that 15 children are killed with guns in this country every day. Only 29% of parents with guns in their house believe that the most important message about gun safety is that "guns kept in the home kill family members more often than they kill in self-defense" (Sutherland, 1999).

Witnessing a violent event can lead to trauma and future violence. Witnessing violence can create aggression and anxiety disorders (e.g., acute and posttraumatic stress) and disrupt the ability to develop empathy for others (Osofsky, 1995). In one study of a major city, up to 90% of elementary school children witnessed violence, and 33% witnessed a homicide (Groves, Zuckerman, Maran, & Cohen, 1993).

Between 1993 and 1999, 429,100 nurses were victims of violent crimes in the workplace annually, according to the Bureau of Justice Statistics (2001). The most prominent incidents are deaths, stabbings, and shootings, but nurses are easy targets for clients who hit, shove, kick, spit, and bite. Because of their high visibility, nurses are also the most likely target of screaming, threatening, and verbally abusive relatives (Hemmila, 2003).

A national survey of registered nurses sponsored by *NurseWeek* and the American Organization of Nurse Executives found that 28% of the nurses who responded had experienced episodes of violence in the workplace within the past year (Hemmila, 2003).

Another survey of emergency room nurses found that 56 had experienced violence in the previous year but that 29% did not report it. Only 2 of the 55 nurses said they felt safe all the time at work, and 73% said being assaulted is part of the job (Hemmila, 2003).

The fact that such a large percentage of nurses believed being assaulted is part of the job demonstrates the depth of the problem. Preventing violence should be a unit's number one goal. Designing safer work settings is a prime example of how to do that.

LEADERSHIP CHALLENGE How could Wanda use this information to show the need for a violence prevention program?

Physical Design Strategies

To protect against violence in the workplace, more hospitals are using physical barriers, electronic surveillance, security guards and metal detectors, doors with access cards, two-way mirrors, panic-bar doors locked from the outside only, and trouble lights or geographic location devices; they are also shortening visiting hours (Hemmila, 2003; National Institute for Occupational Safety [NIOSH], 1996).

Physical separating workers from clients through the use of bullet-resistant barriers or enclosures has been proposed for hospital emergency departments. The height and depth of counters and whether they are bulletproof are also important considerations. Leaders must weigh the safety factor versus the frustration such measures cause for workers and clients (NIOSH, 1996).

Visibility and lighting are important environmental design considerations. Making high-risk areas visible to more people and installing good external lighting can decrease the risk of workplace assaults (NIOSH, 1996).

Access to and egress from the workplace are also important. The number of entrances and exits, the ease with which nonemployees can gain access to work areas because doors are unlocked, and the number of areas where potential attackers can hide are issues to consider (NIOSH, 1996).

LEADERSHIP CHALLENGE Wanda has asked to start a violence prevention committee. What should she suggest in the way of environmental design to the other members?

LEADERSHIP TIP

To prevent violence, sources of stress and strain must be identified first.

Administrative Controls

Causes of workplace violence range from an accident that kills or maims, to an episode or pattern of abuse or harassment, to continuing stress from organizational restructuring. Nurse leaders who are prepared for crisis know that stress directly affects their employees and clients and will be alert to the following danger signals:

- Conflicts occur between employees, or between employees and clients, and include fights, threats, harassment, or the breakdown in work group and nurse-client functioning.
- An increasing diversity in the workforce results in discrimination and sexual harassment claims.
- Downsizing and restructuring occur in a climate of disrespect without expressions of positive gratefulness for employee contributions.
- Drug and alcohol abuse and even domestic violence occur in the workplace.
- Unstable and problematic employee and employer behavior is on the rise.
- Clients or staff are taking antidepressants. (Braverman, 1999; Healy, Herxheimer & Menkes, 2006)

LEADERSHIP CHALLENGE Which of these factors should Wanda pursue first? Give a rationale for your answer.

Increasing the number of staff on duty may be an appropriate first step, as may meeting with small groups in a respectful and encouraging way. The use of security guards or receptionists to screen persons entering the workplace and controlling access to actual work areas has also been suggested by security experts (NIOSH, 1996).

Policies and procedures for assessing and reporting threats and violent incidents must be in place. Such policies should indicate a zero tolerance of workplace violence and provide mechanisms for reporting and handling incidents. Nurses must report violent incidents so the information can allow employers to assess whether prevention strategies are appropriate and effective. Without this information, safety needs will not be addressed. These policies should also include guidance on how to recognize the potential for violence, methods for defusing or de-escalating potentially violent situations, and instruction about the use of security devices and protective equipment. Detailed procedures for obtaining health care and psychological support following violent incidents should also be available (NIOSH, 1996).

A **threat assessment team** must be developed to receive reports of threats and violent incidents. This team should include representatives from human resources, security, employee assistance, unions, workers, management, and perhaps the legal and public relations departments. The mission of this team is to assess threats of violence, to determine how specific a threat is and whether the person threatening the worker has the means to carry out the threat, and to determine the steps needed to prevent the threat from being carried out. This team should also review violent incident reports periodically to identify ways that similar incidents can be prevented in the future. When violence or the threat of violence

> **KEY TERM**
>
> A **threat assessment team** assesses threats of violence, determines how specific a threat is and whether the person threatening the worker has the means for carrying out the threat, determines the steps needed to prevent the threat from being carried out, and reviews violent incident reports periodically to identify ways that similar incidents can be prevented in the future.

occurs between coworkers, firing the perpetrator may or may not reduce the risk for future violence. Retaining control over the perpetrator and requiring counseling may be more appropriate. Whatever is decided, the violence prevention policy should explicitly state the consequences of making threats or committing acts of violence in the workplace and should be available to all employees.

A **violence prevention policy** must state:

- Procedures and responsibilities to be taken in the event of a violent incident
- How the response team is to be assembled and who is responsible for the victims' immediate care
- How to carry out stress debriefing sessions with victims, their coworkers, and perhaps the families of victims and coworkers

> **KEY TERM**
>
> A **violence prevention policy** states procedures and responsibilities to be taken in the event of a violent incident, how the response team is to be assembled, who is responsible for the victims' immediate care, and how to carry out stress debriefing sessions.

Employee assistance programs, human resource professionals, and local mental health and emergency service personnel can provide assistance in developing these strategies (NIOSH, 1996).

Other measures to prevent workplace violence include an analysis of:

- *Relationships in the work setting.* How do workers treat each other? How are they treated by their supervisors and others? Are security and respect promoted?

- *How standards are enforced.* Violence policy should be prominently posted and distributed to staff, identifying inappropriate or abusive behavior, with a zero-tolerance statement. What disciplinary action will be taken if staff show violent behavior? How consistently, impartially, and fairly are the standards enforced?
- *How employee grievances are handled.* Are employee grievances acted on quickly and responsibly and not allowed to escalate? Are human resource and employee assistance personnel or a mental health clinical nurse specialist available for consultation to defuse dangerous situations? Are employees encouraged to seek assistance when needed?
- *How staff is hired.* Do hiring procedures need to be overhauled to pay attention to applicants' past history of violence? Do group screenings and thorough background checks need to be done for signs of hostility, anger tendencies, and problems with conduct? Are there reports of argumentative behavior or multiple transfers and terminations? Should personality tests be used as screening tools?
- *Supervisory and nurse leader training.* Do supervisors and nurse leaders receive special training to identify volatile employees (i.e., those who have temper outbursts, make threats, or are inappropriately sensitive and over-react to criticism) and in using fair and consistent discipline?
- *Violence aftermath counseling.* Is aftermath debriefing instituted within 12 hours following the incident to minimize posttraumatic stress disorder? (Rosch, 1994)

For violence prevention materials, go to http://www.crisisprevention.com/ store/pamphlets.

LEADERSHIP CHALLENGE How can Wanda use this prevention analysis on her unit?

Responding to the Immediate Threat of Workplace Violence

All legal, human resource, employee assistance, community mental health, and law enforcement resources should be used to develop a response to any situation that poses an immediate threat of workplace violence. The risk of injury must be minimized. Threats that refer to a specific time or place may require you to shift workplace procedures and time frames. For example, if a client or employee has leveled a threat such as "I know where you park and what time you get off work!" it may be advisable to change or even stagger departure times.

Training Sessions

Training sessions that teach specific defense strategies must also be available. Some topics to include are:

- How to approach an employee or client suspected of violent or self-destructive behavior
- How to conduct a face-to-face investigation and gather all related information (including asking for permission to talk to a client's past treatment sources)
- How to inform the employee or client that agency policy requires a danger-of-violence assessment and that results will be shared with him or her and with the appropriate human resource, medical, nursing, and mental health representatives
- How to establish a nonpunitive violence education, assessment, or counseling situation that the client/employee manages and finances

Threat-of-Violence Assessment

The **threat-of-violence assessment** includes a process for gathering information and making appropriate decisions. An assessment proceeds step-by-step and involves determining the risk, establishing a time-out period, and engaging the at-risk client or employee as an active, willing participant in the process. Box 22-1 can be used to complete the assessment and decision-making process once an at-risk individual has been identified.

> **KEY TERM**
>
> The **threat-of-violence assessment** includes a process for gathering information and making appropriate decisions.

LEADERSHIP CHALLENGE Should Wanda develop her own threat-of-violence assessment, or should she and her committee develop a customized form? Give a rationale for your answer.

Dealing with the Consequences of Workplace Violence

When someone is injured, it is important to report the incident and document everything right away before details are forgotten. Assault should not be considered part of any job. Nurses must demand protection and better training so they can defend themselves.

Once an attack is reported, hospitals and other organizations should offer follow-up support with debriefing sessions as well as the vigorous pursuit of criminal prosecution.

BOX 22-1   THREAT-OF-VIOLENCE ASSESSMENT AND DECISION MAKING

- Determination of risk
  - Has a weapon been displayed?
  - Has a clear intent or plan been expressed?
  - Does the individual have the means to carry out the plan?
  - How imminent is the threat?

- Involvement of employee or client in the assessment plan
  - If an employee is involved, defer decisions, and put that person on leave with pay.
  - Ask the individual to be an active, willing participant and to meet with the nurse leader and a human resource representative or mental health specialist.
  - Explain that no decision will be made until the conclusion of fact finding.

  - Explain the assessment process.
  - Examine multiple sources of information: the employee's/client's words, other employees or family members with relevant information, medical records, personnel records (but obtain the employee's consent first).
  - Questions to be answered include the following: Where is the record of discipline or client history for past problems? Where is the employee documentation of performance or claims for medical disability? What is the history of changes, morale/emotional issues, or complaints? What is known about what else may be going on in the client's or employee's life?

When clients come in who have been using alcohol or drugs or who have been involved in any kind of resistance with police, they should be put into point restraints, according to Mary Alexander, MSN, RN, director of emergency services at Gnaden Huetten (Hemmila, 2003).

Not everyone may agree with this evaluation. Nurses must tune in to clients who might act out. Someone who is being uncooperative and uses threatening body language should be approached with caution. Nurses often go it alone. They must learn to call for assistance if they cannot calm a client (Hemmila, 2003).

Physical Defense Methods

Many hospitals now require staff members to attend violence management training to learn about potentially dangerous situations and how to defend themselves. A training film may have saved Lori Cline, MNSc, RN, from serious injury. When she leaned over an Alzheimer's client, the women sat up and put her hands around Cline's neck and started to choke her. The nurse remembered how to release herself, something she had seen in a training film. She slipped both of her hands between the client's hands and applied pressure on the inside of the attacker's wrists, giving her leverage to break the hold and call for help. Cline believes hospitals are not doing enough to keep staff safe and blames staffing shortages for increasing nurses' risks (Hemmila, 2003).

Anger Control Skills

Violence is the acting out of anger. Learning communication skills can help reduce the tendency to act out anger. Rules that you should learn and practice include:

- *Taking a time-out whenever you feel yourself getting angry.* Make a contract with yourself to take a time-out. Simply walking away when you're angry will not work unless you clearly communicate with the other person. For example, say, "I'm going to leave before I hurt someone or break something. I will return when I can talk without losing my temper."
- *Practicing prevention by learning to relax.* Listening to relaxation tapes and learning relaxation skills will help your reduce body tension and the tendency to get angry. Some words you can use are "I am not going to let this upset me" and "I can stay in control and keep relaxed."
- *Quitting trying to control other people.* You can let go of an idea and not argue. Some ideas for loosening control include forgetting about trying to make everyone agree; learning to say what you have to say once and only once; realizing that difference is good; making requests or suggestions, not demands and threats; never asking yes-or-no questions unless you can accept the answer; learning to live with other people's choices; and being grateful when you get what you want and being polite even when you don't.
- *Rewarding people when they do what you want.* Examples include praising them, giving them food, letting them use something you have, doing something for them, being understanding, or just listening.
- *Speaking softly without cursing or threatening.*
- *Taking responsibility for everything you say and do.* You can stop saying, "You make me angry" and start saying, "I make myself angry." You can stop giving people the silent treatment and let them in on what you think and feel so you can solve the problems that bother you.
- *Telling others what bothers you in a direct, specific, and polite way.* For example, you can say, "I'm angry that I'm being asked to work overtime again when I'm exhausted and need to get home to my family; please set up a schedule so this kind of thing doesn't happen again."
- *Using "I" statements.* Voice a specific behavior that bothers you ("I want to be listened to when I say I have pain"); report the feeling you're experiencing ("I feel angry when I'm not listened to"); or request a change in behavior ("Please listen to me in the future when I say I'm in pain").
- *Challenging irrational thoughts that keep you angry.* You can avoid "awfulizing" by refusing to turn disappointments into disasters and by asking, "If this were the last moment of my life, would this really matter?" or saying, "Compared to the worst thing that's ever happened to me, this isn't that bad." You can also:

- Realize that the world is neither good or bad, that it just is
- Accept that despite your background, you're responsible for how you behave
- Refuse to make excuses and realize that you can and will control your anger
- Vow to avoid blaming past experiences for your current anger
- Understand that just because somebody makes a request doesn't mean they're bossing you around, that you can say no if you want to
- Challenge your ideas that make you angry because you're in charge of what you think

- *Preventing resentment.* Measures to prevent resentment include sticking to the issue and not bringing in old hurts, asking yourself what the problem is and figuring out what to do to fix it, getting help when you need it, and taking responsibility for your own happiness.
- *Learning to forgive for the sake of your own health, not someone else's.* Make a list of people you need to forgive (including yourself), and start doing it. Write down the reasons you need to forgive, remembering how forgiving those people will help you and how your hatred is hurting you. List the angry thoughts you have most often and the things you do because of your hate (making late-night calls and hanging up, starting rumors, putting sugar in others' gas tank, threatening them, hitting them, avoiding them, etc.). Promise to stop hateful thoughts and actions, and begin to do it with the first person on your list. Write down two or three good things about each person you resent, pray for them, or think of one nice thing that could happen to them. (Potter-Efron, 1994)

LEADERSHIP CHALLENGE How could Wanda use this information with her staff? Give a rationale for your answer.

Research Questions on Workplace Violence

Although research about workplace violence is accumulating, a number of questions remain:

- What are the specific tasks and environments that place workers at greatest risk?
- What factors influence the lethality of violent incidents?
- What are the relationships of workplace assault victims to offenders?
- Are there identifiable precipitating events?

- What safety measures might reduce violence?
- How do victims' actions influence the outcome of attacks?
- Which prevention strategies are most effective?

Summary

This chapter presented information on reducing workplace violence and included violence facts and statistics, physical design strategies, administrative controls, responding to the immediate threat of workplace violence, training sessions, threat-of-violence assessment, dealing with the consequences of violence, physical defense methods, anger control skills, and research questions on workplace violence. The final chapter deals with planning succession.

Key Term Review

■ A **threat assessment team** assesses threats of violence, determines how specific a threat is and whether the person threatening the worker has the means for carrying out the threat, determines the steps needed to prevent the threat from being carried out, and reviews violent incident reports periodically to identify ways that similar incidents can be prevented in the future.

■ The **threat-of-violence assessment** includes a process for gathering information and making appropriate decisions.

■ A **violence prevention policy** states procedures and responsibilities to be taken in the event of a violent incident, how the response team is to be assembled, who is responsible for the victims' immediate care, and how to carry out stress debriefing sessions.

Leadership Development Exercises

■ **Leadership Development Exercise 22-1**

   a. Compare the violence statistics in your hospital or organization with the statistics discussed in this chapter. How does your institution compare?
   b. If you're unable to obtain statistics, interview a nurse leader about violence in your institution or another one.
   c. Share your findings with at least two colleagues.

■ **Leadership Development Exercise 22-2**

Describe any environmental changes your institution has made to reduce violence. If no changes have been made or some are lacking, develop a plan for the ideal violence prevention unit.

■ **Leadership Development Exercise 22-3**

Analyze administrative controls to reduce workplace violence in your institution. If many are missing, devise the controls needed to reduce violence. Share your findings with at least two colleagues.

Optional: Share your findings with a nurse leader in your institution.

■ **Leadership Development Exercise 22-4**

How does your institution respond to an immediate threat of workplace violence? What steps are missing? Which ones would you add to make your institution better prepared for workplace violence?

■ **Leadership Development Exercise 22-5**

Find out how your institution deals with the consequences of workplace violence. Based on this chapter, what other actions would you suggest?

■ **Leadership Development Exercise 22-6**

Discuss measures nurse leaders can use and teach staff to reduce workplace violence.

Advanced Leadership Development Exercises

■ **Leadership Development Exercise 22-7**

Teach a group of less advanced nurse leaders about workplace violence.

■ **Leadership Development Exercise 22-8**

  a. Design a problem statement focused on workplace violence.
  b. Consult with a more advanced nurse researcher.
  c. Revise your problem statement as necessary.

■ **Leadership Development Exercise 22-9**

  a. Prepare a research project focused on some aspect of workplace violence.
  b. Consult with a more advanced nurse researcher.
  c. Revise your design as necessary.

References

Abner, C. (1995). Battering in the womb. *Massachusetts Psychological Association Quarterly*, *38*(4), 8.

Braverman, M. (1999). *Preventing workplace violence: A guide for employers and practitioners.* Thousand Oaks, CA: Sage.

Bureau of Justice Statistics. (2001). *Law enforcement officers most at risk for workplace violence.* Retrieved July 12, 2007, from http://www.ojp.usdoj.gov/bjs/pub/press/vw99pr.htm

Campbell, J. C. (1998). *Empowering survivors of abuse: Health care, battered women and their children.* Thousand Oaks, CA: Sage.

Campbell, J. C. (1999). If I can't have you no one can: Murder linked to battery during pregnancy. *Reflections*, *25*(3), 8–12.

Capaldo, T., & Lindner, L. (1999). Resensitizing society: Understanding the connection between violence toward human and nonhuman animals. *Forensic Examiner*, *8*(7/8), 28–30.

Groves, B. M., Zuckerman, B., Maran, S., & Cohen, D. (1993). Silent victims: Children who witness violence. *Journal of the American Medical Association*, *269*(2), 262–263.

Healy, D., Herxheimer, A., & Menkes, D. B. (2006). Antidepressants and violence: Problems at the interface of medicine and law. *PLoS Medicine*, *3*(9), 372.

Hemmila, D. (2003). Hospitals and staff take precautions to guard against growing wave of violence in health care settings. *NurseWeek News*, 1–4.

National Institute for Occupational Safety and Health. (1996). *Violence in the workplace: Risk factors and prevention strategies.* Retrieved July 12, 2007, from http://www.cdc.gov/niosh/Violcont.html

Osofsky, J. (1995). The effects of exposure to violence on young children. *American Psychologist*, *50*(9), 786.

Potter-Efron, R. (1994). *Angry all the time: An emergency guide to anger control.* Oakland, CA: New Harbinger.

Rosch, P. J. (1994). Preventing workplace violence. *Newsletter of the American Institute of Stress, 6,* 3–4.

Sutherland, M. W. (1999, February). The killing fields: Our schools, small towns and the suburbs. *Nursing Spectrum (Florida),* 2.

Succession Planning

CHAPTER OBJECTIVES

After reading this chapter, answering the leadership challenges, and participating in the leadership development exercises, you will be able to:

- Describe the challenges of succession planning
- Discuss the statistics on succession planning
- Describe different perspectives on succession planning
- Analyze strategies and tactics for effective succession planning

Advanced nurses will be able to:

- Teach less advanced nurse leaders about succession planning
- Design a problem statement focused on succession planning
- Prepare a research project focused on some aspect of succession planning

Introduction

As many as 55% of current nursing leaders will retire between 2011 and 2020. What will happen to the profession if younger nurses, so few of whom seem interested in leadership positions, are not mentored? The success of the profession may hinge on the ability to recruit and develop future leaders (Sherman & Bishop, 2007).

LEADERSHIP IN ACTION

Norm, a current nurse leader, turns 67 next year. If it weren't for health problems, he would continue to work. He knows he may be a little late, but he wants to do all he can to find and train a successor before he leaves.

LEADERSHIP CHALLENGE What advice would you give Norm?

Facts and Statistics about Succession Planning

According to a 2004 survey of 34 nurse executives and 78 nurse managers conducted at the annual Minnesota Organization of Leaders in Nursing conference, three-quarters of nurse managers reported that they had no succession plan. Of the ones that did, most reported having an informal succession plan (Denning & Associates, 2004).

The results are not surprising. Healthcare systems today are challenged by the lack of consistent workforce planning, which affects succession planning. Disruption in leadership continuity can have unfortunate consequences, including reduced confidence from the community and employees and a negative impact on image and financing (Blouin, McDonagh, Nelstadt, & Helfand, 2006).

Not making succession a priority may result from nursing's short-sighted view of the process. Success planning extends well beyond the search for a nurse executive. Succession planning includes leadership development programs, mentoring, performance assessment, and overall workforce planning (Blouin et al., 2006).

KEY TERM

The **clinical nurse leader role** is designed to provide leadership at the critical point of client care.

The Challenge of Succession

With the nursing shortage, the importance of strong nursing leadership at all levels is being recognized. Innovative programs such as the **clinical nurse leader role,** designed to provide leadership at the critical point of client care, is developing momentum (Sherman & Bishop, 2007).

As baby boomers holding leadership roles prepare to retire, younger nurses have clear and mostly negative opinions about leadership, especially about the salary and 24/7 accountability that go with the job. To encourage nurses to take on leadership roles, succession planning must provide adequate compensation and a better work-life balance (Sherman & Bishop, 2007).

Perspectives on Succession Planning

Beyers (2006) interviewed six nurse executives from five different settings about the process of succession planning in nursing. Here is what she learned from a chief nursing officer:

- Ask everyone reporting to a new leader to participate in clarifying the role and in defining attributes for the person who fills that role.
- Ensure that the successor can be self-directed in establishing his or her identity.
- To reduce tension between the incoming leader and the outgoing leader and between staff members, only use overlapping roles for a brief period of time.
- Conduct regular open discussions with the current leader, CEO, and successor about the succession plan experience.
- Negotiate a role for the current leader to assume leadership for special projects, allowing the successor space to learn about his or her talents, strengths, and need for learning.
- Take time to recognize the sense of loss about the outgoing leader's departure.

Beyers (2006) also spoke to an RN who is the vice president of patient care services at a hospital and part of an organization-wide change to succession planning. That interviewee made additional suggestions:

- Appoint a talent manager to support succession processes in the organization.
- Team the identified successor with the talent manager to develop a leadership development plan.
- Work with each of the directors to identify a consistent approach for succession planning and to identify the right nurse leader or nurse manager for those roles.
- Arrange for interested nurse leaders to work with the talent manager.
- Arrange for staff nurses to work with nurse leaders on their own succession-planning processes. (Beyers, 2006)

A nurse with the title of chief quality officer added the following ideas:

- No matter what level of succession, nurses must be encouraged to develop their own leadership style.
- The culture must support succession planning.
- Leaders should engage staff nurses in leadership by encouraging them to participate in special projects and arrange for them to attend workshops and conferences.

A nurse president and CEO added some ideas about barriers to succession:

- Some leaders worry that emerging leaders will become better than they are.
- Succession planning is very time consuming.
- There are currently resource constraints and downsizing.

The same CEO also added her ideas about educating staff nurses:

- Let staff nurses attend finance committee meetings and help prepare documentation for a waiver and other papers that are important to the organization.
- Nurses have to learn to put their plans into executive jargon that businesspeople can understand. They understand client safety, but the same connection business has made between viewing human resources as assets to be invested in must be made continuously.

Beyers (2006) concluded that succession planning is a complex set of processes that must be tailored to the specific organization. According to her, succession planning is about developing nurses as leaders wherever they are in the organization.

Strategies for Innovative Succession Planning

Strategies and tactics for effective nursing succession can be learned from business examples. Colgate-Palmolive, for example, starts formal leadership evaluation in the first year of employment (Charan, 2005). Other organizations have found essential skills for tomorrow's leaders in health care. Those skills include knowing how to affect strategic growth and improve revenues; managing quality, cost, and service expectations; using effective communication and negotiation; balancing human and capital investment requirements; managing physicians and community relationships; and developing leaders for the future (Conger & Fullmer, 2003).

KEY TERM

Demand forecasting is when an organization anticipates the leadership workforce that it will need to carry out its mission.

Demand forecasting is when an organization anticipates the leadership workforce that it will need to carry out its mission (Pynes, 2004). Nursing leaders must use demand forecasting to know where, when, and what type of leaders are essential. High-performing nurse leaders should be visible in the organization and take on challenging assignments that expand their responsibilities as they mature in the leadership role (Blouin et al., 2006).

Although many organizations believe they can find more qualified candidates outside the organization, research has shown that internally developed and promoted candidates are more successful in the long term (Charan, 2005). Why? Perhaps because internal candidates understand the organization's cultural norms and values and have long-standing loyalty and support networks (Blouin et al., 2006).

Mentoring and coaching are crucial components of succession planning. **Career broadening** is a gift senior leaders can bestow on future leaders by giving them the time, energy, advice, and experiences needed to gain competencies (Blouin et al., 2006).

Examples of career-broadening activities include sitting on a key task force or committee, presenting key initiatives to the hospital board, taking the lead on an important project, participating in an internship or fellowship, taking a leadership position in a professional organization, and participating in an advanced continuing education leadership program (Blouin et al., 2006).

Sherman and Bishop (2007) suggested four strategies for developing leaders:

> **KEY TERM**
>
> **Career broadening** is a gift senior leaders can bestow on future leaders by giving them the time, energy, advice, and experiences needed to gain competencies.

> **LEADERSHIP TIP**
>
> Organizations must be willing to invest in career-broadening paths for high-performing individuals or risk losing them to positions in other settings (Blouin et al., 2006).

1. *Create expectations of leadership.* Work in collaboration with each staff nurse to create a development plan, including leadership expectations in job descriptions; incorporate leadership behaviors into annual performance evaluations; and make employees part of career planning.

2. *Assess leadership potential during job interviews.* Evaluate candidates' ability to communicate and build relationships, plan, be accountable, provide examples of leading, and show interest in leadership positions.

3. *Expose new graduates to leadership.* Let them attend nursing leadership meetings and continuing education sessions, sit on task forces for unit-based projects, cochair committees with seasoned nurse leaders, and take part in residency programs that give them visibility; help them become known in the organization. Let them vie to attend the Aspiring Nurse Leader Institute sponsored by the American Organization of Nurse Executives.

4. *Identify and develop talent.* Give nurses feedback on their strengths and areas for development, discuss behaviors that can derail a nursing career, and provide them with a mentor.

Summary

This chapter focused on succession planning and included statistics and facts about succession, the challenge of succession, perspectives on succession planning, and strategies for innovative succession planning. Part V, "Nurse Leaders Speak," provides a rare view of how real-life nurse leaders handle leadership challenges.

Key Term Review

- **Career broadening** is a gift senior leaders can bestow on future leaders by giving them the time, energy, advice, and experiences needed to gain competencies.
- The **clinical nurse leader role** is designed to provide leadership at the critical point of client care.
- **Demand forecasting** is when an organization anticipates the leadership workforce that it will need to carry out its mission.

Leadership Development Exercises

- ### Leadership Development Exercise 23-1

  a. Interview a nurse leader about his or her succession plan.
  b. Share your findings with at least two colleagues.

- ### Leadership Development Exercise 23-2

  a. Pair off with a classmate, and role-play a job interview to develop a nurse leader using suggestions found in this chapter.
  b. Obtain feedback from the other person about what you played well and what you need to improve.
  c. Replay the scene.
  d. Switch role and discuss.
  e. Replay the scene again, if needed.

- ### Leadership Development Exercise 23-3

  a. Identify which of the four strategies suggested by Sherman and Bishop (2007) operate in your organization.
  b. Devise a plan to integrate the missing strategies in your organization.
  c. Share your findings with at least two colleagues.
  d. **Optional:** Identify a plan to help integrate the missing strategies in your organization.

Advanced Leadership Development Exercises

- ### Leadership Development Exercise 23-4

  a. Teach a group of less experienced nurse leaders about succession planning.
  b. Obtain feedback from your learners.
  c. Share your findings with at least two colleagues.

■ **Leadership Development Exercise 23-5**

a. Develop a problem statement for a research study related to succession planning.
b. Share your problem statement with a more skilled nurse researcher, and obtain feedback.
c. Revise your problem statement, if necessary.
d. Share your problem statement with at least two colleagues.

■ **Leadership Development Exercise 23-6**

a. Develop a research project for testing some aspect of succession planning.
b. Share your project with a more experienced nurse researcher, and obtain feedback.
c. Revise your project as necessary.

References

Beyers, M. (2006). Nurse executives' perspectives on succession planning. *Journal of Nursing Administration, 36*(6), 304–312.

Blouin, A. S., McDonagh, K. J., Nelstadt, A. M., & Helfand, B. (2006). Leading tomorrow's healthcare organizations, strategies and tactics for effective succession planning. *Journal of Nursing Administration, 36*(6), 325–330.

Charan, R. (2005). Ending the CEO succession crisis. *Harvard Business Review, 83*(2), 72–81.

Conger, J. A., & Fullmer, R. M. (2003). Developing your leadership pipeline. *Harvard Business Review, 81*(12), 76–84, 125.

Denning, D. R., & Associates. (2004). *Nurse executive/nurse manager survey, evaluation results.* Retrieved January 9, 2007, from http://www.moln.org/files/NurseSurveyRevised4-29-2004.ppt

Pynes, J. E. (2004). The implementation of workforce and succession planning in the public sector. *Public Personnel Management, 33*(4), 389–404.

Sherman, R. O., & Bishop, M. (2007, January). Grooming our future leaders. *American Nurse Today,* 24–25.

Part V

Nurse Leaders Speak

Marion G. Anema, PhD, RN
Robin Arnicar, RN
Ellen Cram, PhD, RN
M. Louise Fitzpatrick, EdD, RN, FAAN
Jane E. Hirsch, MS, RN, CNAA–BC
Jeanne Jacobson, MA, RN
Bonnie T. Mackey, PhD, AHN–BC
Shirley A. Smoyak, PhD, RN, FAAN
Sandra Swearingen, PhD, RN
Ann Marriner Tomey, PhD, RN, FAAN
Sharon M. Weinstein, MS, RN, CRNI, FAAN
Gracie S. Wishnia, PhD, RN C

Nurse Leaders Speak

Faculty/Student Conflict

MARION G. ANEMA, PhD, RN
Associate Director, Nursing Programs
Western Governors University
Wimberley, TX

It was a busy day in the dean's office at the school of nursing. I had several meetings and was trying to respond to phone calls and e-mails. The faculty meeting had turned into a complaint session focusing on students' lack of preparation for class and clinical, their lack of preparation for tests, and the fact that they challenged faculty in class. My assistant alerted me that a group of junior students needed to see me. They had major issues with the faculty in their medical-surgical course.

During my administrative experience as a dean of a nursing school, there were situations where students and faculty had issues that were not resolved. There were negative interactions between students and faculty. Students in the BSN program would schedule appointments with me to share their concerns. Faculty, in groups or individually, shared their concerns with me about student behaviors.

There were 6 faculty and 60 students involved in sharing their concerns and issues during one semester.

What exactly happened: Complaints/issues from students included that faculty:

- Did not respond to e-mails or phone calls in a timely manner
- Started class late or ended early

433

- Included confusing questions on exams
- Gave lectures that were disorganized and did not follow the syllabus or textbooks
- Allowed too little time for questions or comments in class
- Expected students to know how to do everything in clinical
- Were unresponsive to students' problems or emergencies

Faculty had continuing issues/problems with students and generalized them to entire classes. Students:

- Were not prepared for class or clinical and had not read the assigned readings or practiced skills in the lab
- Were tired in clinical because of working the evening before
- Earned low grades on weekly quizzes
- Asked for specific answers rather than using critical analysis
- Blamed faculty for their course and clinical problems

The goals: The goals were to find ways to change behavior, promote positive communication, and empower both students and faculty to sustain positive changes.

The outcomes: The outcomes were to initiate strategies that addressed the problems/issues identified by students and faculty. A sustainable plan was implemented so both groups were empowered to achieve results to their immediate concerns and to engage in ongoing communication.

Elements of nursing leadership involved: I used the Kotter model to start the process of resolving the issues:

- There was a **sense of urgency** because the issues distracted students and faculty. Instead of focusing on learning, they continuously found fault with each other. Negative patterns of behavior were being established within the group. The students and faculty were ready to make the effort to resolve their issues.
- My **leadership role** was to serve as a facilitator for both groups so they could find a common ground for looking at the issues and behaviors.
- It was essential that everyone involved had a **shared vision** and that specific strategies were developed. The shared vision was to find ways to resolve the issues and change behaviors.
- The vision was **communicated** so both groups could agree on the strategies.
- Students and faculty wanted some immediate changes to feel empowered and know that **change** was possible.
- Strategies were implemented to produce **short-term wins.**

  - Strategy 1: I met with the students and faculty to clearly identify the specific issues and resulting behaviors. The vision of what everyone wanted to accomplish was discussed and clearly identified. Two lists were developed. The lists were compared for similarities and differences. The group prioritized the issues.

- Strategy 2: The faculty and students were randomly divided into groups so there was one faculty and 10 students. The task for each group was to address one of the top five issues/concerns from the differences list.
- Faculty agreed to start and finish class on time.
- Students agreed to stop blaming faculty for class and clinical problems; they would reflect on what actually caused specific problems/issues.
- The groups discussed the similar issues, and that started the process for working together.

■ Students and faculty wanted to **continue** the new behaviors and **create more change.**

- Strategy 3: A shared online classroom space was created. Students posted questions in a Q&A section. Faculty rotated the monitoring of the site and responding to students within 24 hours. Students had common questions, so responses were posted so that everyone could see them. Faculty posted reminders and tips about clinical and classroom activities. Students knew they could send e-mails to their clinical faculty and expect a response before the next clinical day.
- Strategy 4: Students scheduled study groups at times convenient for them and helped each other focus on learning the material and preparing for clinical.

■ A **goal** was to sustain the changes and ensure that a culture of transformation continued.

- Strategy 5: Shared governance was formalized with monthly meetings to determine which changes were positive. A prioritized list of changes was reviewed at each meeting and posted on the class Internet site.
- Examples of resolving problems included reviewing examinations to determine why some questions were problematic, revising classroom activities to allow time for questions, providing outcomes of content, and incorporating active student learning activities.

It is essential to create a positive student learning environment and allow faculty to focus on their teaching and mentoring. Both groups need to have a common understanding of expectations and of how to develop communication processes. In this situation, the students and faculty did not take the initiative to address and resolve the issues. My leadership strategies included several tactics to start the process. The strategies provided sustainable ways to communicate and resolve issues.

Resource

S. Austin, M. Brewer, G. F. Donnelly, M. A. Fitzpatrick, G. Harbeson, P. S. Hunt, et al. (2003). *Five keys to successful nursing management.* Philadelphia: Lippincott, Williams & Wilkins.

Helping Nurses Function as a Team

ROBIN ARNICAR, RN
Past Director of Nursing
Maryland Long-Term Care Facility

In 2000, after being recruited to a director of nursing position at a reputable long-term care facility in Maryland, it became abundantly clear that the nursing leadership was not functioning as a team but rather lending itself to ineffective care delivery, poor staff morale, and an overall sense of chaos for both the staff and the residents.

While most of the necessary nursing administration positions were filled, I focused on this vital group of leaders. After gaining a clear understanding of each team member's current role and tasks, I set out to gain a sense of their commitment to the changes that were about to happen and their desire and willingness to support the goals set before them. The goal was not only to have the right team members but also to ensure that they were in the right positions, given their strengths and weaknesses.

I started with my immediate support team:

- **The assistant director of nursing.** While she was more than capable and extremely supportive, she acknowledged that she only accepted the position out of a sense of loyalty to the facility. Her true love was managing a unit.
- **The quality improvement coordinator.** She was a dedicated employee with an eye for detail—perfect!—except for one small shortcoming: her negativity. Oh well, that would change as things improved, right?
- **The nurse assessment coordinators.** The coordinators shared one full-time position equally. One coordinator clearly worked the position because it worked well for her family life. That was important, but was it effective? The other coordinator was taking on two tasks: being the part-time assessment coordinator and the part-time staff development coordinator. It was certainly a big task for one person and for a facility that needed so much training. I learned that she was formerly the staff development coordinator on a full-time basis, and for reasons I disagreed with, the position was made part-time. I was able to convince upper management that training was to be a big part of our future success, and the position was made full-time again.
- **The staff development coordinator.** Formerly part-time, she was reinstated as full-time. I realized she worked very methodically and taught very passionately. People liked her and would confide in her. I pondered whether this was a mission accomplished or whether she was an underutilized resource.

- **The nurse managers.** Both had the tendency to micromanage their respective units because they were not comfortable with delegation. One was definitely more receptive to change than the other. The receptive manager was willing to learn and showed great potential for advancement. The other consistently resisted and constantly verbalized that it "wouldn't work."

Armed with a better understanding of my immediate team, I laid out my priorities:

- The nurse assessment position must be, for consistency, full-time. The current assessment coordinator (the one who did not also handle development) not only lacked the desire to work full-time but also lacked the knowledge to be successful in the position. She was offered an alternate staff position, and a replacement was sought. Through an employee referral, we were able to obtain a dynamic, talented nurse assessment coordinator. She brought years of expertise and a much-needed sense of "change is good" to our team.
- The nurse managers must be dynamic frontline leaders. After several attempts to teach delegation and management skills to the managers, it was clear that one manager was not going to make the necessary changes and decided to seek employment elsewhere. The other manager was trying very hard to change and showed a lot of desire to learn. It also became very clear that she had a keen eye for detail and a love for quality improvement.
- While the quality improvement coordinator was technically excellent, her negativity was not improving, and it became clear that she was burned out. She decided that a career outside of long-term care could suit her well and resigned. With openings in both the quality improvement (QI) and nurse manager positions, we took advantage of the opportunity to get the right people in the right positions. I accepted an offer from my assistant director of nursing (ADON) to move her to her much-loved nurse manager position. We moved the remaining manager to the QI position that she seemed well suited to. We then hired a replacement nurse manager. This left only the ADON position open. I analyzed my own leadership style and the team's needs and came to realize that the current staff development coordinator would be a perfect complement. She accepted the position, and after a few attempts, we were able to secure a complementary staff development coordinator.

With the immediate team completed, we were ready to take on the challenges of implementing programs and policies that would improve the quality of life for both our residents and coworkers. Our team went on to work collaboratively to achieve many successes, including improving employee morale, decreasing staff turnover, eliminating the need for temporary agency staff, improving resident satisfaction, and achieving greater regulatory compliance, including a deficiency-free nursing survey.

Nursing leadership presents many challenges and opportunities. Often, the most immediate challenge comes in the form of developing an effective team. Effective team building means having the right people in the right positions. To do this, the leader must have a clear understanding of the goals of the overall team as well as that of each individual team member. Be sure that each team member knows what the goals are. Don't be afraid to make changes that you know will benefit the overall team. A good team will follow a good leader anywhere. While change is difficult for everyone, not making the necessary changes can be a leadership nightmare!

Decreasing Work–Related Injuries

ELLEN CRAM, PhD, RN
Associate Professor
College of Nursing
University of Iowa
Iowa City, IA

When and where the event occurred: 2001, at a teaching hospital with involvement and support from the broader university

Who was involved: Me, a clinical nurse specialist (Karen Stenger, MA, RN), a human resources representative who was also the point person for the Americans with Disabilities Act (Jan Gorman), an orthopedic surgeon (Dr. Ernest Found), and several people in physical therapy and environmental engineering.

We had noticed and were becoming increasingly concerned about the number of musculoskeletal injuries nurses were sustaining. These nurses were off work for long periods of time, were often having repeat injuries, and were sometimes depleting all their sick time. We required nurses to be able to push, pull, and lift 40 pounds before they were allowed to return to work.

We looked at the literature for cumulative joint stress and nursing injury. Recognizing that this is a widespread problem, we wanted to capitalize on the knowledge and innovation in other nursing centers. We used work from industrial engineering, vocational rehabilitation, and human resources as well as nursing scholarship to help guide our plans.

We developed a coalition of resources to design a comprehensive program. Our program included preventing injuries while moving patients; it incorporated nursing education, bedside equipment review and redesign/relocation, and infusion or ergonomic lifting/moving of equipment. Nurses who had injuries were enrolled in an intensive rehabilitation program that included physical therapy, coping skills, and returning to work much more quickly than had been past practice.

Nurses were returned to work in roles other than direct patient care as soon as they were physically able to sit or stand for 4 hours or more without requiring prescription pain medication. The types of work nurses did included chart review for documentation standards compliance, quality improvement, staff education, and community outreach. Nurses' responses were generally that they learned a lot, felt valued, and were much less depressed than when they had been home for a prolonged recovery.

The goals:

- To decrease work-related injuries for nurses
- To minimize the negative impact of an injury for a nurse
- To capitalize on the skills and capacity that the injured nurse could bring to the organization

The outcomes: A significant reduction in injuries, significant reduction in lost workdays, high degree of satisfaction of the nurses involved in the rehab program

Elements of nursing leadership involved: Collaboration, coalition building, change planning and management, innovative thinking, cost reduction, and enhanced staff satisfaction

Lessons learned from this event: There is great benefit from working with colleagues outside of nursing who have knowledge that is applicable to nursing work. The perspectives shared greatly benefited all those involved. People in other disciplines also came away with a much greater appreciation of the work of nurses and how much physical labor is involved.

The flexibility for injured nurses to do work other than direct care has opened some of their eyes to other possible roles for them in nursing. It has encouraged several people to go back to school. We have seen great growth in some of these staff. Rather than retiring on full disability, these nurses are fully contributing to the profession!

This program has continued to morph and grow. Ergonomics is a key issue with not only keeping the aging nursing workforce active in the field but also with retaining and protecting new nurses from cumulative musculoskeletal stresses.

Aid for Muslim Students after 9/11

M. LOUISE FITZPATRICK, EdD, RN, FAAN
Connelly Endowed Dean and Professor
College of Nursing
Villanova University
Villanova, PA

The world stood still for a split second on September 11, 2001, and then erupted into the chaos that the tragedy ignited. Our suburban Philadelphia campus, 70 miles from New York City, was gripped by the shockwaves that followed. Parents of students; large numbers of Villanova alumni (many of them young or at their prime); and friends, relatives, and colleagues of faculty and staff worked in the financial district in Lower Manhattan. We learned later that 15 alumni lost their lives in the destruction of the World Trade Center. Relatives of alumni and then current students increased that number significantly.

In a faith-based institution, tragedy and celebrations often revolve around community worship, so it was not surprising that an immediate rallying point for mutual support, comfort, and solace was our campus church. For me, priorities were different. Immediately, I realized that my task was not to participate in the normal community response and activities related to the disaster but to concern myself with interpreting this event to 20 young Muslim nurses who had arrived to study with us only 5 weeks earlier.

Our experience with Muslim students from the Middle East was considerable, but this situation was unprecedented; and although the embassy staff in Washington and the ministry of health in the nurses' country knew Villanova well, this was a new cohort of students. They came from various regions of the same country but did not necessarily know one another well. They were adjusting to life in a new environment, a new academic experience, a new cultural experience, and one another. The students resided in apartments a few miles from campus, which had been secured for them by our college of nursing, and commuted to campus by suburban train. A large supermarket, drugstore, and discount store were proximate to the apartments. When disaster struck, I initially isolated myself in my office to try to think through a strategy. My goals included:

- Creating a safety net and haven for Muslim students who were frightened and concerned about incidents that might be directed at them
- Creating an atmosphere of trust, despite the students' recent acquaintance with us
- Serving as a communication link between the students, the embassy in the United States, and the ministry of health, which was the sponsoring agency for the educational program
- Attempting to calm students so that they could interpret their situation accurately to their families at home, who were panicking and phoning them
- Supporting the students in their decisions to remain in the United States or to leave (their embassy was advising students that they were free to leave for home, if they wished to do so)
- Educating the university's neighbors in this suburban community as well as local businesses concerning the identity of these students and their association with the university (the young women in the group were particularly visible since they all wore *hijab*)

The first step was to gather the students together in the college of nursing and to create a secure atmosphere. This was accomplished through an initial group meeting with me and key faculty in the college. However, the important ingredient was my phone call to an Arab Muslim colleague in our business school, who is also a personal friend, requesting that he come to the gathering and address the students in their native Arabic. The outcome was the students' willingness to express their concerns and develop confidence in us. Very helpful in achieving this result were the characteristics that my colleague was able to provide: cultural identity, religious congruence, language, and the maturity and position that older males typically assume in Middle Eastern Islamic societies.

That initial conversation led to a series of meetings with the students and our faculty as they weighed the consequences of returning home or remaining with us for study. My direct telephone conversation with both the minister of health in their country and the cultural attaché in Washington, with whom we had developed a good working relationship over several years, was of great benefit. They were satisfied that we had the interests of the students and the situation in hand. Despite the continuing distress that permeated American life following the September 11th tragedy, the embassy was able to address the needs of other students from its country who were scattered in universities or in small groups of twos and threes where there was not an adequate support infrastructure.

Throughout the process, the posture of colleagues, faculty, and administration was one of support and interpretation, rather than direction or attempts to influence the students' decisions to return to their country or to remain. Simultaneously, I made personal contacts with the offices of our university and, most important, the business community and neighbors who assured me of their watchful attention for anything negative that might affect the students. Of great significance was the natural leadership within the student group that began to emerge and influenced individual members' decision making.

The result of our intervention was the independent decision of all 20 students to continue their educations with us, uninterrupted. An unanticipated and culminating experience occurred later, when key members of the student group, representatives of faculty, and I developed a proposal to share our experiences at a program at the National Student Nurses' Association convention in Philadelphia. At that convention, these students shared their lived experience of September 11th with American nursing students and faculty from schools throughout the United States. They candidly answered questions from the audience about what that tragedy had been like for them and the fears they had as Muslim students from the Middle East during and after September 11th.

The outcome of the presentation was cathartic for our students and brought the situation to some resolution and closure. However, the added value was educating the American nursing students about appreciating the dilemmas and fears that September 11th had created among these Muslim students and their families, who were thousands of miles away from them. In retrospect, several elements of leadership surfaced:

- Defining the problem and its parameters, gathering relevant data, and developing a strategy that articulates and prioritizes specific goals
- Recognizing and engaging culturally competent tactics to work through the strategy
- Creating an atmosphere of safety with the objective of developing trust
- Supporting individuals in their own decision-making process and supplying facts for them to consider without unduly influencing them
- Encouraging natural leadership within the group
- Assuming responsibility and accountability
- Recognizing the importance of investing in and building relationships with collaborating and cooperating sponsorship groups to build trusting partnerships when situations require them
- Providing the opportunity for sharing different perspectives to develop cultural awareness

There were many lessons learned. While the September 11th event could be considered unique and hopefully will not reoccur, it underscored the need to plan for crises and to recognize the situations associated with the larger dilemma that might not be immediately obvious.

The related advice that should be shared is the importance of understanding what obligations and commitments we take on (over and above the ordinary) when we bring international students onto our campuses, as well as the importance of what we learn from these students and their lived experiences with us.

As a nurse educator of many decades and a dean for nearly 30 years, I encourage others to embrace the opportunity to collaborate with other countries and their students and to appreciate and celebrate differences as well as those characteristics that motivate all of us and make us human.

Closure of a Healthcare Facility

JANE E. HIRSCH, MS, RN, CNAA-BC
School of Nursing
University of California, San Francisco
San Francisco, CA

As the chief nurse executive at the University of California, San Francisco (UCSF) Medical Center, I was actively involved in the closure of one of our facilities: Mt. Zion, a small, primarily community-based facility that had been an acute care hospital in San Francisco for over 100 years. UCSF had merged with this facility in 1990, but by 1999, the original goals for Mt. Zion had not been achieved in terms of volume and revenue; and on the heels of the failed merger between UCSF Medical Center and Stanford Hospitals and Clinics, it was determined that the best course of action would be to close this facility from an acute care perspective and use the space for outpatient activity only. The decision was made to close this hospital by September 1999.

UCSF Mt. Zion had an incredibly rich history in San Francisco: it had been opened by Jewish physicians who were denied admitting privileges in other city hospitals. As a community teaching hospital, Mt. Zion had an extremely loyal patient base and many long-term physicians and staff. The decision to close the hospital was met with extreme disappointment, sadness, and anger from staff and patients alike.

A planning committee was established to represent all disciplines; I represented nursing and patient care services. Other key UCSF Medical Center leaders, both administrators and physicians, also participated. A timeline was established, and the work began with communicating to staff, patients, the community at large, San Francisco city leadership, and the department of health services.

While the primary goal of the hospital closure was to save money, we also thought that we could improve efficiencies by consolidating all inpatient activities at the main hospital site. Inpatient volume was already running high in the main hospital, and the emergency department (ED) was also already very busy. Since the ED at Mt. Zion would be closing, we needed to determine how much of that volume, as well as the inpatient volume, would transfer to the main hospital. I participated in multiple community meetings, presenting information to patients, community members, and staff about how the closure and transition of patients would occur.

Our nursing and patient care employees are represented by unions, so although the two hospitals were separate in terms of patient populations (and acuity), another goal was that any Mt. Zion staff member who wished could transfer to the main hospital. This entailed multiple staffing plans for the main hospital units and departments and determining how many positions to hold open and not recruit for, pending the potential transfer of our Mt. Zion employees. This process caused much anxiety, distress, and fear; a significant number of the Mt. Zion employees had worked there for years and were concerned about working at the much larger, much busier, and more acute main hospital. Less senior employees at the main Medical Center feared being laid off and replaced by someone who might not have had the same level of expertise or experience with their patient populations. Managers, while understanding the situation, were frustrated about not being able to actively recruit for open positions and were also concerned about potentially having to orient transferred employees to much sicker patient populations.

As the nursing leader, I was closely involved with almost every aspect of the closure but played a key role in working with the staff. Morale had already been damaged by the failed merger with Stanford and subsequent loss of some key administrative leaders, so I made every effort to be as visible as possible, attend staff and physician meetings, make rounds, talk personally with individual staff members about their concerns, and try to assist them with decision making. A key element was working closely with our human resource department, which did an incredible job of calculating seniority, assisting us with determining placements, and working with individual employees who had many questions and concerns. A significant number of the longer-term Mt. Zion employees elected to retire, rather than transfer to the "unknown" and perhaps more frightening atmosphere of the main Medical Center. Nurses and unit-specific patient care personnel who decided to transfer were asked to identify their top three choices of patient care units, and much diligence went into determining placement so that most needs were met.

I worked closely with the medical staff on all aspects of patient—and physician—transfer. We worked out new block-time allocations in the operating rooms, which involved reviewing and verifying past use of operating room time. New locker space, new office space, and additional conference space had to be created in an already space-challenged environment. A transition plan was created so that various patient populations were transferred gradually, along with staff, and we obviously had to keep in mind emergency procedures and patient and staff safety as the inpatient population dwindled.

An enormous amount of effort occurred in a few short months, and the hospital was successfully and safely closed. From a nursing perspective, every leadership skill I possessed was needed and used. Hospitals are "homes" or "villages" for many patients and staff, and dealing with the anger and grief with understanding and caring was incredibly intense. From a business perspective, my financial, planning, and human resource expertise was essential. Multiple timelines, business plans, and volume projections and revisions occurred. Communication and collaboration were paramount with staff, physicians, and our community. Visibility, providing as much information as possible as often as possible, and projecting optimism without seeming Pollyannaish was critical. Through this incredibly difficult and emotional project, I realized as never before the importance and necessity of the patient care and staff advocacy perspective that nursing brings to the table—and how to use those abilities to bring about a successful outcome to a most stressful situation.

Communication Cards

JEANNE JACOBSON, MA, RN
Educator
Metro State University and St. Catherine's College
St. Paul, MN

A complex medical-surgical unit at a midwestern university hospital was having difficulty communicating effectively to nurses who floated onto the unit from the float pool. The unit was composed of 31 beds, had a 90% occupancy rating, and had a very diverse patient population. In addition, the average length of stay was 3.5 days, making the intensity on the unit very high. Students from many disciplines had a constant presence on the unit. The unit was well organized and had a seasoned staff who worked well as a team. The challenge was that staff nurses floating to the unit for a day were faced with many aspects of patient care that were not familiar to them.

The unit assigned a buddy to each float nurse to serve as a resource. Both the unit nurse and the float nurse had very busy patient care assignments and had little time to communicate with each other during the shift. The charge nurse on the unit was another resource for the float nurse but was also very busy.

I was the nurse manager for the patient care unit and was receiving feedback from the float pool nurse manager that float nurses did not want to come to the unit because of the complexity and diversity of patients. The float nurses also reported that the nurses on the unit were welcoming but that the busyness of the unit made them less available to help others.

The unit had a nurse practice council, composed of six staff nurses and the assistant nurse manager, that focused on performance improvement issues. The nurse practice council agreed to address the float nurses' communication concerns. It used feedback that the unit had already received and surveyed additional float nurses for their input. In addition, the members of the practice council solicited feedback from the unit staff.

The goal was to provide information that float nurses needed to be able to function effectively on the patient care unit and to help ensure nurse satisfaction. The float nurses needed to receive this information concisely and immediately upon their assignment to the unit.

After gathering input from staff and float nurses and reviewing the goal, the nurse practice group proposed a tool that became known as "float cards." The float cards were organized by the diverse patient population mix and were succinct in content. The cards contained critical information for each patient population group as well as helpful hints in delivering care for the variety of patients. All this information was placed on two 5 x 7 inch cards that fit into the Kardex that the unit used for care plans.

The content of the cards was reviewed by staff and float nurses for authenticity and clarity. Revisions were made from the feedback. The float cards were posted on the staff education bulletin board and sent to the float pool nurse manager for review at staff meetings.

The charge nurse gave the float cards to nurses upon their arrival on the unit along with a patient care assignment. Nurse buddies continued to be assigned, and the charge nurse continued to serve as a resource.

The float cards were immediately successful. Float nurses received information they needed to successfully care for their patients and were more satisfied with their experience on the patient care units. Staff on the unit felt less overwhelmed by questions from the float nurses.

One unexpected outcome was that the float nurses communicated the success of the float cards to other patient care units, and those units requested copies so that they could develop their own cards. A second unexpected outcome was that float nurses began to request being assigned to our unit because they enjoyed their experiences. Patients received more consistent care from the same unit and float nurses.

The learnings included the concept that nurses at the bedside are best able to make patient care decisions and that nurse managers need to provide the environment in which that can happen. Also, lessons learned can be shared and transferred to other patient populations. Lastly, keeping the solution simple was the best solution to this issue.

Adjusting Care Units to Meet Client Needs

JEANNE JACOBSON, MA, RN
Educator
Metro State University and St. Catherine's College
St. Paul, MN

In the late 1980s, healthcare costs were skyrocketing, patient care outcomes remained constant, and patient satisfaction was fluctuating at a large Midwest medical center. One group of patients that entered the acute care center required relatively minor surgical procedures but needed ventilators for respiratory support either at home or in long-term care centers. The acute care center had previously established a criterion that all adult patients requiring ventilator support be cared for in an ICU environment. In the late 1980s, the medical center proposed that it was safe to change the criterion and that this group of patients be cared for outside the ICU. A medical-surgical unit was designated with the goals of decreasing ICU costs and length of stay and improving patient satisfaction.

I was the nurse manager on the unit selected to care for these patients, who were ventilator dependent and respiratory stable. An interdisciplinary team was formed to plan for the care of these patients. The team consisted of unit staff nurses, respiratory therapists, an ICU staff nurse, a social worker, a nursing supervisor, and me. The team planned all aspects of care for this patient population, including criteria for admission to the unit, education for the staff who would care for the patients, and an assessment of the type of ventilator that would support the patients while in the hospital.

The team proposed that a specific number of nursing staff be orientated to care for this group of patients because of the relatively few patients it expected to see annually. Staffing patterns were explored to ensure that sufficient numbers of staff who were educated to care for these patients were scheduled 24/7. The respiratory care department also scheduled specific staff that would support the nursing staff on the unit and come to the unit immediately if an emergency arose. Nursing staff and respiratory staff evaluated three types of ventilators and chose the model that would best serve this group of patients.

A competency checklist was developed, and an education plan was put in place to cover the staff's educational needs. Education was given to all the staff who would care for these patients, including the nursing supervisors who would be available to help the unit staff troubleshoot problems.

Following the staff education sessions that occurred several weeks before a patient meeting, the criteria for this type of care was discussed. We determined at that time that a mini review course was needed. During this review session, we observed that staff were focusing on troubleshooting the ventilator rather than on meeting patient needs. As a result of the review session, the educators were able to redirect staff on patient priorities and encourage them to beep the on-call respiratory therapist to troubleshoot any ventilator issues.

Initially, patients received 1:1 care on the unit, and, as staff became more familiar and comfortable with caring for these patients, the nurse-to-patient ratio increased to 1:3 or 1:4. With support from the social worker, patients were discharged from the unit earlier than they had been from the ICU. The patients were consistently placed in private rooms near the nurse's desk to ensure adequate visibility. Patients identified that they were comfortable being cared for in a non-ICU environment and were more satisfied with their overall hospital course. The cost to care for these patients certainly decreased, although at the time we did not do a formal cost analysis.

Establishing the National Association of Nurse Massage Therapists

BONNIE T. MACKEY, PhD, AHN-BC
Director
Mackey Health Institute
Fernandina Beach, FL

Holistic nursing encompasses a wide array of healing modalities. Specialty organizations have been formed to support advanced education specific to these healing modalities. As a holistic nurse practitioner, I completed advanced training in various energy-work interventions, herbology and the use of plant-based medicine, visualization and healing, color therapy, acupressure, massage therapy, and other healing modalities. When I joined the American Holistic Nurses Association, I realized there was little representation for nurse massage therapy in that organization.

In 1987, I learned about a group of nurses who had taken advanced training in massage therapy and who had formed a loosely assembled organization known as the Georgia Association of Nurse Massage Therapists. Their purpose was to gather together those nurses who brought their nursing knowledge, skills, and caring hearts into the practice of traditional massage therapy. The association was looking to expand because of the many nurses across the United States who wanted to be associated with a nursing-based massage therapy organization.

History of the National Association of Nurse Massage Therapists

In 1990, I joined with a group of four nurses to form the first nonprofit nurse massage therapy organization: the National Association of Nurse Massage Therapists (NANMT). Because the NANMT was early in its developmental stages, many task-based initiatives were set forth. The first task at hand was to establish standards of practice, a formal document that detailed standards of practice for nurse massage therapists. Although there were five board members, in reality there were primarily two members who were committed to carrying out the copious amount of work. Hence, the NANMT Standards of Practice for Nurse Massage Therapists was co-authored by Bonnie T. Mackey, PhD, AHN-BC and Bobbi Harris, RN, LMT.

Because a nurse leader takes the initiative to garner support from other national nursing organizations, the initiative was taken to petition two national organizations for membership into their organizations: the National Federation of Specialty Nursing Organizations (NFSNO) and the American Nurses Association's National Organization Liaison Forum (NOLF). The NANMT was seated in both organizations. Together these two initiatives, establishing the standards of practice and garnering support from national organizations, provided a stronger presence for the NANMT as a national nursing specialty organization. Our next step was to gain approval as a continuing education provider.

I assumed the position of Director of Education. One major role of this position was to design and develop educational programs for nurse massage therapy. Program development meant that the state boards of nursing needed to be educated about nurses as massage therapists so that the practice could be understood as such. Three massage-therapy-related courses requisite to the application process mandated by the Florida Board of Nursing (http://www.doh.state.fl.us/mqa/nursing/) were developed. Approval was granted in 1992, giving the NANMT the ability to distribute credits for continuing education courses in nurse massage therapy.

Nursing leadership in this case encompassed being aware of the rules and regulations that governed the practice of massage therapy *and* the practice of nursing in each state. Massage therapy is a licensed and/or nationally certified profession that may or may not be regulated by a massage-based governing board. For example, states may be regulated by various boards: Board of Medicine, Board of Health, Board of Physical Therapy, or Board of Massage. Several states do not regulate the massage therapy profession. The NANMT was aware that most state boards that governed the licenses of physical therapists and massage therapists misunderstood the nurse massage therapist role. Because the rules and regulations of the massage therapy profession varied tremendously from state to state, the volunteer position of NANMT State Representative was developed.

State Representatives were identified within the NANMT membership for the purpose of educating the state boards or agencies about nurse massage therapy as a recognized specialty. Leadership in nursing for NANMT also meant stepping in and being the voice for nurses in a time of need. In several cases, the individual's nursing license was suspended, and in one case, a nursing license was revoked. As a nursing leader in an emerging specialty where nurses' roles are being defined and continually evolving, experience in the specialty field is advantageous. Investing time reviewing each case and spending hours on legal and political research can allow the nurse leader to provide guidance and support to nurses in need. Furthering this role entails studying and identifying the common theme in all cases where licensure was threatened and then taking action to deter future license-related issues.

One common theme that each nurse massage therapist presented with was the lack of documentation. In most cases, the nurse massage therapist did *not* keep a client record that stated the focused problem, intervention, evaluation, and overall plan of care. This created a problem. Due to a lack of documentation, there was no way any board or legal entity could determine what the nurse massage therapist was doing and why. Knowing this, *The Client Health Record: A Documentation Manual for the Nurse Massage Therapist* was authored and published in 1995. The documentation manual provides a level of ongoing client management that reflects nursing assessment, nursing diagnosis, scientific rationale for holistic nursing and massage-therapy-related interventions, evaluation, and total plan of care.

The nurse leader empowers nurses through awareness and education. In the case of NANMT, a documentation course for continuing education credits was designed and taught at the NANMT conference. The course educated nurse massage therapists on the importance of documentation and provided documentation formats that they could use. The documentation manual still serves as a tool for nurse massage therapists that drives the quality of care, minimizes the likelihood of misunderstandings and misinterpretations, and supports the unique roles that nurse massage therapists assume. Since implementation of NANMT documentation guidelines, there has not been any nurse massage therapist who has had his or her license threatened.

Discovery of and advancing a new specialty warrants the study of other nursing organizations that share similar aims and visions. Not all board members may agree with the nurse leader's viewpoint. Persistence and open communication when dealing with a new idea is a process and is recognized as such. It takes time for board members to reach general consensus. Adapting to differences in understanding an opinion is also part of the process.

Many board discussions centered on the importance of joining hands with other sister organizations. The American Holistic Nurses Association (AHNA; http://www.ahna.org) was one organization that was identified as a collaborative affiliate. Recognizing that separateness within nursing has always been an issue, letters were written and open discussions took place with various AHNA board members about the possibility of uniting. One shared endeavor was developing the nurse massage therapy part of the AHNA certification program.

Understanding the importance of certification and the need to undertake the task by the specialty organization is reflected in the nursing leadership role. The certification process is arduous, expensive, and labor intensive. The NANMT did not have the funds of its own to develop nurse massage therapy certification. An enormous amount of work went into the research of a joint certification venture with the AHNA. This did not come to fruition. The NANMT still does not offer certification. It was decided that those who wanted certification could obtain it through the National Certification Board for Therapeutic Massage and Bodywork (NCBTMB). While the NCBTMB track is a solid pathway to certification, it does little to address the *nursing* aspects of massage therapy.

Regardless of specific outcomes, nursing leadership entails working as a team member on projects outside the specialty organization with the aim of advancing nursing. One outcome of the AHNA-NANMT vision was an invitation to serve on the corresponding committee sponsored by the AHNA that provided content validity data for the development of the AHNA core curriculum and the AHNA certification examination in holistic nursing. Although the NANMT was not involved in the certification process, its sister organization, the AHNA, was. Involvement with sister organizations allows the nursing leader to recognize the field of nursing as a whole entity, greater than the sum of its specialties. The nurse leader participates as a leader regardless of the separate specialty organizations because the leader recognizes that nurses are the cohesive force of all nursing organizations. Leadership in nursing acknowledges participation in nursing-related projects while advancing the field of nursing across all nursing organizations.

Accepting an invitation to speak at international and national conventions is part of the nursing leadership role. In May 1995, the NANMT was represented at the First Annual International Congress on Alternative and Complementary Medicine; the subject was *Nurse Massage Therapy: Touching the Spirit of*

Humanity. This opportunity permitted a strong voice in the nursing revolution for advancing nursing massage therapy as a basic science, healing art, and learned profession on an international level.

Nursing leaders recognize that organizations are always dynamic and are engaged in forever changing processes that facilitate membership and organizational adaptation [m8]. In August 1995, reapplication for continuing education providership through the Florida Board of Nursing was denied. The course, Principles and Practice of Massage Therapy for Nurses Level I, was denied because the "subject matter was not appropriate for continuing education for nurses" (Rule 59S-5.003 [2] . . . a rule which outlines subject categories appropriate for continuing education for nurses). The nurse leader represents the nursing specialty by appealing state decisions and attending state nursing meetings. At one Florida Board of Nursing meeting, a Florida massage law was stated and used to support the legal right for nurses to practice massage therapy. In the 1945 Biennial Report of the Attorney General, *as stated under the exempt clause*, Massage Registration Law, Chapter 480, provisions of Section 480.03, Florida Statutes, 1941, affirms: "a registered nurse can legally practice massage therapy." I stated that nurse massage therapy as a nursing specialty is derived from standardized education for nurses through specific nurse massage therapy programs and continuing education programs, thereby protecting the public through providing a standard for quality of care. The application for continuing education was still denied.

A nurse leader studies the politics of various governing boards to understand the decision to deny continuing education providership. Some states recognize national certification for massage therapists obtained through the National Certification Board for Therapeutic Massage & Bodywork. Other states only recognize massage therapy licensure through their Board of Massage Therapy. Most states recognize dually held licensure and certification. Many nurse massage therapists were licensed as a both a nurse and massage therapist. Since the NANMT does not offer a certification track specific to nurse massage therapy, all NANMT licensed nurse members held a massage licensure, massage certification or both.

Nursing leadership means self-introspection in relation to the board. Recognition that the organization may move forward and take new direction with new spirit and energy promulgates the decision to step away from the board. Building a new nursing specialty comes in phases. When an incoming nurse leader assumes new roles, the outgoing nurse leader stays close to that nurse to afford a gentle and informative transition into new roles, offering information, guidance, and support during the learning process.

Stepping away from the NANMT board in 1995 when everything was moving forward was an accomplishment. Maintaining individual membership while serving as an adviser to the board signifies leadership by being available. Two years later, in 1997, a telephone call was received from the founder of the NANMT, stating that the new NANMT president dissolved the NANMT in an attempt to create a privately held organization. NANMT members were dispersed, funds were drained, and office equipment was under siege. The nurse leader brings expertise, wisdom, energy, faith, and devotion forward when asked at a time of great need.

The nurse leader brings knowledge and skills to create a strategy to provide direction while clearing out what is not effective. Contacting individuals in national nursing organizations (i.e., NFSNO and NOLF) resulted in their being sympathetic to the NANMT's cause. These organizations carefully guided the NANMT through the necessary legal processes. Based on trust, qualifications, and devotion, a new board was installed.

The nurse leader steps into new roles that the leader is qualified to assume, knowing that expertise and wisdom will guide the leader through the rebuilding of a shattered organization. In a time of trauma when emotions are heightened, the nurse leader is sensitive to the cause at hand and recognizes that a sense of betrayal felt by the organization and its members may shift again to faithfulness and loyalty.

Repair work through rebuilding organization visibility was accomplished by accepting an invitation to write a vignette entitled the "National Association of Nurse Massage Therapists" in the third edition of *Policy and Politics in Nursing and Healthcare*. All nurses must be mindful of contemporary issues in professional organizations. Nursing leadership continues to support nurses by creating exposure for the organization that represents them.

In 1999, it was time to rally again for the NANMT to link with the AHNA, since both organizations shared a common vision in holistic nursing. It was proposed that the NANMT create specialty interest groups within the AHNA. The vision was based on the NANMT sharing organizational, financial, and educational initiatives as well as conference-related activities with the AHNA. As a result, the NANMT attended the AHNA conference as an organization and held shared meetings to discuss concerns. Before this conference, courses were developed and continuing education credits applied for through the North Carolina Nurses Association. Continuing education providership was assigned to the NANMT. The outcome? Conference educational initiatives were fulfilled, but linkage with the AHNA did not occur. A nurse leader holds strong to the vision and realizes that it unfolds step-by-step. A nurse leader also realizes that there is a collective whole to consider and that the nurse leader is a part of that whole.

After the NANMT-AHNA conference, the NANMT president was killed in an accident. The nurse leader who has the expertise of the operations and management of the organization identifies nurses who meet the qualifications to fill board positions. The nurse leader also guides the new president until competence is demonstrated. The nurse leader then moves on, maintains membership in the organization, and continues to advance the nurses' knowledge through providing education for credit at national nursing conferences.

Experienced nurse leaders know that any event in nursing is never a single event, but an ongoing timeline-based event that unfolds as the organization and the people who serve it develop. Leadership involves growing with the project or organization. It takes vision, devotion, commitment, perseverance, patience, time, motivation, focused intention, teamwork, honest communication, future forecasting, intuition, insight, and a generous heart to be a nursing leader who is willing to forge through the unknown territory of a newly emerging nursing specialty or project. It also takes knowing when to get involved and when to let go. Nursing leadership is about forming an idea that evolves and gives shape to the direction of future endeavors that promote all possibilities for nurses and the nursing profession.

Encounters with a Dean: How to Survive

SHIRLEY A. SMOYAK, PhD, RN, FAAN
Professor II
Division of Continuous Education and Outreach
Rutgers, the State University of New Jersey
New Brunswick, NJ

Editor
Journal of Psychosocial Nursing and Mental Health Services
Slack, Inc.
Thorofare, NJ

The College of Nursing at Rutgers, the State University of New Jersey, recently celebrated a gala billed as marking 50 years since graduating the first baccalaureate class. I was a member of the class of 1957, which theoretically should have been the class being honored. This was not the case. The current dean, Felissa Lashley, insisted that the first class was actually 1956—and that the celebration just happened to be in 2007. My big sister, from nursing school days, is Marilyn Potts Nusbaum. She kindly provided her diploma, which announced that she graduated from the Rutgers-Newark College of Arts and Sciences with a major in nursing. My diploma states that I graduated from the Rutgers University College of Nursing. The board of governors had voted in the spring of 1956 to make the former department into a college. The actual designation of the unit as a college did not occur until the following year.

Is this really a big issue? Yes, if you choose to understand it in the context of other events.

During the summer of 2006, my classmates and I met in Surf City, home of Marie Varrelman Melchiori, who had hosted various members of our class over the past 50 years. We discussed ways to make this a really special event and promised to find old photos from our student days to share. The group also decided that providing some historical memories would be wonderful.

Dorothy DeMaio, one of the former deans of the college of nursing, who served for 14 years (the longest tenure as dean) beginning in 1984, offered to supply some of the historical documents that she had collected for a book she was writing about the history of nursing at Rutgers. Nursing at Rutgers actually began in 1918, at the then New Jersey College for Women. Dorothy, using minutes from the boards of trustees and governors meeting, constructed a timeline of the attempts to move nursing into a university setting.

In the fall of 2006, I proposed to Dean Lashley that I do a documentary for the upcoming gala, using my classmates' materials, old photos, and data from the university archives. I planned to interview those key figures who were still living and who were knowledgeable about the history of nursing at Rutgers. I had completed a documentary on Mary Harper, using the Rutgers iTV studio, with Hebert Peck as director. This DVD has won awards, and I offered this as evidence of my expertise.

In the months that followed, Lashley threw up one roadblock or barrier after another. She insisted on a written plan, which I provided. She wanted it written differently using words that I did not use. She wanted a budget. I provided this and reminded her that I had contributed $5,000 to be used for the 50th celebration.

During this time, our communication occurred through a member of the Rutgers University Foundation (RUF) staff, who was assigned as a development officer for the college of nursing. My e-mails and phone calls to the dean were never answered by her. Instead, the response would come from the staff member.

For the spring semester, one of my assignments from the head of my unit, Ray Caprio (vice president for continuous education and outreach), was to do the nursing documentary, which was given a three-credit load (actually, six credits of time and effort). I developed an advisory committee and a plan for the work with the iTV team. These were shared with Lashley, who refused to participate.

Her refusal to participate then became outright interference with the documentary efforts. She locked the lounge in the building where photos of former deans were hanging. She directed staff to block any efforts of mine to get historical documents from the files. She told faculty that they were to refuse to give me any access to current students in classrooms or clinical areas. When I arrived at the nursing building, announcing my plan to her beforehand (thinking she would change her mind when she saw how far along the project had come), she called campus police and told them that she was in danger! The iTV team and I left to go to the law school to tape one of the interviewees. The team had lights and other equipment on a cart, which was wheeled past the nursing building on the way to the law school. She called campus police again, saying she needed an escort to her car because "those people are all over the campus."

In spite of all this, the planned documentary was completed on time for the gala and DVDs were made for all those who were coming to the event. I was told by the RUF staff member that the dean had forbidden them to be distributed and had ordered her staff to confiscate them if attempts were made to give them to the guests.

My classmates and I had anticipated a bit of a confrontation. But we did not expect to be greeted by Franklin Township police, who had been hired to keep me from distributing the DVDs.

There, of course, are details that are better told over a glass of wine (like one of my classmates hiding the cart with the boxes in the ladies' room, while I "discussed" the matter with the police). In the end, I was told by the officer that if I did not turn over the DVDs so that they could be confiscated and properly locked up for "safety" (it's unclear who or what was in danger), he would have no recourse but to jail me. He quickly added that I probably could post bail and go home because Franklin municipal judges were reasonable and friendly. I would be arrested for "disturbing the peace."

The alternative was to turn over the DVDs immediately. In exchange, I would be allowed to stay and participate in the evening's events. Considering the facts that I had paid $300 to attend and that my classmates were there also, I said I wished to stay. The officer actually went into the ladies' room to get the cart because my classmate refused to do so. He did not threaten her with arrest.

A final strategy of mine was to attempt to enlist the aid of our university president, Richard L. McCormick. I approached him and suggested that if he spoke with the police, the DVDs would be allowed to be distributed. My best persuasive efforts were for naught. He refused to get involved. Finally, I said to him, "OK, Dick, I think I understand. To you, I am just a very tiny pea (gesturing to the tip of my pinky fingernail) on your enormously large platter (gesturing—with the widest sweep I could manage with my arms) of academic troubles." He half-smiled and said, "That's right!"

So hereafter, when people ask me how I would like to be introduced, I will just say, "Tell them that I am a very small pea on a very large academic platter. That should do it."

Patient Satisfaction Scores

SANDRA SWEARINGEN, PhD, RN
Nursing Leadership Development
Florida Hospital
Orlando, FL

I had assumed a new position as a nurse manager of a troubled unit. The patient satisfaction scores had been a problem for many quarters. I had been there less than

3 months when the patient satisfaction scores were returned. Although they had gone up slightly, they were still well below the desired mean. The administrator of the facility, a nurse, called me down to her office and proceeded to admonish me for the low scores. I was floored. I had been there fewer than 3 months in a troubled unit with many open positions, and I was being chewed out for low patient satisfaction scores. Needless to say, I was upset and angry that I was being held accountable for something that I had not had sufficient time to impact.

I went to my chief nursing officer and told her about the conversation and how I thought the administrator wasn't being reasonable about the change in patient satisfaction scores. She told me that the administrator was "passionate" about patient satisfaction, and although she agreed that the comments were not appropriate, she understood the source—the administrator's passion. As I continued to work there and develop a relationship with the administrator, I began to understand what being passionate about something means.

Being passionate means that everything you do focuses on, or relates to, one specific goal. In the administrator's case, it was patient satisfaction. She truly was passionate about patient satisfaction, and everything that was done in the operations of the facility was always tempered with "How will it impact the satisfaction of the patients?"

People with passion accomplish their goals even in the shadow of overwhelming odds. I know that administrator did. She was able to garner high patient satisfaction scores just by making sure everyone knew that was her passion.

Through the years, I have been able to identify persons with passion and have seen the difference they can make. From the physician who is passionate about the quality of care that his patients receive to the unit clerk who is passionate about the quality of the work she produces, people with passion make a difference. They won't accept less than the best in themselves and in those whom they associate with. They love to see people grow and blossom. They are the change agents in a troubled organization. They never give up on their passion.

I have a passion for teaching nurses to lead. I have always thought that the reason so many nurses fail as leaders is that they have never been taught the skills necessary to lead. Although I have always tried to teach others in nursing leadership skills, it wasn't until I assumed a position in Nursing Leadership Development that my passion found an outlet. I find myself consumed with developing nurses to lead. I have finally figured out that the achievement of goals I feel passionate about is one of the greatest areas of self-satisfaction . Everyone strives to achieve goals, but when passion is attached, the internal reward is like nothing else. Every nurse who succeeds in leadership fuels my passion. Passion makes people try harder, work harder, and not give up on people.

The thing with passion is that it is contagious! The more passionate that I am about leadership development, the more passionate others become. I once read that if you set yourself on fire, others will come to watch you burn. By watching you burn, they seize some of your heat and head off to start their own fires. This is what passion is all about.

I highly recommend that everyone finds what he or she is passionate about and works toward achieving it. It makes such a huge difference in your life and will impact the lives of others. You will be excited and be ready to start each and every day with that inner burn that is your passion. And you just never know what spark of interest you might fuel in others!

Mentoring a Nursing Supervisor

SANDRA SWEARINGEN, PhD, RN
Nursing Leadership Development
Florida Hospital
Orlando, FL

In my mid-20s, I took a job as a nursing supervisor at a 250-bed acute care hospital in rural Virginia. The chief nursing officer at that facility, Pat, became a life-long mentor for me. I had been a nurse for about 6 years when I took the job but had really never found anyone who took the time to form a mentoring relationship with me. Pat was the first nurse whom I truly considered a leader in her field. Although I have met many leaders in nursing since then, she is the one nursing leader who has impacted my career and shaped my destiny in nursing leadership.

Nurses in the early 1980s in rural Virginia were still thought of as being hand-maidens to physicians. At that time, a lot of what you did was based solely on the direction of the physicians. Nurses were not encouraged to have independent thoughts, and autonomy in practice was unheard of. Under Pat's direction and leadership, my beliefs about the importance of being a nurse soon changed.

Pat is a formidable woman who has always understood the importance and the need for nursing. She is an excellent organizer and one of the best at securing the resources that nurses need to do their job. She has been extremely successful as a nurse leader and has taught me the following characteristics of nurse leadership that I carry with me today.

Having a vision: To be a nurse leader you have to have and emanate a vision to your followers. Pat's vision was simple—"to make a difference" —but everything that she did was directed at making that difference. From securing adequate numbers of staff to caring for her patients, training her staff in the latest techniques and nursing roles, making sure that the patient received the best possible care, and standing up and calling for a nursing voice in a physician-dominated culture, Pat lived her vision daily and imparted her vision to all those who worked for her. Everyone who worked for her knew where she was taking them and followed her willingly.

Being able to make hard decisions: Pat could make those hard decisions that every nursing leader has to make at one time or another. If you as a nurse didn't or wouldn't follow Pat's vision, you didn't stay in her employment. If you didn't truly care for patients and meet their needs, you didn't stay. If you were not able to work within the restraints of the system and still deliver quality care and work, you didn't stay. She truly cared for her employees, but she was the first to show me that some people are not really cut out to be high-quality nurses. She understood that one bad apple can spoil the whole bunch and worked hard to keep those bad apples out of her staff.

Setting parameters of acceptable behavior for your employees: I once heard Pat tell an administrator after he had changed the way he wanted something done without notifying those it impacted, "You can't expect people to play the ball game if they don't know the rules." She was a leader who clearly stated the parameters of acceptable behavior for her staff. Sometimes, she came off as gruff and dictatorial, but she never held people accountable for something that they were not aware of. I have seen her go toe-to-toe with an administrator or physician who wanted to discipline her nurses for not doing something that they were unaware needed to be done. She led with clarity and did not tolerate those who did not do the same.

Nurturing your staff: Never, ever, forget that your nurses are people first. Be there for them at work and in their personal life, if needed. Pat taught me that no matter what, life interferes with work sometimes. People can't just leave their emotions at the door, so as a leader, it is your responsibility to make sure that they are still able to function and care for your patients. She was there for her employees in life, in death, and in crisis. She was always willing to be a point of strength in their life and strove to make sure that their lives were the best that they could be. She attended weddings, showers, and funerals. She celebrated and she mourned with her employees. Whatever was important in the life of her employees, she was part of it.

Serving as the role model for your staff: Pat taught me that you can't expect your staff to do something that you won't. From how you behave to how you respond, you are in a fishbowl as a leader, and everyone is watching. They might not remember your triumphs, but they will surely remember your failures.

Rolling up you sleeves and jumping in: Pat taught me that sometimes the best way to really see what is going on is to roll up your sleeves and jump in the middle of the situation. Perspective from the inside of a situation is always different than it is from the outside. You might need to experience what your employees are going through to understand how to fix it.

Pat is retired now, but I still keep in contact with her. I still seek and listen to her advice and guidance. Because of her, I actively mentor others. Mentoring is the door to making a difference. Pat taught me that it is part of your professional responsibility to help those coming up in the nursing profession. It is the right thing to do. The only way that nursing is ever going to be able to make a difference is to stand together as one strong, directed, and united body.

Leadership or Friendship?

SANDRA SWEARINGEN, PhD, RN
Nursing Leadership Development
Florida Hospital
Orlando, Florida

Most nurses are promoted up through the ranks to a leadership level. Being a leader in nursing and having friends who work for you is a difficult situation, but it's one that most nursing leaders face. Through years of working alongside other nurses and sharing their lives, successes, and failures, most nurses create a strong bond with other nurses. You cry together, you rejoice together, and you mourn together. Just being a nurse includes you in the ranks of being a friend.

So what happens when, all of a sudden, you are promoted to being a leader? Do you maintain those same relationships, or do you have to discard them to perform the duties of a leader? The caring and close bonding that make you a nurse and a friend don't always convert well to leadership roles. It is human nature to gravitate to a leader in hopes that he or she can help you move along your own career path. What happens when you become the person whom people gravitate toward to reach their own goals? Do you let your friendship get in the way of making tough decisions? Do you cut your friends breaks? Do you turn a blind eye to their unacceptable behaviors? Most of us would say no and try to treat everyone equally. Unfortunately, that is easier said than done.

I have personally struggled with this throughout my career and have watched many other nurse leaders face the same struggle. Sometimes, the result of the struggle makes the leader; sometimes, it ruins the leader. Throughout the years, I have learned one undisputed rule of leadership: it can be lonely at the top.

Having friends at work in the staff ranks can lead others to accuse you of unfairness, partiality, and special favors—even if that's not happening. The leader in nursing must remember that she or he is under a microscope. Any friendship between the leader and a staff member or a lower-level leader can and will be seen as favoritism. In actuality, you will probably expect more of your friends, be harsher with them, and demand that they perform at a higher level than others in your staff. It doesn't matter whether they are good employees; it's the perception of the masses that count. The masses will perceive favoritism just because those employees are your friends.

Don't think just because you don't associate at work that no one will know you are friends. One little slip, such as the friend asking you what you thought of the sermon you both heard on Sunday, is enough to start the negative wheel of perception turning: "You were friends before, and you attend church together. Therefore, you must still be friends."

The other side of this equation, besides what friendship does to your stance as a leader, is what it does to the friend. Throughout the years, I have seen those perceived as being friends of the leader also bear the consequences of the friendship. It is as if they are wearing a big scarlet *F*—for *favoritism*—on their shoulder. They are mistrusted, ostracized, and overall punished for being the leader's friend. Jealousy abounds, and relationships with others break down. Every move they make suggests that they use their friendship to get ahead. They are talked about and soon find themselves in a very lonely position.

Leadership *is* lonely at times. Making the decision to lead should not be taken lightly. If you as a leader can't stand to break those friendship ties, don't head down the leadership path. There is a huge difference between being friendly and having friends. You must be friendly to do your job well, but if you have friends in the ranks, it will hurt your ability to lead at your highest level. We all need friends, but a leader must cultivate new ones at each level of leadership. Your peers become your new pool of friends. Or you can look outside of work to develop friendships—they may not truly understand what you are going through daily, but if they are a good friend, they will listen and help you as they can. After all, that is what friendship is about—lending a hand and being there for someone, even if you don't understand where that person is coming from.

Helping Staff Grow

SANDRA SWEARINGEN, PhD, RN
Nursing Leadership Development
Florida Hospital
Orlando, FL

I had over 20 years in turning around for-profit healthcare institutions that were not meeting quality standards or that were experiencing issues with quality of care delivered. I was physically and emotionally worn out from those turnaround activities. I decided that I needed to see how the other half of the healthcare industry functioned—the nonprofit side—and possibly take a position that didn't require 70 or more intense hours of work a week. I soon realized how naive I can sometimes be!

I assumed a nursing operations manager position in a large multisystem nonprofit. At the time of my orientation to the facility, I quickly realized that the position had been open for an extended period of time (a small fact not imparted to me during the interview process). The unit of 60 beds had 27 RN openings, staff that reminded me of abused women, poor patient satisfaction, and a poor reputation in the institution.

After observing the situation for a while, it became evident that the staff had been poorly led. The previous nurse manager had been overwhelmed by the task of being interim nurse manager of this unit and the full-time manager of a PCU and an ICU. This nursing operations manager's large span of control had set her up for failure. Unfortunately, it also set the staff up for failure because of a lack of leadership direction. In addition, as so often happens, because the unit was a medical-surgical unit, it was not considered to be as important as the specialty units. Since the interim nurse manager was from a PCU and an ICU, the nurses of the medical-surgical unit were well aware that they were thought of as step-children.

As I watched these nurses work, I developed a deep respect for what they were trying to do. Staffing ratios were high, equipment was scarce, and help was non-existent, but each and every nurse truly did his or her best given the daily circumstances. Because of the previous leadership, the staff demonstrated a sense of hopelessness, a fear of being reprimanded for the slightest thing, a feeling of not being worthy to work in the institution, and a definite sense of mistrust of management. In addition, the finances were horrendous, and the patient satisfaction was not good. Evidently, I had landed myself right back in another turnaround situation!

The first thing that I did was to meet with the employees and find out what they thought was wrong with their unit and how they thought it could be fixed. Things such as scheduling, working short-staffed, and not being appreciated were some of the top themes that ran through the nursing staff. It had become acceptable to float nurses off the unit to cover shortages in other units, even though floating them rendered the medical-surgical unit short. It was OK for the medical-surgical unit to work short as long as the other units were up to optimal staffing levels. That was the first thing that was stopped. After much discussion, I finally got hospital administrators to understand that the lack of planning on their part should not make our unit suffer. The medical-surgical unit shouldn't have to work short just so the other units could be up to optimal staffing levels.

The next mountain that was tackled was the treatment that the medical-surgical nurses received when they were appropriately floated. Evidently, the whole organization thought that the medical-surgical nurses were less important, and staff had taken to treating them that way. After numerous meetings and discussions, the nursing management team finally saw that each nurse was a professional and should be treated as such, no matter where he or she worked. This was coupled with the fact that because of construction in the PCU, nurses were floated to medical-surgical to maintain their full-time status. This was an eye-opener for many of the PCU nurses. They began to see what it takes to be a medical-surgical nurse—guts, determination, and expert organizational skills. The PCU nurses gained a whole new level of respect for the medical-surgical nurses and their abilities to handle up to eight patients a day.

Education of the staff to ensure their skills were top shelf was undertaken. Some of the staff, because of their low self-esteem, had not kept up with their skills as well as they should have, and in addition, I had a lot of new nurses without a lot of experience. I was lucky to have a top-notch educator who knew what needed to be done but was never afforded the time necessary to educate the staff. I turned her loose and supported her in what she thought needed to be done. In 6 months, the self-esteem and skill level of the staff started to show dramatic differences. By the end of a year, the unit was able to take those patients who required a higher level of skill delivery, therefore relieving some of the burden on the PCU.

As for finances, as the staff became more self-assured and began participating in the actual management of the unit, the finances began to improve. The fact that I stopped the practice of nurses who floated to other units being paid out of my cost center also helped improve the bottom line dramatically!

The overarching principle that I used in the unit—the one that made the most difference to the employees—was that I truly cared about each and every one of them and wanted them to be the best that they could be. I stood up for them, I fought for them, and I made them see their importance in the scheme of the hospital operations. All that the staff needed was someone to believe in them. Once they had that, they blossomed and grew at a rapid pace.

As for patient satisfaction, I have always thought that "happy nurses make happy patients." At the end of 2 years, the patient satisfaction was high, the nurse satisfaction was high, and the finances were good. I look back on it, and I know that I am not the one who made the change in the unit; I was only the catalyst for allowing the staff to do what they do naturally. By supporting the staff and breaking down barriers for them, I empowered them to remedy their own problems. After all, they are professionals, and they know what needs to be done; we in management just need to give them the support and resources to get the job done.

Leading a National Organization

ANN MARRINER TOMEY, PhD, RN, FAAN
Professor Emeriti
College of Nursing
Indiana State University
Terre Haute, IN

I served as the public relations officer of a chapter of Phi Kappa Phi from May 2001 to May 2003, served as vice president from May 2003 to September 2003, and then precipitously became president when the then president resigned and served from September 2003 to May 2005 in that role. There was predominately one induction a year, in the spring. A list of faculty Phi Kappa Phi members was circulated to faculty asking for nominations of other faculty members before the induction. There was little response to that. Students who were eligible for induction were sent a letter of invitation from the university president's office. Faculty were not informed of the students who would be inducted, and very few attended inductions. Phi Kappa Phi officers were given a script for induction.

Consequently, I knew very little about the organization when I became president. I was president for many months before I learned there was an operation manual. I had to request one because no one provided me with it. I initiated some service activities the first year I was president. We officers of Phi Kappa Phi chapter held a meeting for students with some leaders of volunteer community organizations. Three students, some Phi Kappa Phi officers, and several community members attended the meeting. Two students committed to community service. Faculty learned about the community's needs, became involved themselves, and started getting their classroom students involved. A community needs grant resulted from the connection with the previous president of the chapter who is an English teacher and a librarian.

Fortunately, I had the opportunity to attend a national convention in the summer of 2004. I then learned much about the organization and the opportunities available. I read the available literature and took information back to campus for the officers. At the beginning of the 2004–2005 academic year, I circulated information to the officers and an agenda that itemized the many activities we could do. At our first officer meeting, we set goals to encourage graduate fellowship applications (one had been submitted some years before but was not awarded), to encourage study abroad grant applications, to apply for a new grant, and to collaborate with other organizations. We identified who was responsible for addressing which goal.

As president, I sent a call for nominations for graduate fellowships to all faculties and encouraged the deans to support those efforts. A psychology professor nominated a student; she applied and received a $2,000 national graduate fellowship for her graduate education. That was a first for our chapter.

I contacted the coordinator for academic programs abroad, informed her of the qualifications and applications needed for those study abroad grants. I requested that she watch for students who would qualify and encourage them to apply. She persuaded four students to apply for the grants. Three of the four were awarded $1,000 study abroad grants from the national office to recognize and assist undergraduate scholars as they sought knowledge abroad. Those were 3 of the 38 national awards given and the only ones awarded to Indiana students. Those were first-time accomplishments for our chapter.

The public relations officer agreed to work on the goal to collaborate with other organizations. He facilitated the cosponsorship of a blood drive with Epsilon Phi

Tau in January 2005 and the Phi Kappa Phi sponsorship of a $250 award to the Undergraduate/Graduate Research Showcase in the spring of 2005, both first-time accomplishments for our chapter.

The past president agreed to apply for the new national literacy grant. He and a local librarian submitted "Cultural Literacy for English Language Learners" to support the public library's English as a second language program with $1,612.20 that resulted from the literacy project started the previous year as a result of the community service learning meeting. Phi Kappa Phi members served as facilitators at a kickoff cultural literacy event that focused on reading and discussing world and local news and as facilitators in additional English conversation clubs.

Principles used to facilitate the accomplishments included the following. I, as president, made meetings efficient by circulating reports, research results, necessary facts, and proposals for actions and an agenda before the meetings. Agendas identified who was responsible for which actions. Officers could volunteer to work in their areas of interest. Key university people who could facilitate goals were contacted and asked to help. I contacted the officers periodically to inquire about their progress with their commitments to keep them motivated. People were recognized, praised, and rewarded for their participation. Succession planning was done by providing the new president with the operations manual and other materials.

Directing a Partnership between the United States and Nations of the Former Soviet Union

SHARON M. WEINSTEIN, MS, RN, CRNI, FAAN
President
Global Education Development Institute
Hawthorn Woods, IL

With the dissolution of the former Soviet Union in the 1990s, a plethora of newly independent states (NIS) evolved, and at the same time, something ended. Members of the healthcare community, once linked by a common country, were no longer able to communicate with their former colleagues through international conferences and symposia.

Early in 1992, nursing emerged as a key issue throughout the NIS and central and eastern European (CEE) countries. Cognizant of the need to tackle nursing issues within the context of a partnership model, US nurse leaders developed nursing task forces to meet the challenges of nurses at an institutional level and to provide a forum for the exchange of ideas and lessons learned. The task forces were the driving force behind the nursing agenda. In my capacity as director of the partnership program between US hospitals and their counterparts in the NIS/CEE countries, I created a cadre of nurse leaders who composed the infrastructure for nursing education, practice, and process within their respective countries. These nurse professionals, formerly classified as "middle-level personnel" rose to excellence, and nurses and nursing have benefited.

As the program director, I created task forces representing nurse leaders from our US hospitals and the chief nurses of the ministries of health of the republics of Armenia, Georgia, Belarus, Moldova, Ukraine, Russia, Kazakhstan, Kyrgyzstan, Uzbekistan, Turkmenistan, and Tajikistan, as well as the CEE countries of Latvia, Croatia, Albania, Romania, and Lithuania, among others.

Our outcomes exceeded our initial expectations and focused on three main areas: education, clinical practice, and leadership.

Education

A series of in-country conferences focused on education and curriculum reforms. Local nursing resource centers (NRCs) provided nursing faculty, students, and practitioners with alternative forms of learning. Each site was equipped with computers, textbooks, videotapes, anatomical models, and educational posters addressing the clinical, managerial, and psychosocial aspects of health care. The centers encouraged independent learning and enhanced traditional teaching methodologies. Nurses attest to the impact of the nursing initiative and the NRCs on their profession.

Basic nursing education in the NIS/CEE has traditionally been viewed as vocational training, rather than university-based training. With a faculty composed primarily of physician nurse educators, a move toward developing a cadre of nurse faculty evolved. The natural starting point was the creation of a baccalaureate-level model. Traditionally, baccalaureate and advanced practice nursing was not available in all these countries. Nursing education has since expanded from a 2-year program to advanced clinical and management training. Four-year baccalaureate nursing programs and continuous learning have become commonplace; such programs include skill laboratories, postgraduate training, and the extensive use of the NRCs.

International nursing conferences have extended the learning process, and NIS/CEE nurses attended the International Council of Nurses meetings in London and Copenhagen. Truly, second-generation leaders have evolved.

Clinical Practice

Changes in clinical practice occurred with the introduction of clinical practice guidelines, nursing standards, policies, and procedures. Process workshops introduced practice patterns that have transformed nursing's role and image. Countries such as Kyrgyzstan and Russia have seen the development of new nursing roles for clinical nurse educators, clinical managers, and nurse teachers.

Leadership

The first nursing association in Russia was founded in 1992 as a voice for the nursing profession before the government, other nongovernmental organizations, and the public at large. Although delegates from 44 regions of the Russian Federation emerged as fledgling leaders, they lacked the experience and advocacy skills necessary to enter into a policy dialogue with local officials. Training in organizational development and strategy formulation to influence policy change that supports the nursing profession contributed to the success of these associations, which now exist in all the former NIS/CEE countries. The All-Russian Nursing Association, which follows the federation model, has been accepted for membership in the International Council of Nurses.

Elements of nursing leadership included mentoring, negotiation skills, communication skills, and novice to expert. Our nurse leaders were also inducted as community leaders into Sigma Theta Tau International Honor Society of Nursing and recognized as leaders within their own countries.

Leaders have historically helped others integrate their personal values with the values of the workplace—and explain the paradoxes when values collided. Because senior nurses in the NIS/CEE countries have always taken a backseat to physician administrators within their respective institutions, it was essential that they develop the skills associated with senior leadership roles. Many participants in the initiative had traveled to the United States and had seen their counterparts in practice environments. The partnership model set the stage for early development and helped identify emerging nurse leaders in each country and in each region. Over a 3-year period, these early leaders became presidents and executive directors of local nursing associations and chief nurses of their respective health ministries.

Providing Leadership for Students Abroad

GRACIE S. WISHNIA, PhD, RN C
Associate Professor, Gerontology
Spalding University
Louisville, KY

The leadership event occurred a couple of years ago when I had the opportunity to lead a group of nurses to visit the University of Quito as part of our university's partnership with Catholic University of Ecuador.

During the trip, students and faculty from the United States got to visit hospitals, clinics, and health centers in Quito and the surrounding rural areas. The students had to do an environmental assessment of their host family as well as the areas they visited.

Nursing faculty were to compare educational programs and standards in other countries and to identify different standards of practice. Faculty exhibited leadership by communicating with, motivating, and managing students in unfamiliar and potentially threatening situations. For example, not knowing the language makes a person feel powerless in a situation that otherwise may be very familiar. Also being in an environment where the food, temperature, customs, and habits are different makes a person feel as if he or she does not have control. Each of these instances are leadership challenges.

Students and faculty visited hospitals and health centers. Students observed the levels of care, organizational patterns of nurses on the floor, team nursing in some places, and total quality assurance with total quality management models in other places. Students observed the care of older adults in day care as well as in tertiary facilities. In many situations, nursing leaders demonstrated how to provide quality care, sometimes without having adequate resources.

The goals of the program were to analyze health care to vulnerable populations in a less developed nation with fewer resources and under stressors other than just staffing patterns. Study abroad is valuable not just for the content of the course but for the nonverbal observations in the field that students and faculty discuss and analyze.

The outcomes of the program were presentation papers and posters that students shared with others in the United States upon their return. Students learned that nursing as a profession has the same goals all over the world, that a vulnerable individual who is ill has the same needs all over the world. The valuable outcomes are observations about and discussions of how outcomes are achieved when resources are scarce and when nurses' educational preparation is not necessarily at the MSN or doctoral level. Evidence practice is an area that nurses are hungry for, and language is a barrier for nurses in other countries to get advanced preparation. Nurses in other countries valued the visit and would like to come and observe in this country.

Elements of nursing leadership included motivation, communication, delegation, and observing the active role ancillary personnel have in Ecuador. The physician and the nurse manager work hand in hand, but the hierarchy of the professionals differs from the models in this country, which was valuable for students to see.

Trips with students abroad can open the eyes of our healthcare providers to the advantages and disadvantages of services elsewhere and bring the world closer to collaborate and learn from various models of practice.

Index

and food sources, 86–87
and stress, 86
vitamin C
  and food sources, 86
  and stress, 86–87
vitamin E
  and food sources, 87
  and stress, 87

W

Watson-Glaser Critical Thinking Appraisal, 115
Wehr's model for conflict mapping, 164
Weiss's model of conflict patterns, 168
work environment
  and health, 20–21
  and injuries, 438–439
  and job satisfaction, 331–332

and peak healing, 353–354
and supervision, 331
working with colleagues outside of nursing, 439
workplace violence
  and administrative controls, 412
  and aftermath counseling, 414
  and anger control skills, 417
  and causes, 412
  and danger signals, 412
  and dealing with the consequences of violence, 415
  and employee grievances, 414
  and employer–employee collaboration imperative, 410
  and facts and statistics, 410
  and materialism, 410
  and physical defense methods, 416
  and physical design strategies, 411

and prevention policies, 413
and procedures for reporting threats and violence, 412
and relationships in the work setting, 413
and research questions, 418
and response to immediate threats, 414
and staff hiring procedures, 414
and standards enforcement, 414
and supervisory and nurse leader training, 414
and threat assessment team, 413
and threat of violence assessment, 415
and training sessions topics, 415

Y

"You" statements, 170

Z

zero tolerance for workplace violence, 412